Ob/Gyn Sonography

AN ILLUSTRATED REVIEW

Ob/Gyn Sonography

AN ILLUSTRATED REVIEW

MARIE DE LANGE, BS, RT, RDMS, RDCS, FSDMS
Diagnostic Medical Sonography Program Director
Ultrasound Vascular Laboratory Manager
Loma Linda University Medical Center
Loma Linda, California

GLENN A. ROUSE, MD
Clinical Professor of Diagnostic Radiology
Loma Linda University School of Medicine
Chief of Inpatient Ultrasound Services
Loma Linda University Medical Center
Loma Linda, California

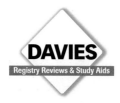

To all the students and sonographers who, through the years, have learned and worked in our facility. To work with them has made me a better sonologist, and a better person.

—Glenn A. Rouse, MD

To my awesome family, George, Nicole, Gina, Tom, Kit, Mom, and Dad, who supported, encouraged, and loved me. To all of my family and dear friends who cheered me on. And to all my coworkers and colleagues who have so positively impacted education at Loma Linda University and made working there such a pleasure. Special thanks to my incredible daughter Nicole for her editorial assistance.

—Marie De Lange, BS, RT, RDMS, RDCS, FSDMS

Library of Congress Cataloging in Publication Data

00-000000

Copyright © 2004 Davies Publishing, Inc.

All rights reserved. No part of this work may be reproduced, stored in a retrieval system, or transmitted in any form or by any means, electronic or mechanical, including photocopying, scanning, and recording, without the written permission of the publisher.

Davies Publishing, Inc.
Ultrasound Education & Test Preparation
32 South Raymond Avenue
Pasadena, California 91105-1935
Phone 626-792-3046
Facsimile 626-792-5308
E-mail info@DaviesPublishing.com
Website www.DaviesPublishing.com

Cover, interior design, and art direction by Satori Design Group
Editorial production by Janet Heard and Christian Jones
Index by Bruce Tracy, PhD
Prepress production by The Left Coast Group

Printed and bound in the United States of America

ISBN 0-941022-59-5

Preface

We wrote this book to serve several purposes:

- A topic-by-topic review for the ARDMS specialty exam in ob/gyn sonography.
- A concise text for those in training.
- A clinical reference for practicing sonographers.
- A resource for interpreting physicians.
- A convenient and inexpensive means of earning continuing medical education (CME) credit.

A complete CME application and exam at the end of the book also make it possible to earn SDMS-approved continuing medical education credits toward satisfaction of ARDMS, ICAVL, and other requirements for professional registration and facility accreditation.

It is with great pleasure that we offer this new book to you. We hope that it will provide a strong educational foundation upon which those with less experience can build and those with more experience can expand. It is our hope that *Ob/Gyn Sonography: An Illustrated Review* will be of great immediate help to you as well as remaining a valuable reference for you in the years ahead.

You have our best wishes for success.

Marie De Lange, BS, RT, RDMS, RDCS, FSDMS
Loma Linda, California

Glenn A. Rouse, MD
Loma Linda, California

Contributing Authors

Kathy Munson, BS, RDMS, RDCS, RVT
Staff Echocardiographer
Pediatric Echocardiography Laboratory
Loma Linda University Medical Center
Author of Fetal Echo Section

Curtis Serikaku, BS, RDMS
Staff Sonographer
Ultrasound Vascular Laboratory
Loma Linda University Medical Center
Coordination of Images

Phil-Ann Tan-Sinn, RT, RDMS, RDCS, RVT
Staff Sonographer
Ultrasound Vascular Laboratory
Loma Linda University Medical Center
Development and Organization of Review Questions

Contents

Preface

Color Plates

Part I Obstetrics 1

AIUM Guidelines 2

Chapter 1 First Trimester 3

Gestational Age 3

Fertilization/Embryology 4

Sonographic Findings in Early Intrauterine Pregnancy 8

Abnormal First Trimester (Failed Pregnancy) 15

Sonographic Signs of Abnormal Early Pregnancy 16

Ectopic Pregnancy 20

Sonographic Findings Related to Ectopic Pregnancy 23

Chapter 2 Second/Third Trimester (Normal Anatomy) 25

Face 27

Cranium 29

Thorax 32

Heart 33

Spine 34

Extremities 36

Fetal Abdomen and Pelvis 38

Summary 40

3 Placenta 41

Growth and Development (Embryology) 42

Placental Size and Shape 43

Abnormalties of Placental Shape 43

Intraplacental Lesions 45

Placental Grading 46

Placenta Previa 47

Placental Abruption 48

Marginal and Subchorionic Hemorrhage 49

Placenta Accreta 49

Chorioangioma 52

Placental Doppler 52

Umbilical Cord 53

4 Assessment of Gestational Age 59

First Trimester 60

Second and Third Trimester 64

5 Complications 73

Intrauterine Growth Restriction 73

Multiple Gestations 80

Maternal Illness 91

Fetal Therapy 98

Antepartum/Postpartum Considerations 102

6 Amniotic Fluid 111

Amniotic Fluid Volume 111

Fetal Pulmonic Maturity Studies 113

7 Genetic Studies

Diseases Arising From a Single Gene 115

Maternal Serum Testing 116

Chorionic Villus Sampling 119

Fetal Demise 121

8 Fetal Abnormalities   123

Abnormalities of the Fetal Head and Face   123

Embryology of the Fetal Face   124

Fetal Brain and Cranium   130

Abnormalities of the Fetal Neck   139

Neural Tube Defects   139

Abdominal Wall Abnormalities   144

Thoracic Abnormalities   152

Genitourinary Abnormalities   159

Gastrointestinal Abnormalities   170

Skeletal Abnormalities   177

Cardiac Abnormalities   189

Syndromes   201

9 Coexisting Disorders   213

Pelvic Masses   213

Cystic Masses   214

Complex Masses   216

Solid Masses   216

Coexisting Maternal Disorders Presenting Primarily with Pain   218

Trophoblastic Disease   219

Part II Gynecology   225

10 Pelvic Anatomy   227

Embryology   227

Development of Female Pelvic Organs During Childhood   228

Normal Adult Pelvic Anatomy   229

Sonographic Technique   234

Sonographic Appearance of Normal Pelvic Organs   235

Indications of Pelvic Sonography   236

Contraindications to Endovaginal Sonography   236

11 Physiology 237

Menstrual Cycle 237

Pregnancy Tests 239

Human Chorionic Gonadotropin 239

Fertilization 239

12 Pediatric Abnormalities 241

Sexual Ambiguity 241

Precocious Puberty 242

Hematometra/Hematocolpos 242

Other Abnormalities 243

13 Infertility 245

Indications for Sonography in Infertility 246

The Infertility Work-Up 246

Causes of Infertility 246

Medications and Treatment 250

Assisted Reproductive Technology 251

14 Postmenopausal Pelvis 253

Anatomy and Physiology 253

Indications for Sonography 254

Pathology 254

Therapy 255

15 Pelvic Pathology 257

Uterine Pathology 257

Vaginal Pathology 266

The Ovary 266

Endometriosis 279

Polycystic Ovary Disease 279

Inflammatory Pelvic Conditions 280

Other Pelvic Masses 281

Urinary Masses 281

Sonographic Imaging of Contraceptive Devices 282

Upper Abdominal Findings Associated with Pelvic Disease 283

Part III Patient Care Preparation and Techniques 285

16 Patient Care Preparation and Techniques 287

Sonographer's Interaction with the Patient 287

Performing the Examination 288

Supine Hypotension 288

Infectious Disease Control 288

Physical Principles 289

Artifacts 289

Bioeffects 290

Part IV Case Studies for Self-Assessment 293

17 Case Studies for Self-Assessment 295

Obstetrics 295

Gynecology

Answers and Explanations 317

Appendix A
AIUM Guidelines for Performing Routine Obstetrical Examinations **345**

Appendix B
AIUM Guidelines for the Gynecological Examination **351**

Appendix C CME Quiz **355**

Suggested Reading 369

References 371

Index 381

Color Plates

Color Plate 1.

Fetal gallbladder. Transverse sonogram. Note that the gallbladder (arrow) does not show blood flow. sp = spine, A = aorta, I = inferior vena cava, Uv = umbilical vein.

Color Plate 2.

Succenturiate lobe. Sagittal sonogram demonstrates succenturiate placenta. The posterior placental segment is separate from the anterior portion of the placenta, and there is a vessel crossing from the placenta to the succenturiate lobe.

Color Plate 3.

Placenta accreta. Sagittal view of the placenta demonstrates increased color Doppler flow posterior to the placenta. This indicates invasion of the bladder wall by placenta.

Color Plate 4.

Battledore placenta. Sonogram of the placenta. Note color flow of the cord insertion at the margin of the placenta.

Color Plate 5.

Vasa previa. **A** Sagittal view demonstrates the cord below the head in the lower uterine segment. Note the placenta nearby anteriorly. **B** Transverse view shows multiple vessels crossing the internal os.

Color Plate 6.

Umbilical Doppler. **A** Normal umbilical diastolic flow. **B** Abnormal reversal of diastolic flow.

Color Plate 7.

TRAP Doppler. Doppler of the umbilical cord of the acardiac twin in Figure 70 shows that arterial flow (**A**) and venous flow (**B**) are reversed. FA=fetal abdomen.

Color Plate 8.

Cleft lip. Three-dimensional sonogram of a fetus different from that in figure 87, also showing unilateral cleft lip.

Color Plate 9.

Gastroschisis. **A** Transverse sonogram of the pelvis of a fetus with gastroschisis. Note bowel (B) outside of fetal pelvis. The bladder (BL) is also visible. **B** Transverse sonogram of the abdomen shows the intact umbilicus at the cord insertion (arrow).

Color Plate 10.

Pulmonary sequestration. **A** Transverse sonogram of a fetal chest showing an echogenic pulmonary sequestration. Note the artery arising directly from the aorta supplying the sequestration. **B** Sagittal sonogram of the same fetus with pulmonary sequestration. Note again the aorta (blue) supplying a vessel to the sequestration (red).

Color Plate 11.

Ebstein's syndrome. **A** Short-axis view at the level of the papillary muscles. Note the anterior leaflet of the tricuspid valve visualized within the dilated RV. **B** M-mode in a long-axis view. Note the tricuspid valve easily visualized within the RV. **C** Short-axis M-mode view at the level of the aortic valve (AoV). Note the tricuspid valve low in the RV outflow tract. **D** Apical four-chamber view in diastole. Note atrialization of the RV (arrows). **E** Apical four-chamber view in systole. **F** Color apical four-chamber view. Note the severe tricuspid valve regurgitation (arrow) and atrialization of the RV.

Color Plate 12.

Truncus arteriosus. **A** Apical five-chamber view in systole. Note the truncal valve (arrows). **B** Apical five-chamber view. Note the outflow (color). **C** Apical five-chamber view demonstrating regurgitation (arrow). **D** Left parasternal short-axis view in diastole. Again note the valve within the main truncus. **E** Suprasternal notch (SSN) long-axis view demonstrates the aortic arch of the truncus and both branches of the pulmonary artery.

Color Plate 13.

Atrial ventricular canal. Apical four-chamber view in systole. Note atrial ventricular canal.

Color Plate 14.

Twin pregnancy with mole. **A** Note that the cord vessels (arrow) in yellow insert into only the normal placenta (NP) and not the hydatidiform mole (HM) **B** Another view of the same case shows molar tissue (HM) adjacent to normal placenta (NP).

Color Plate 15.

Corpus luteum cyst. **A** Transverse sonogram of the right ovary. Note the thickened walls of the corpus luteum cyst. **B** Increased blood flow surrounding the corpus luteum cyst.

Color Plate 16.

Hemorrhagic cyst. **A** Transverse sonogram of the right ovary. Note the complex mass within the ovary (cursors). **B** Minimally increased blood flow.

Color Plate 17.

Ovarian torsion. **A** Sonogram of the torsed left ovary. Note the large size of this ovary. **B** Sonogram of the normal right ovary with follicles. **C** Sonogram and Doppler of the abnormal left ovary. Note absence of diastolic flow. **D** Sonogram and Doppler of the normal right ovary. Note normal systolic and diastolic flow.

Color Plate 18.

Cystadenocarcinoma. Sagittal (**A**) and transverse (**B**) sonograms of cystadenocarcinoma. Note the solid masses and blood flow within the tumor.

COLOR PLATES xvii

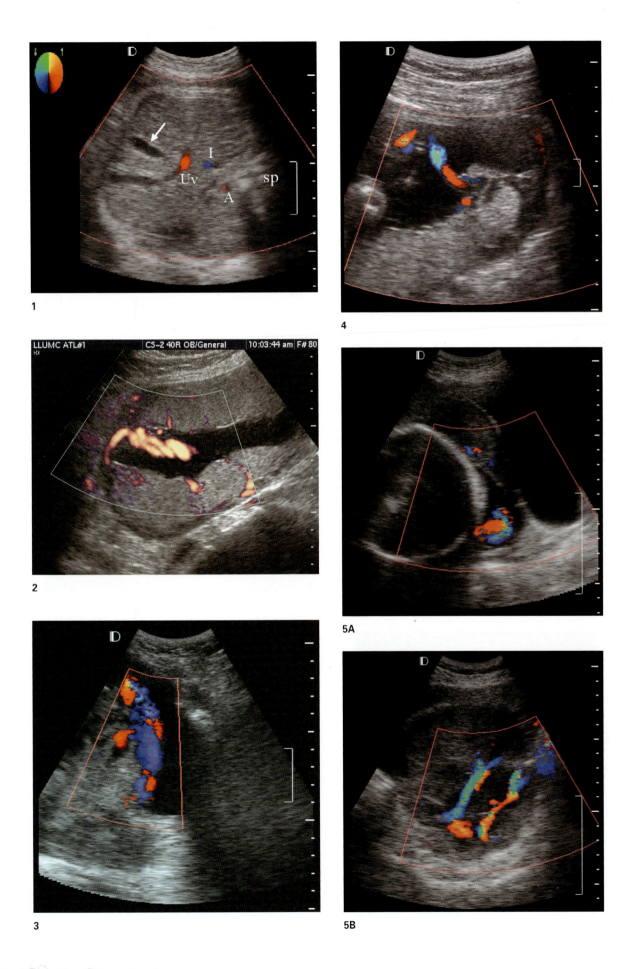

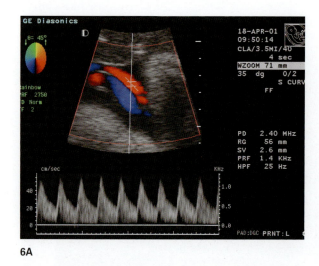

6A

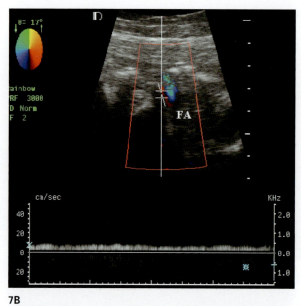

7B

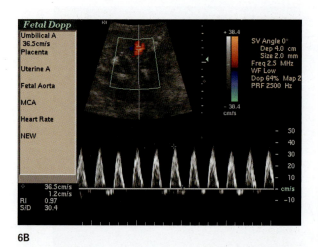

6B

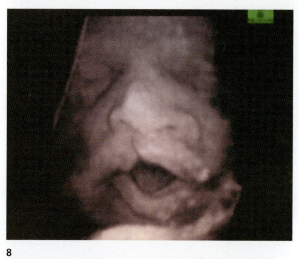

8

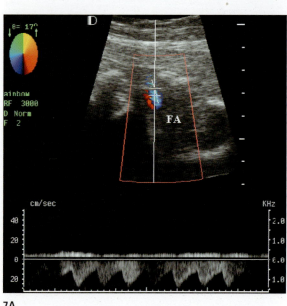

7A

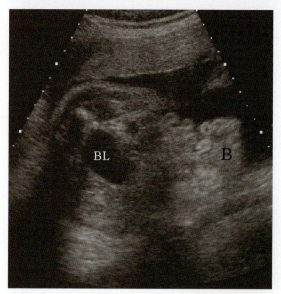

9A

COLOR PLATES xix

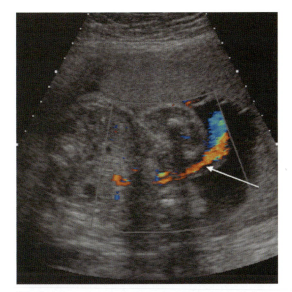

9B

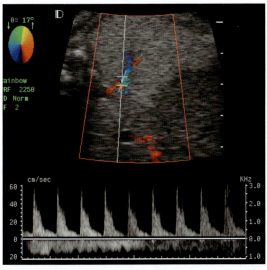

10A

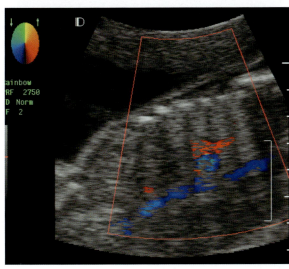

10B

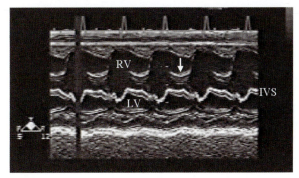

11A

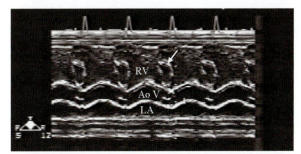

11B

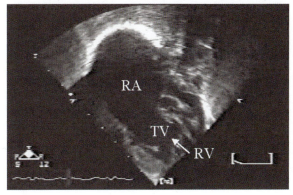

11C

11D

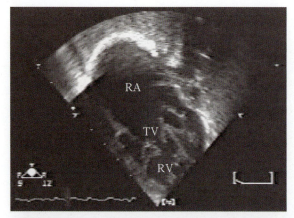

11E

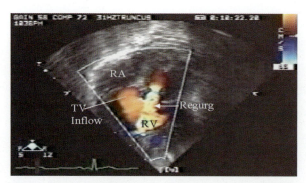

12C

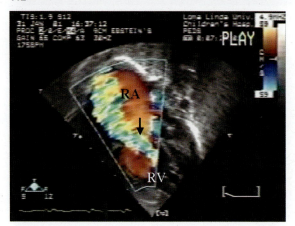

11F

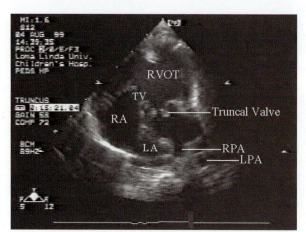

12D

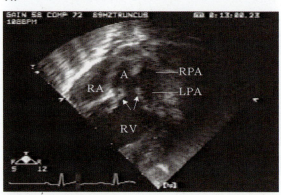

12A

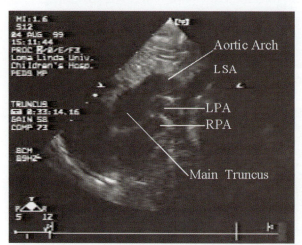

12E

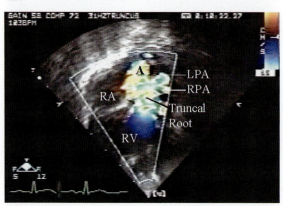

12B

COLOR PLATES   xxi

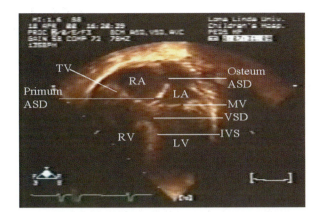

13

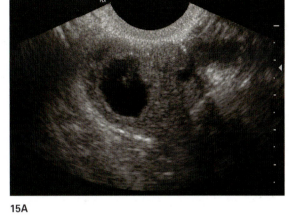

15A

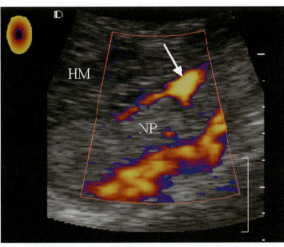

14A

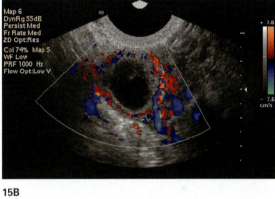

15B

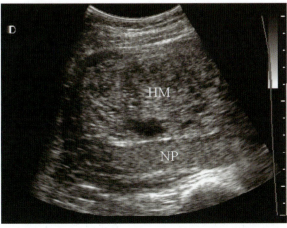

14B

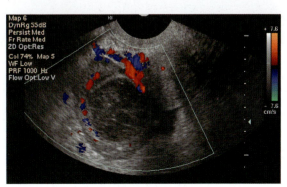

16A

16B

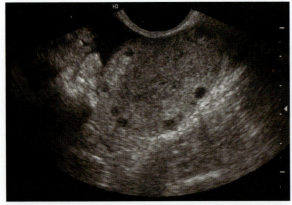
17A

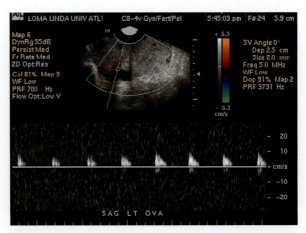
17D

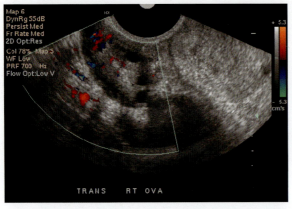
17B

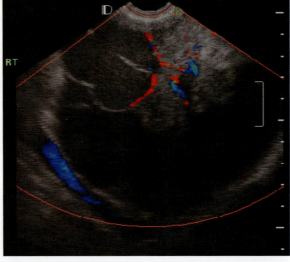
18A

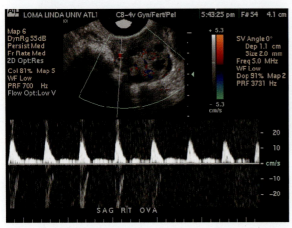
17C

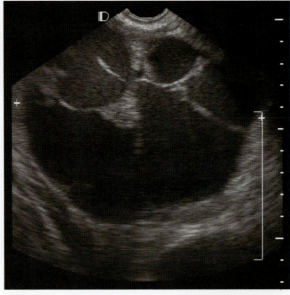
18B

Obstetrics

PART I

AIUM GUIDELINES

FIRST TRIMESTER

SECOND/THIRD TRIMESTER (NORMAL ANATOMY)

PLACENTA

ASSESSMENT OF GESTATIONAL AGE

COMPLICATIONS

AMNIOTIC FLUID

GENETIC STUDIES

FETAL DEMISE

FETAL ABNORMALITIES

COEXISTING DISORDERS

The introduction of ultrasound to the practice of obstetrics has greatly improved the clinical management of the fetus and mother during pregnancy. Endovaginal sonography has made possible very early visualization of pregnancy and implantation. Today in North America approximately 60–100% of mothers receive an obstetrical sonogram in the antenatal period.[1]

The benefits of obstetrical ultrasound include:

- Accurate assessment of gestational age
- Confirmation of fetal viability
- Assessment of multiple pregnancy including chorionicity (number of placentas) and amnionicity (number of amniotic sacs)

- *Localization of placenta*
- *Diagnosis of intrauterine growth restriction/retardation (IUGR) and fetal anomalies*
- *Observation of fetal biophysical behavior*
- *Detection of uterine or adnexal masses*
- *Guidance for chorionic villus sampling (CVS), amniocentesis, and percutaneous umbilical blood sampling (PUBS)*

While performing an obstetrical sonogram, the sonographer can directly visualize the internal and external anatomy of the fetus and detect malformations. Sonographic assessment provides the parents with information necessary to make informed decisions about the pregnancy. As more pregnant woman receive obstetrical sonograms and participate in prenatal screening programs, a greater number of fetal anomalies will be detected.

AIUM Guidelines

The American Institute of Ultrasound in Medicine (AIUM) has established minimum guidelines for performing routine obstetrical sonograms. These guidelines have become an informal minimum legal standard for obstetrical sonography.[2] (See Appendix A for a copy of the guidelines.)

CHAPTER 1 — First Trimester

Gestational Age

Fertilization/Embryology

Sonographic Findings in Early Intrauterine Pregnancy

Abnormal First Trimester (Failed Pregnancy)

Sonographic Signs of Abnormal Early Pregnancy

Ectopic Pregnancy

Sonographic Findings Related to Ectopic Pregnancy

. . . .

Gestational Age

There are two different methods for calculating gestational age. Embryology books calculate gestational age beginning with ovulation and fertilization of the ovum. In clinical obstetrical practice, the date of ovulation is usually unknown, and obstetricians and sonographers typically calculate the gestational age from the first day of the last menstrual period (LMP). The first day of the last menstrual period is a known event that usually precedes ovulation by about two weeks. *In this book we always use gestational age calculated from the first day of the last menstrual period.* When calculated from the last menstrual period, weeks of gestation are usually expressed as *menstrual weeks.*

Figure 1.

Summary of the first week (third menstrual week). Summary of the ovarian cycle, fertilization, and human development during the first week. Stage 1 of development begins with fertilization and ends when the zygote forms. In stage 2 (days 2 to 3 following conception/15 to 16 days since last menstrual period) the early stages of cleavage occur (from 2 to about 32 cells)—[morula]). In stage 3 (days 4 to 5 following conception/17 to 18 menstrual days) the blastocyst becomes free. Stage 4 (days 5 to 6 following conception/ 18 to 19 menstrual days) is characterized by the blastocyst attaching to the wall of the uterus. The blastocysts are sectioned to show their internal structure. Reprinted with permission from Moore KL, Persaud TVN: *Before We Are Born: Essentials of Embryology and Birth Defects*, 6th edition. Philadelphia, Saunders, 2003, p 36.

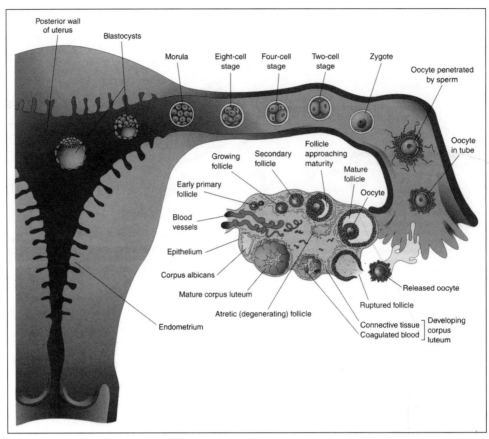

Fertilization/Embryology

At the beginning of the third week after the first day of the last menstrual period, ovulation occurs, and fertilization of the ovum usually follows within a day or two. The early development of the conceptus/embryo can be summarized as follows:

1 The Conceptus Period: Weeks 3–5

- Week 3 (Days 14–21): Early development of the conceptus (figure 1)

    Day 14: Ovulation and fertilization of ovum.

    Days 14–18: Zygote traverses the fallopian tube.

    8-cell stage.

    12- to 16-cell stage: *morula.*

    Day 18: Morula enters uterus.

    Days 18–21: Blastocyst cavity and inner cell mass form; blastocyst cavity becomes primary yolk sac; amniotic formation begins.

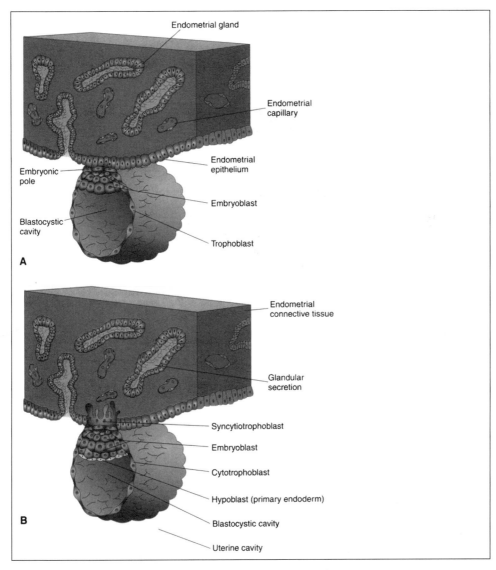

Figure 2.
Attachment of the blastocyst to the endometrial epithelium and the early stages of its implantation. **A** At six days (19 menstrual days) the trophoblast is attached to the endometrial epithelium at the embryonic pole of the blastocyst. **B** At seven days (20 menstrual days) the syncytiotrophoblast has penetrated the epithelium and has started to invade the endometrial stroma (framework of connective tissue). Reprinted with permission from Moore KL, Persaud TVN: *Before We Are Born: Essentials of Embryology and Birth Defects,* 6th edition. Philadelphia, Saunders, 2003, p 34.

- Week 4 (Days 21–28)

  Implantation of the blastocyst in the uterine wall and formation of the *syncytiotrophoblast* (placental precursor) (figure 2). Vaginal bleeding may occur at this time.

  Bilaminar embryonic disc: Transformation of inner cell mass into bilaminar embryonic disc (figure 3).

  Amnion and *chorion:* Regression of primary yolk sac and formation of secondary yolk sac and the surrounding *chorionic cavity* (figure 4). The *amniotic sac* enlarges on the side of the embryo opposite the chorionic cavity. The adjacent amnion and secondary yolk sac are sometimes visible sonographically within the chorionic cavity. This finding is called the "double bleb" sign. At the beginning of the 4th week, the gestational sac is about 1 mm in diameter.

Figure 3.
Implanted blastocyst. Drawing of a section through a blastocyst of about 9 gestational days (22 menstrual days) implanted in the endometrium. Note the lacunae appearing in the syncytiotrophoblast. The actual size of the conceptus is about 0.1 mm. The type of implantation illustrated here, in which the blastocyst becomes competely embedded in the endometrium, is called *interstitial implantation*. Reprinted with permission from Moore KL, Persaud TVN: *Before We Are Born: Essentials of Embryology and Birth Defects,* 6th edition. Philadelphia, Saunders, 2003, p 38.

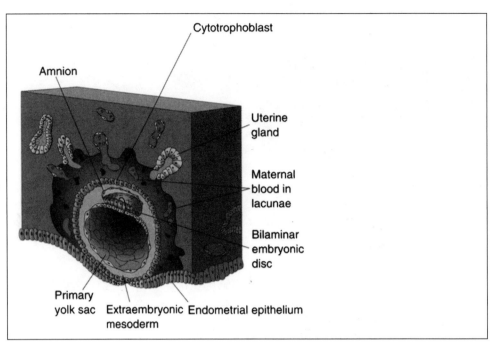

- Week 5 (Days 29–30)

Gastrulation: Formation of the trilaminar disc, comprising the three primary germ layers: ectoderm, endoderm, mesoderm; formation of the primitive node and streak (*mesenchyme*) and formation of *notocord*. The notocord forms within the embryonic plate between the amnion and the secondary yolk sac. The notocord induces development of the

Figure 4.
Implanted embryo. Drawing of a section through an implanted human embryo at 14 gestational days (27 menstrual days), showing the newly formed secondary yolk sac and the location of the prechordal plate in its roof. Reprinted with permission from Moore KL, Persaud TVN: *Before We Are Born: Essentials of Embryology and Birth Defects,* 6th edition. Philadelphia, Saunders, 2003, p 40.

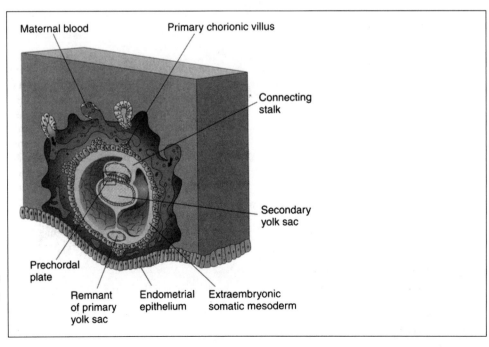

structure of the early embryo and later develops into the vertebral bodies of the spinal column.

- Week 5 (Days 31–42)

    Neurulation: Formation of the neural plate and neural tube and somites, which develop into the central nervous system (figure 5).

    Day 35: Neural tube formation begins.

    Day 40: Closing of the *rostral* (head) end of the neural tube.

    Day 42: Closing of the *caudal* (sacral) end of the neural tube.

    If the neural tube does not close properly, neural tube defects will be the result.

    Angiogenesis and *hematogenesis:* Formation of primitive blood cells and blood vessels, heart, and placental vascularity.

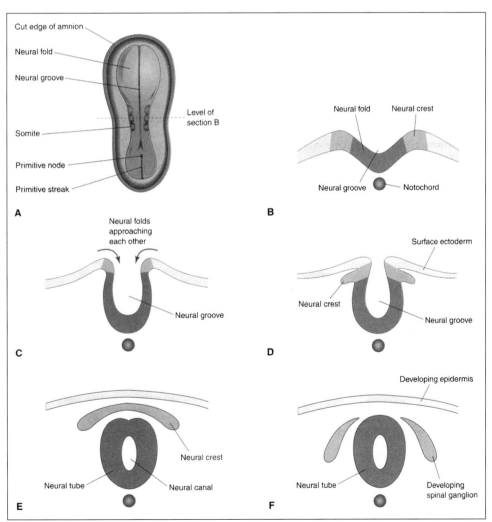

Figure 5.

The developing embryo. Diagrammatic transverse sections through progressively older embryos, illustrating formation of the neural groove, the neural tube, and the neural crest up to the end of the 6th menstrual week. Reprinted with permission from Moore KL, Persaud TVN: *Before We Are Born: Essentials of Embryology and Birth Defects,* 6th edition. Philadelphia, Saunders, 2003, p 55.

2 The Embryonic Period: Weeks 6–10: Formation of All Permanent Internal and External Structures of the Individual

- Cardiovascular system

    6 weeks: Unidirectional blood flow.

    8 weeks: Formation of the heart is complete.

    10 weeks: Formation of the peripheral vascular system is complete.

- Gastrointestinal system

    6 weeks: Formation of the primitive gut.

    8–12 weeks: Herniation of the midgut into the umbilical cord.

    8 weeks: Separation of the rectum from the urogenital sinus.

    10 weeks: Perforation of the anal membrane.

- Urogenital system

    8 weeks: Formation of the primitive kidney (*metanephros*) in the pelvis and ascension into the abdomen.

    11 weeks: Kidneys in adult position, external genitalia similar in males and females; genitalia differentiate by 14 weeks.

- Musculoskeletal system

    5.5–6 weeks: Formation of limb buds.

    7.5–8 weeks: Digital rays develop; arms bent at elbow.

    8 weeks: Clavicle begins to ossify.

    9 weeks: Mandible, palate, vertebral bodies, and neural arches begin to ossify.

    11 weeks: Long bones begin to ossify.

Sonographic Findings in Early Intrauterine Pregnancy

1 Decidual Thickening

The earliest sonographic sign of pregnancy that has been described is focal thickening of the echogenic decidua at the site of implantation.[3] This finding is quite subtle, and the predictive value of the finding has not been established.

2 Gestational Sac

- The fluid-filled gestational sac is first visible at about 4.5–5 menstrual weeks, and it is the first definitive sign of pregnancy. With the use of endovaginal scanning, it can be visualized at a mean sac diameter (MSD)

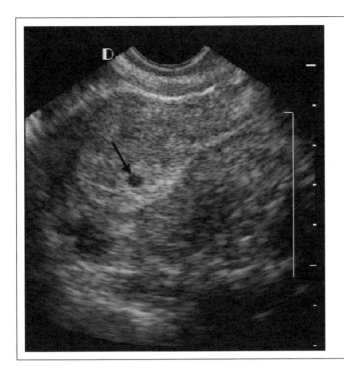

Figure 6.
Early intrauterine pregnancy. Longitudinal view of a pregnant uterus containing a small echolucency (arrow) most likely representing an early intrauterine pregnancy.

of 2–3 mm and on transabdominal scanning at approximately 5 mm mean sac diameter. It appears as a small fluid collection surrounded by an echogenic rim. The central fluid is the chorionic cavity. The surrounding echogenic rim represents the developing chorionic villi and adjacent decidual tissue. The normal position for the gestational sac is in the upper- to mid-uterus.

- Intradecidual sign: The sonographic presence of a small gestational sac (figure 6) within the decidua at approximately 4.0–4.5 weeks, with a mean sac diameter of approximately 2.5 mm, is known as the *intradecidual sign*. To distinguish a true intradecidual sign from a decidual (endometrial) cyst, the sonographer must be sure that the gestational sac is directly adjacent to the endometrial canal. Because the intradecidual sign can sometimes mimic a pseudogestational sac of ectopic pregnancy, its value appears somewhat limited.

- Double decidual sign: The echogenic ring formed by the decidua vera (parietalis) and decidua capsularis is called the *double decidual sign*. The *decidua basalis* (future placenta) may be visualized as an area of echogenic thickening on one portion of the sac. This sign can typically be visualized by 5.5–6 menstrual weeks (figure 7), when the mean sac diameter is approximately 10 mm. With the extensive use of high-resolution transvaginal sonography, the double sac sign plays a less significant role in the determination of pregnancy.

Figure 7.

Gestational sac. Note the thickening of deciduas basalis (large arrow) and "double sac" area (multiple small arrows).

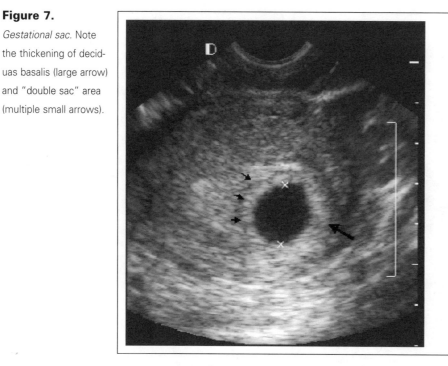

- The gestational sac is measured by imaging the sac in the long axis (figure 8) and taking the A-P, longitudinal, and transverse measurements, then averaging the three measurements to get the mean sac diameter. The early gestational sac is elliptical and may be distorted by a focal myometrial contraction (FMC). The gestational sac is measured as a part of the obstetrical sonogram until about 10 menstrual weeks. After about

Figure 8.

Measuring the gestational sac. Longitudinal view of a gestational sac demonstrating measurements in the long and A-P axes (cursors).

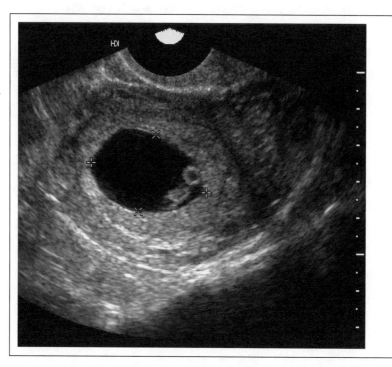

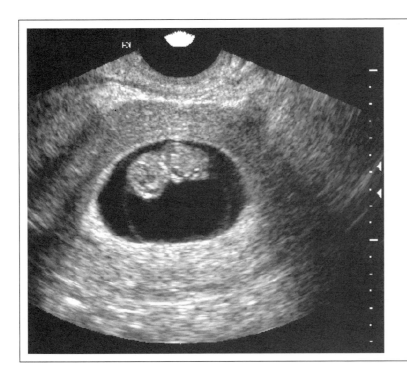

Figure 9.
Crown-rump length. Sonogram of an embryo (crown-rump length) at approximately 7 menstrual weeks.

7 menstrual weeks, the gestational sac measurement is no longer used as the primary means of determining gestational age. Once the embryo is large enough to measure accurately, the crown-rump length (CRL) (figure 9) becomes the primary measurement for determining age. The comparison of embryo size and gestational sac size is helpful in assessing the risk of miscarriage.

3 Yolk Sac

● The yolk sac is the first structure visualized within the gestational sac. The sonographically visualized yolk sac is the secondary yolk sac. It is spherical in shape, with a sonolucent center and clearly defined echogenic wall (figure 10). On transvaginal sonography it is often visualized when the mean sac diameter of the gestational sac is approximately 5 mm (5 menstrual weeks) and normally should always be visualized when the mean sac diameter is 8 mm (5.5 menstrual weeks). High-frequency transvaginal sonography (7–10 MHz) is required to consistently visualize yolk sacs in 8-mm gestational sacs. On transabdominal sonography the yolk sac should always be visible at approximately 20 mm mean sac diameter or 7 menstrual weeks.

● While the placenta is developing, the yolk sac transfers nutrients to the embryo. Hematopoiesis occurs in the wall of the yolk sac in the 5th week before the liver takes over that function at about the 8th week. The upper limit of the yolk sac is 5.6 mm at approximately 5–10 weeks.

Figure 10.

Yolk sac. Sonogram of a gestational sac with yolk sac (arrow) situated normally between the amnion and chorion.

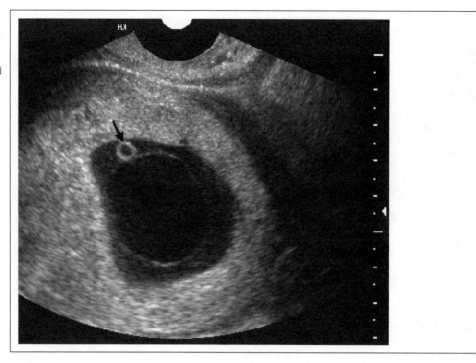

4 Double Bleb Sign

At 5.5 menstrual weeks, the developing amniotic sac measures about 2 mm in diameter and becomes visible adjacent to the yolk sac. (See figure 11.) This double sac appearance is called the *double bleb sign*. At this time the bilaminar embryonic disc lies between the yolk sac and the amnion. The double bleb sign is no longer visible by 7 menstrual weeks.

Figure 11A.

Double bleb sign. Transverse view through gestational sac. Note the amnion (black arrow) and yolk sac (white arrow) with embryo situated between.

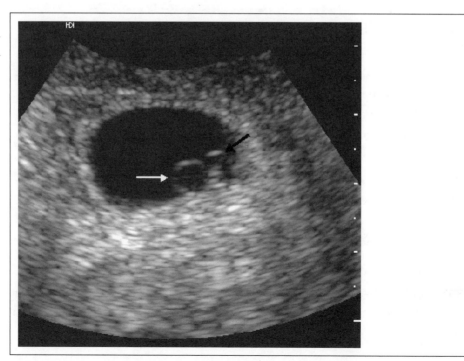

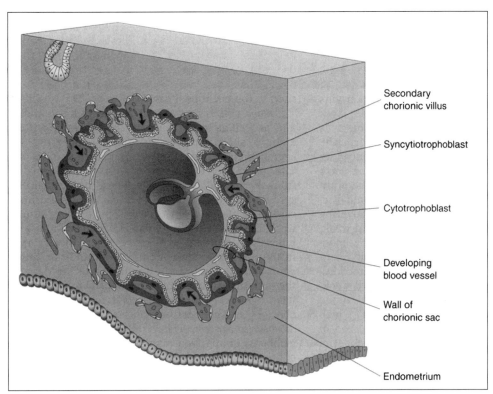

Figure 11B.
The embryo. Sagittal section of an embryo (about 29 menstrual days/16 gestational days). Reprinted with permission from Moore KL, Persaud TVN: *Before We Are Born: Essentials of Embryology and Birth Defects*, 6th edition. Philadelphia, Saunders, 2003, p 59.

5 Embryo

● With the use of endovaginal sonography (EVS), the embryo is often visible at 5–5.5 menstrual weeks, measuring 1–2 mm in crown-rump length, adjacent to the yolk sac. Embryonic cardiac activity may be visualized when the crown-rump length is approximately 2–4 mm and will be observed in normal embryos greater than 5 mm in length. In normal pregnancies when the gestational mean sac diameter is greater than 16 mm, the embryo and heartbeat will also be visualized. High-frequency (7–10 MHz) endovaginal sonography probes, appropriate focusing, and low-persistence settings are needed to adequately image the embryo and heartbeat.

● Cardiac activity: Embryonic cardiac activity may sometimes be detected between 5 and 6 weeks' menstrual age (figure 12), and the rate is relatively slow. Most investigators have reported a normal range of 100–115 bpm between 5 and 6 weeks' menstrual age. The mean heart rate increases to approximately 140 bpm by 9 weeks' menstrual age. There appears to be a correlation between slow heart rates and miscarriage in embryos: less than 100 bpm before 6.2 menstrual weeks and less than 120 bpm between 6.3 and 7.0 weeks.[4] If the embryonic heart rate is abnormally low, follow-up sonography is advisable.

Figure 12.
Embryonic cardiac activity. M-mode sonogram of gestational sac with cursor demonstrating embryonic cardiac activity.

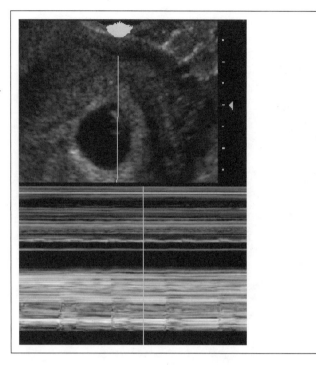

6 Amnion

Gradually the amnion grows to fill the chorionic cavity by approximately 12–16 weeks. With high-resolution equipment, occasionally, diffuse low-level echoes may be observed filling the chorionic cavity (figure 13). The cause of the low-level echoes is unknown but most likely represents the thick proteinaceous material contained within the cavity.

Figure 13.
Amnion. Gestational sac containing amnion (arrow). Note the subtle echoes located between the amnion and chorion representing proteinaceous material.

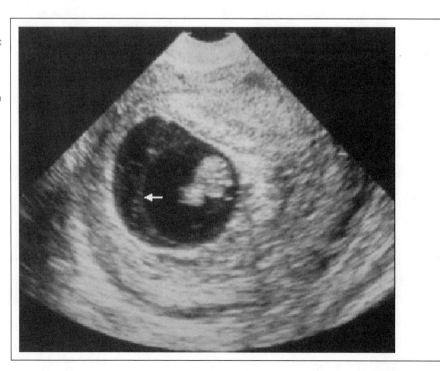

7 Beta-Human Chorionic Gonadotropin and Sonographic Findings

The serum beta–human chorionic gonadotropin hormone (serum hCG) level can be correlated with sonographic findings in early pregnancy. Two different systems have been used to measure beta-hCG. The International Research Preparation (IRP) measuring system was developed first, and later the Second International Standard (SIS) came into use. In samples that have equivalent beta-hCG levels, the numerical result using the SIS system will be approximately double the result using the IRP system. At this time, most laboratories have reverted to using the IRP system. Recently a third standard, the Third IRP (3IS), has been introduced. The 3IS system yields levels similar to the initial IRP. A correlation can be made between sonographic identification of the gestational sac in early pregnancy and maternal serum beta-hCG levels. The gestational sac must be visualized normally:

	IRP or 3IS	**SIS**
Endovaginal sonography	1000–2000 IU/ml	500–1000
Transabdominal sonography	3600 IU/ml	1800

Abnormal First Trimester (Failed Pregnancy)

Wilcox and others have demonstrated a 20–31% rate of early pregnancy loss after implantation in the normal healthy volunteer.[5, 6] Overall, 75% of pregnancies will fail. Vaginal bleeding is not uncommon and occurs in approximately 25% of patients during the first few weeks of pregnancy. Often the bleeding is temporary and likely due to implantation of the conceptus into the endometrium. Sonography plays a major role in assessing the patient who has first trimester bleeding to diagnose early pregnancy failure.

Threatened abortion can be defined as spotting, bleeding, or cramping in the 1st trimester with a closed cervical os. About half of such patients will have a normal outcome and half will subsequently abort. Loss rates are influenced by maternal age, smoking, and alcohol or caffeine consumption, as well as other causes, such as failure of the corpus luteum sufficiently to support the implanted conceptus. The corpus luteum secretes progesterone to support pregnancy until the placenta takes over the hormonal function. It forms during the secretory phase of the menstrual cycle and during pregnancy is usually less than 5 cm in diameter with a variety of appearances. The corpus luteal cyst usually regresses or decreases in size at approximately 16–18 weeks. When the corpus luteal cyst persists beyond 18 weeks it should be followed.

In a *complete abortion,* all the gestational tissue, including the embryo, has passed out of the uterus, and the uterine cavity is empty. If gestational tissue remains within the uterus and bleeding persists, the appropriate term is *incomplete abortion* or *abortion in process*. The term *missed abortion* is vague and has fallen out of use.

If a gestational sac is present in the uterus but no embryo is identified in a sac large enough to require one, the condition is called *blighted ovum* or *anembryonic pregnancy*. In *embryonic demise*, an embryo greater than 5 mm is observed without a heartbeat. Some have suggested the general term *failed pregnancy* to describe all these conditions.

Sonographic Signs of Abnormal Early Pregnancy

1 Abnormal Gestational Sac

- Reasonably reliable early findings that suggest an abnormal pregnancy include:

1. Gestational sac greater than 8 mm without a yolk sac.
2. Gestational sac greater than 16 mm without an embryo or heartbeat.
3. Amniotic sac noted within the gestational sac and absent embryo.
4. Embryo greater than 5 mm without a heartbeat.
5. Mean sac diameter minus crown-rump length less than 5 mm between 5.5 and 9 weeks.
6. Gestational sac much larger than the embryo.

Many physicians allow 2- or 3-mm leeway in mean sac diameter as a margin for error.

- Signs of abnormal pregnancy that are less reliable or not as well established include:

1. Irregular shape of the gestational sac.
2. Missing double sac sign.
3. Weak decidual echoes at the edge of the gestational sac.
4. Low position of the sac in the uterus.
5. Yolk sac less than 2 mm or greater than 5.6 mm, irregular shape, or calcified.
6. Growth of the gestational sac mean sac diameter of less than 0.6 mm per day. (Normal growth is 1.13 mm per day.)
7. Embryonic bradycardia.

In one study, embryos less than 5 mm in size had 100% mortality if the heart rate was less than 80 bpm, 64% if the heart rate was 80–90 bpm, 32% if the heart rate was 90–99 bpm, and 11% if the heart rate was 100 bpm or more.[4]

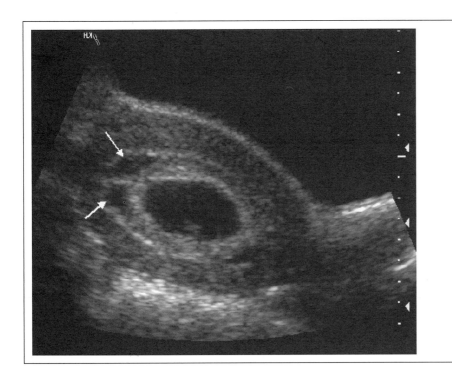

Figure 14.

Subchorionic hemorrhage. Longitudinal view through the uterus demonstrating the gestational sac with hypoechoic area superiorly (arrows) representing hemorrhage.

2 Intrauterine Blood

Blood within the uterine cavity and outside the gestational sac is a marker for an increased risk of miscarriage. The blood collection may be adjacent to or opposite the placenta (subchorionic hemorrhage) (figure 14), or it may be partly or completely retroplacental. During early pregnancy the blood visualized may be due to implantation of *chorion frondosum* (the fetal contribution to the placenta) as it penetrates into *decidua basalis* (the maternal contribution to the placenta). The risk of miscarriage increases with the size of a subchorionic hemorrhage. Abruption is more likely to result in miscarriage than is subchorionic hemorrhage.

3 Fetal Anomalies

- As *endovaginal sonography* has become more widely used, many physicians and sonographers are imaging various anatomical structures in embryos and fetuses late in the first trimester. *Normal fetal structures* that can be confused with abnormality include:

1. Normal herniation (i.e., physiological herniation) of bowel into the base of the umbilical cord. The herniation occurs at about 8 weeks and should return to the abdomen before 14 weeks (figure 15).

2. Prominent rhombencephalon. The early appearance (7–9 menstrual weeks) of the fourth ventricle resembles a posterior fossa cystic mass (figure 16).

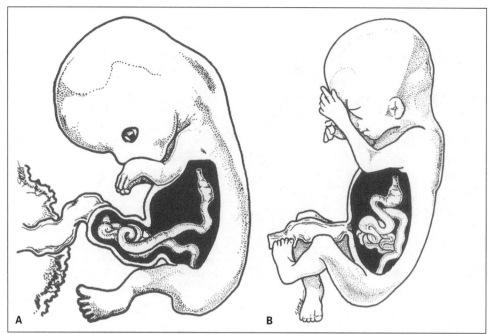

Figure 15.
Physiological herniation. **A** Drawing of a fetus at 9 menstrual weeks demonstrating normal herniation of bowel into the cord. **B** Drawing of a fetus at 14 menstrual weeks showing return of bowel into the abdominal cavity. Reprinted with permission from Cyr DR, Mack LA, Schoenecker SA, et al: Bowel migration in normal fetus: US detection. *Radiology* 161:119–121, 1986.

- *Anencephaly* cannot be detected in the first trimester. Many physicians have observed normal-appearing late first-trimester fetuses that later demonstrated anencephaly.

- *Nuchal translucency.* In late first trimester an important part of fetal evaluation is assessment of the thickness of the posterior nuchal translucency, found along the posterior neck of most embryos. The nuchal translucency is a hypoechoic area between the posterior soft tissues of

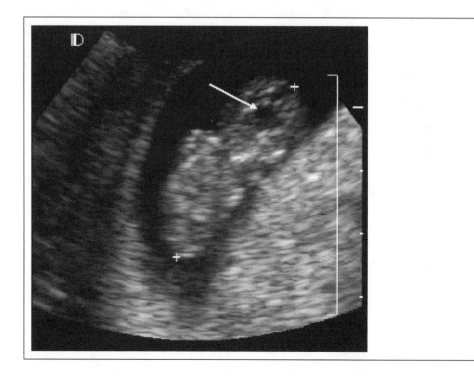

Figure 16.
Rhomboencephalon. Coronal view of an embryo showing the normal rhomboencephalon (arrow).

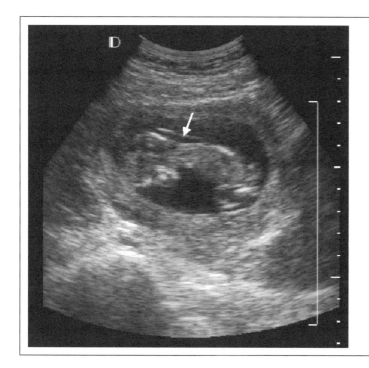

Figure 17.
Nuchal translucency. Sagittal sonogram of a fetus demonstrating abnormal nuchal translucency (arrows).

the neck and the overlying skin. The measurement includes only the translucent portion; it is an inner-to-inner measurement that does not include the thickness of the overlying skin (figure 17). This translucency usually becomes visible by about 10 weeks and is present in normal individuals. The thickness changes during the first trimester, peaking at 13 to 14 weeks, then becoming thinner.

Normal values for nuchal translucency have been established.[7] The 95th percentile for normal fetuses in early pregnancy is 2.2 mm at 11 weeks to 2.8 mm at 14 weeks. Nuchal translucency measurements over the 95th percentile are generally considered to be abnormal. Careful technique is important, for this is a small structure. Enlarging the image makes it easier to accurately measure the translucent area, and the measurement should be taken with the neck of the fetus flexed. A common error is confusing the unfused amnion with the fetal skin, so it is helpful to observe the fetus as it moves away from the edge of the amniotic sac. Both transabdominal and transvaginal techniques have proven successful for assessing the nuchal area. A fetus that has an abnormally thick nuchal translucency will be found to have an abnormal karyotype in 46% of cases overall.[8] The most commonly encountered abnormalities are trisomy 18, trisomy 21, and Turner's syndrome (45,XO). When the translucency contains septations, there may be even higher risk of aneuploidy.

The clinical management of pregnancies with thickened nuchal translucency is still evolving. Most investigators combine the nuchal translucency measurement and biochemical testing when deciding if chromosome testing is required.

Some investigators recommend karyotyping above the 95th percentile, while others would not recommend additional genetic testing unless the nuchal translucency measurement is over 2.5 or 3.5 mm. In most cases, the nuchal translucency will resolve. *Resolution of an abnormally thickened nuchal translucency does not indicate the fetus has normal chromosomes.*

In the case of a normal karyotype with thickened nuchal translucency, the fetus remains at risk. A complete, detailed sonogram in the second trimester is essential in these cases. Most experts have noted a good outcome when both karyotype and follow-up detailed fetal sonogram are normal. Others, however, cautioned that these fetuses remain at increased risk for poor outcome as a result of preterm delivery or growth restriction.

Ectopic Pregnancy

An *ectopic pregnancy* is one that occurs outside the uterine cavity. This may happen because the fallopian tubes are unable to function normally as a result of scarring, intrinsic embryonic abnormalities, pelvic masses, an intrauterine device (IUD), or because of in vitro fertilization. The incidence has been increasing since 1970. Today, sensitive tests such as serum beta-hCG accompanied by physical exam and high-resolution ultrasound exam allow earlier diagnosis of previously unsuspected cases. It is therefore possible to take a more elective approach to management and treatment in these patients. Laparoscopy is considered the gold standard for the diagnosis of ectopic pregnancy. Currently, clinical assessment includes both transvaginal sonography and beta-hCG testing.

The clinical presentation associated with ectopic pregnancy sometimes includes "the classic triad"—pain, bleeding, and palpable adnexal mass—but this combination of symptoms is present in only 45% of patients who have ectopic pregnancy.

Other conditions that can have similar clinical presentation include:

- Symptomatic ovarian cysts.
- Pelvic inflammatory disease (PID).
- Dysfunctional uterine bleeding (DUB).
- Spontaneous abortions.

1 Incidence

Patients who have an increased risk for ectopic pregnancy include those with a history of:

- Previous ectopic pregnancy.
- Pelvic inflammatory disease.
- Previous tubal surgery.
- Use of IUD.
- In vitro fertilization.

Although some patients are at higher risk for ectopic pregnancy, any pregnant woman may have an ectopic pregnancy.

2 Serum beta-Human Chorionic Gonadotropin

Correlating the clinical presentation, sonographic findings, and serum beta-hCG is very important. A negative beta-hCG essentially excludes the diagnosis of a live pregnancy, although a chronic, nonliving ectopic pregnancy may have a negative beta-hCG. Serum beta-hCG is a widely available blood test, which becomes positive at approximately 23 menstrual days (9 days postconception). This occurs before the first missed period and before a gestational sac can be visualized with transvaginal sonography. If the beta-hCG level is less than 1000–2000 IRP, sonography may be negative in a normal pregnancy. In such cases, serial hCG levels or repeat sonograms can be helpful. In a normal pregnancy, the serum beta-hCG doubles every 2 days (1.2–2.2 days), whereas in ectopic pregnancy, the beta-hCG level does not usually rise as quickly.

3 Treatment

Patients suspected of having an ectopic pregnancy may be treated surgically with laparotomy or laparoscopy. Currently, some patients who have early ectopic pregnancy are being treated with systemic methotrexate to inhibit trophoblastic cell growth. Treatment with methotrexate seems to be most effective in early pregnancy, before the embryo appears.

4 Early Intrauterine Pregnancy vs. Ectopic Pregnancy

A small cystic sac may be visualized within the endometrium and represent a:

- Small normal intrauterine pregnancy
- Decidual cyst
- Pseudogestational sac of ectopic pregnancy

Visualization of an intrauterine fluid collection with double sac sign is a more reliable indicator of normal early intrauterine pregnancy than the intradecidual sac. However, the double sac sign does not absolutely rule out a pseudogestational sac. The presence of the yolk sac and embryo further confirm the diagnosis of a normal intrauterine pregnancy. In any case, it is important to evaluate the adnexa, particularly in those patients who have undergone in vitro fertilization.

Scan technique: Some examiners begin with a transabdominal sonogram to evaluate any masses that may not be visualized by transvaginal sonography. In an emergency situation when the bladder is not full, the endovaginal scan can be performed alone, but in those cases upper pelvic masses may be missed. Endovaginal sonography will usually give much better detail of the uterus and endometrium than is possible with transabdominal sonography. Visualization of early intrauterine pregnancy, which is not visible transabdominally, would greatly diminish the likelihood of ectopic pregnancy.

5 Sites of Ectopic Pregnancy

Ectopic pregnancy occurs in the ampullary portion of the fallopian tube approximately 80% of the time and in the isthmic or interstitial portions 10–15% of the time. Rare locations include the cervix, abdomen, and ovaries (figure 18). It is important to scan above and below the ovary and between the ovaries and uterus because the tube is the most common location for ectopic pregnancy. If an adnexal mass is visualized, it should be examined for yolk sac, embryo, and cardiac activity. If a thick-walled cyst is visualized in the adnexa, differentiation must be made between a corpus luteum cyst and tubal ring of ectopic pregnancy.

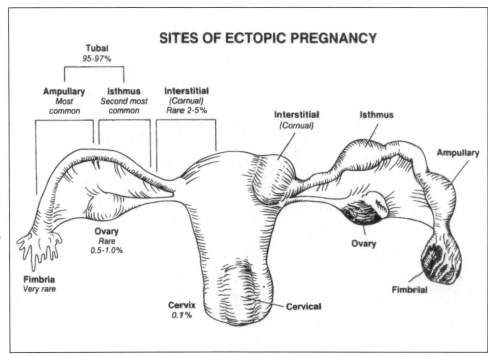

Figure 18. *Sites of ectopic pregnancies.* Common locations of ectopic pregnancy. Note that 95% to 97% of ectopic pregnancies occur somewhere along the course of the fallopian tube. (Modified from Benson RC: *Handbook of Obstetrics & Gynecology,* 8th ed. Los Altos, CA, Lange Medical Publications, 1983; Schoenbaum S, Rosendorf L, Kappelman N, et al: Gray-scale ultrasound in tubal pregnancy. *Radiology* 127:757, 1978.)

The *cul de sac* must also be evaluated for free fluid. Complex fluid is suggestive of blood and possibly ectopic pregnancy. A small amount of fluid is seen in both normal and abnormal pregnancies; however, large amounts of fluid, particularly complex fluid, increase the likelihood of ectopic pregnancy.

Sonographic Findings Related to Ectopic Pregnancy

1 The *endometrium* has no specific findings for ectopic pregnancy. The thickness of the endometrium in ectopic pregnancy seems to vary from thin to thick. A thin-walled, simple-appearing decidual cyst can be seen with ectopic pregnancy or normal intrauterine pregnancy. In a stable patient at risk for ectopic pregnancy, a serial hCG can be obtained as well as a follow-up sonogram.

2 *Fluid* is a nonspecific finding for ectopic pregnancy, though a large amount of fluid is suggestive of ectopic pregnancy. Complex fluid (figure 19) is consistent with hemoperitoneum and is associated with ectopic pregnancy but not necessarily rupture of the fallopian tube.

3 If an *extrauterine adnexal ring, yolk sac,* and *heartbeat* (figure 20) are visualized, these findings are consistent with ectopic pregnancy. Also, a complex adnexal mass separate from the ovary is quite suspicious for ectopic pregnancy in a patient with a positive pregnancy test. Approximately 25% of patients who have an ectopic pregnancy have a completely normal sonogram.

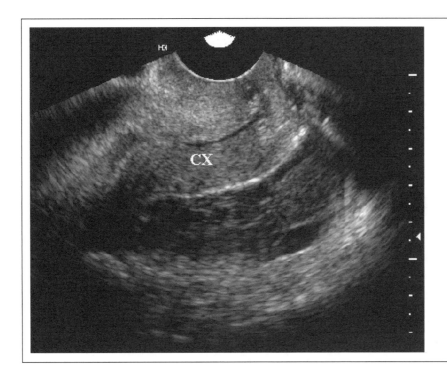

Figure 19.
Complex fluid. Longitudinal midline sonogram of cul de sac area. Note the complex echoes posterior to the cervix (CX) representing hemorrhage.

When a patient is pregnant and has no identifiable intrauterine gestational sac, one of the following is most likely:

- The pregnancy is too small for definitive identification.
- A recent spontaneous abortion has occurred.
- Ectopic pregnancy is present.

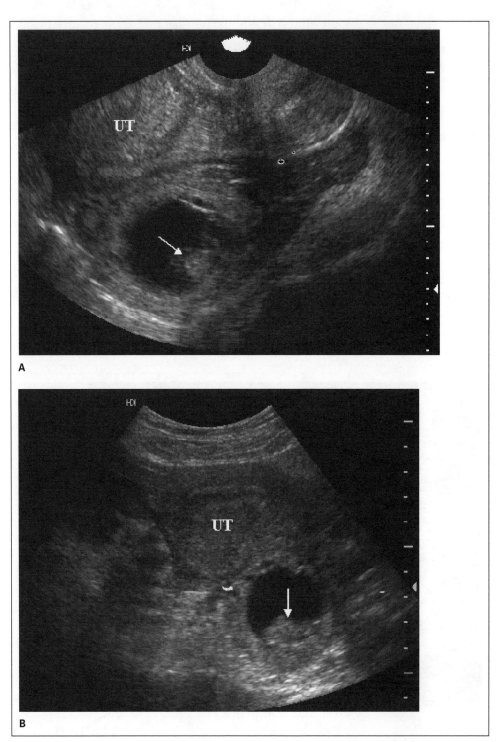

Figure 20.
Ectopic pregnancy. Longitudinal (**A**) and transverse (**B**) views through the uterus (UT). Note the gestational sac with embryo (arrow) located posterior to the uterus.

CHAPTER 2

Second/Third Trimester (Normal Anatomy)

Face

Cranium

Thorax

Heart

Spine

Extremities

Fetal abdomen and pelvis

Summary

. . . .

Since the early days of sonography, steady advances have been made in understanding normal fetal anatomy. Instrumentation has improved, yielding images of high resolution and clarity of detail. The clearer images have led to improved understanding of anatomy. Also, imaging premature neonates, who are the equivalent of third trimester fetuses, has helped improve our understanding of fetal anatomy.

Problems still exist, however. If the fetus is in a suboptimal position, we will be unable to get good images of some fetal parts. Also, if the mother is obese or if the amniotic fluid volume is too low or too high, the quality of the images will be dramatically altered.

With a little effort, it is usually possible to image most of the important fetal structures in most cases. In order to accomplish this, the sonographer must:

1. Assess the fetal position.
2. Decide if the anatomic part of interest is best visualized in long or short axis of the fetus.
3. Use the appropriate transducer, find the best acoustic window to image a particular fetal part, and adjust appropriate imaging parameters, including time-gain compensation, to optimize the image.

Real-time imaging is helpful in rapidly surveying the fetal position and in adjusting for changes in fetal position.

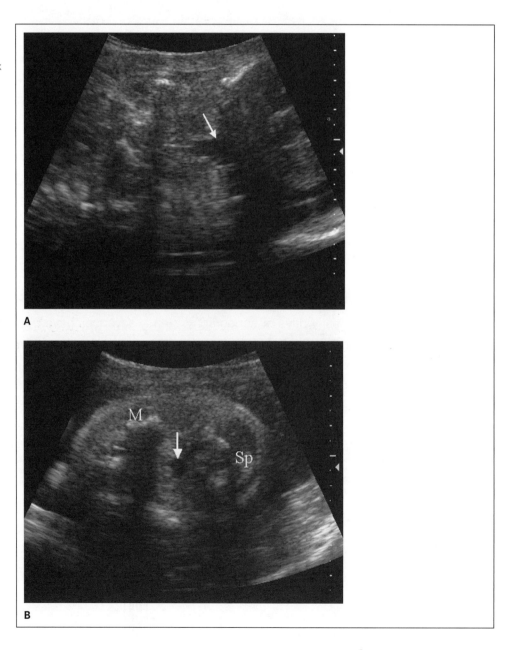

Figure 21.
Fetal neck. **A** Coronal sonogram of fetal neck demonstrating the oropharynx (arrow). **B** Axial sonogram also shows the oropharynx (arrow). Sp = spine, M = mandible.

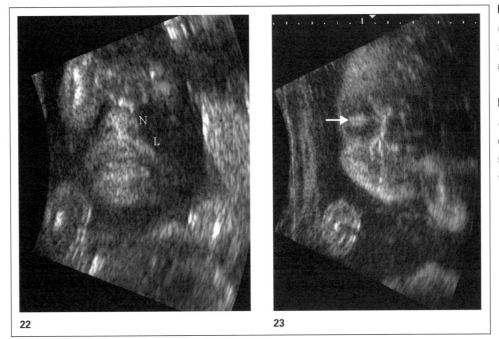

Figure 22.
Coronal view of a fetal face. Note the nose (N) and lips (L).

Figure 23.
Fetal face. Note the eyelid (arrow) in this sonogram of the fetal face.

Face

The fetal face can be visualized with considerable clarity. If detailed imaging of facial anatomy is required, the following views should be obtained:

- Axial views of the orbits, nose, lips, anterior palate, tongue, and oropharynx (figure 21).
- Coronal views of the orbits, nose, lips (figure 22), maxilla, and anterior portion of the mandible.
- Profile view of soft tissues and facial bones, including the nasal bones and mandible.
- Views of the ears.

The brow, cheeks, eyelids (figure 23), lenses, nose, lips, and chin can be consistently imaged. Detailed imaging of the nose and lips (figure 22) is necessary to exclude cleft lip. The nasal bridge, alae, nares, and philtrum (figure 24) can also be visualized.

In the older fetus, detail of the intraorbital contents can be visualized, including globe, lens (figure 25), and sometimes optic nerve. The maxilla, mandible, and tooth buds are also visualized sonographically (figure 26). The gingival ridge with tooth buds is seen commonly in fetuses of 20 weeks or more. The fetal mouth and fetal tongue (figure 27) can be observed. The tongue is identified most easily during swallowing movements. In some second trimester fetuses, the hard palate can be evaluated (figure 28) if the fetal position is favorable.

Figure 24.
Philtrum. Coronal view of fetal face demonstrating the philtrum (arrow). The philtrum is the midline notch in the upper lip between the nostrils.

Figure 25.
Lens. Coronal view of fetal face demonstrating the fetal lens in the fetal orbit.

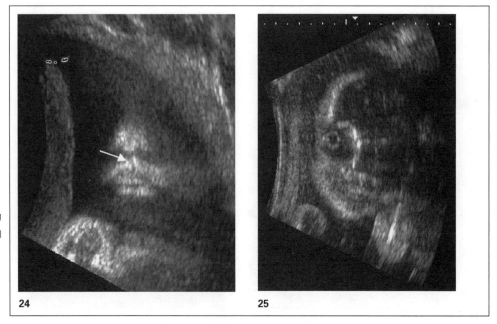

Figure 26.
Maxilla and mandible. Axial sonogram of the maxilla (**A**) and mandible (**B**). The maxilla has a rounder contour anteriorly and the mandible is more pointed anteriorly. Note the hypoechoic toothbuds in the anterior maxilla and mandible (arrows).

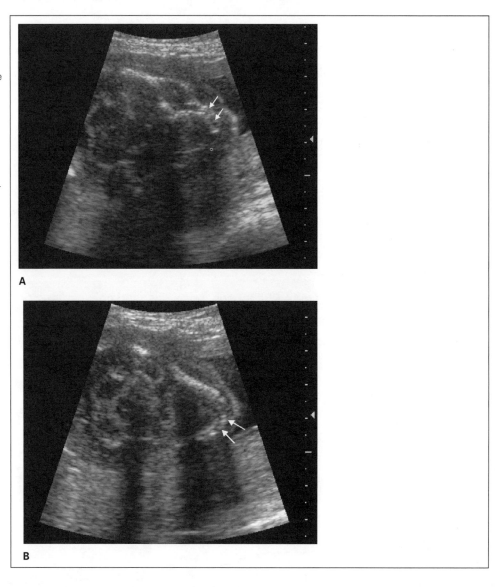

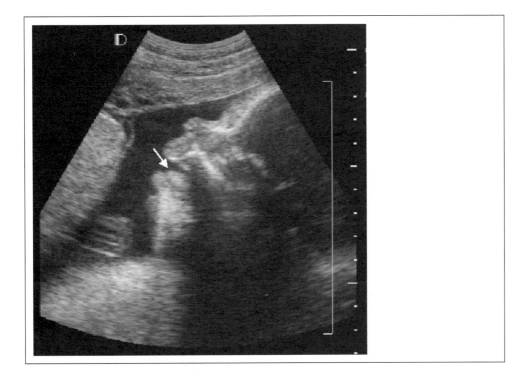

Figure 27.
Tongue. Sagittal sonogram of fetal face. Note the tongue (arrow).

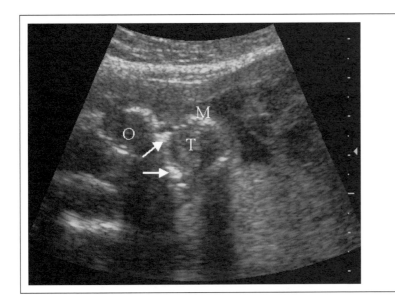

Figure 28.
Hard palate. Coronal sonogram through the fetal face demonstrating the hard palate (arrows). T = tongue, O = orbit, M = mandible

Cranium

The fetal brain was one of the first areas of investigation in the diagnosis of fetal anomalies. This most likely occurred because:

1. Sonographic evaluation was being done on the neonatal head and correlated with fetal sonography.

2. The fetal head was routinely evaluated to obtain a biparietal diameter (BPD) for determination of gestational age.

3. CNS anomalies were among the most significant of birth defects.

Initially only gross anomalies were detected prenatally. Currently, many malformations of the brain can be diagnosed with accuracy even before 20 weeks of development.[9–14] In order to detect anomalous brain development, one must have a clear understanding of normal anatomy. Fetal brain images are usually obtained in axial planes, which are appropriate for both biparietal diameter and head circumference. Scan sweeps from superior to inferior assist in evaluating normal anatomy.

Important dural structures that are visible sonographically include the falx and tentorium.

Occasionally, neural structures generate high-amplitude reflections. This is particularly true of the cerebellar vermis. The surface tissues of the cerebellar hemispheres also appear quite bright.

The lateral ventricles are visualized in the transaxial view, and by 18–20 weeks the occipital and temporal horns are easily recognizable. The middle and anterior portions of the lateral ventricles vary in shape during fetal development; however, throughout the period of observation of fetal lateral ventricles (from 13 to 40 weeks), the size of the atria remains largely unchanged. The transverse diameter of the ventricular atrium (figure 29) shows an average dimension of approximately 7 mm and an upper limit of 10 mm throughout the second and third trimesters. It is important to note that the anterior and occipital horns of the lateral ventricles do not normally contain choroid plexus.

The fetal cerebellum (figure 30) should be routinely imaged in a transverse plane that includes the cavum septum pellucidum anteriorly and the cerebellum posteriorly. The cavum septum pellucidum is a fluid-filled midline structure between the lateral ventricles in the developing fetal

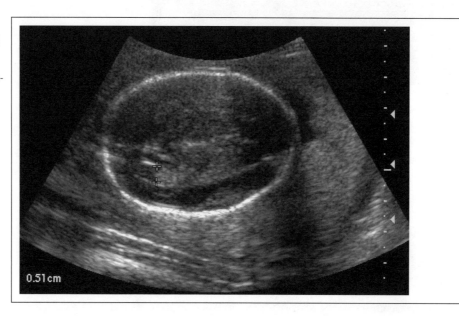

Figure 29.
Ventricular atrium. Axial sonogram of the fetal ventricles showing measurement of the atrium (cursors).

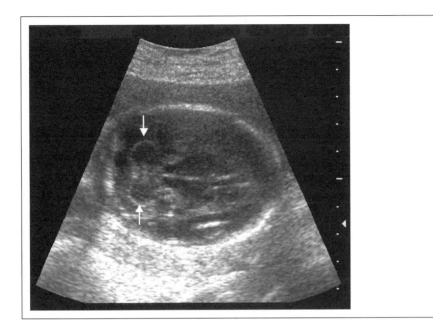

Figure 30.
The fetal cerebellum (arrows).

brain. This structure usually disappears by the end of pregnancy. Fluid is normally visible between the occipital bone and the cerebellar hemispheres. The thickness of the soft tissues of the nape of the neck can also be evaluated.

The ears can be visualized quite well and their progressive maturation noted (figure 31). The external auditory canal, helix, lobule, and tragus can be depicted, but the relative position of the ear is difficult to judge. The ear may be protuberant and may sometimes be mistaken for an abnormality, such as an encephalocele.

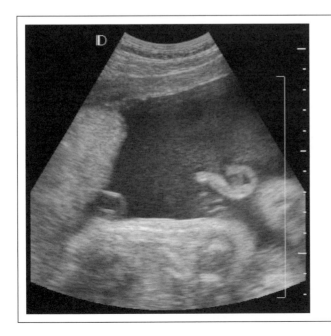

Figure 31.
Ear. Parasagittal view of a fetal ear.

Scalp hair is recognizable in some third-trimester fetuses. Hair is usually easiest to visualize on the nape of the neck, appearing as bright linear echoes at the back of the neck. In fetuses that have tight curly hair, a hazy halo of hair may be observed surrounding the head and should not be confused with scalp edema.

Thorax

The great vessels of the thorax can be visualized from a transverse axial view of the upper mediastinum (figure 32) by moving the transducer cephalad from the four-chamber view of the heart. In this view, one can often identify the superior vena cava, the ascending and descending thoracic aorta, the pulmonary artery, and the ductus arteriosus (coursing from the pulmonary artery to the descending thoracic aorta). In a sagittal plane, the vessels arising from the aortic arch are often visible, including the brachiocephalic, left common carotid, and left subclavian arteries. The common carotid arteries and jugular veins are also commonly seen in the neck of an older fetus.

In some fetuses, the mid and distal esophagus may be visible on ultrasound. The key to identification of this structure is the descending thoracic aorta, a structure fairly easily visualized. The mid and distal portions of the esophagus lie immediately anterior to the descending thoracic aorta. The aorta is first visualized in a longitudinal coronal plane. The transducer is then slowly moved anteriorly. As the aorta disappears from view, the esophagus comes into view but is much more difficult to recognize.

The larynx is virtually always visible when the hypopharynx is filled with fluid. The larynx is recognized as a superior constriction of the tracheal fluid column

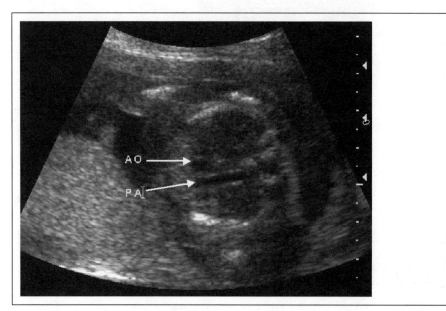

Figure 32.
Great vessels of the heart. Transverse sonogram just above the four-chamber view. Note the aorta and pulmonary artery (arrows). In this example, the superior vena cava and right pulmonary artery are not demonstrated.

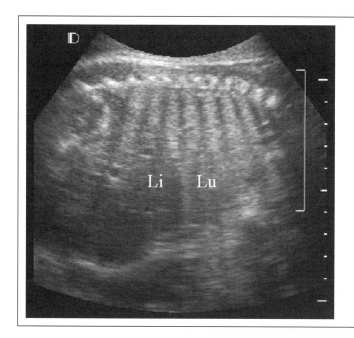

Figure 33.
Diaphragm, lung, and liver. Sagittal view of the fetal chest and abdomen demonstrating the location of the diaphragm. The lung (Lu) is more echogenic than the liver (Li). The position of the diaphragm is indicated by the interface of the liver and lung.

protruding into the hypopharynx. The trachea is sometimes visible and is consistently fluid filled. The trachea, along much of its length, is flanked by conspicuous pulsations of the common carotid arteries. The trachea usually can be traced to its distal end, passing posterior to the aortic arch.

The diaphragm separates the chest from the abdomen and is visible sonographically (figure 33). The diaphragm becomes progressively more visible with fetal growth. The lungs are visualized from the late first trimester onward and early on are defined by adjacent structures: the ribs superolaterally and the heart medially. The lung and liver are initially equal in echogenicity, but as pregnancy progresses, the lung becomes more echogenic than the liver.

Heart

The fetal heart can be most clearly imaged if the fetus is in a supine position within the uterus. If the fetus is lying on its side, the heart can still be imaged fairly well through the ribs. If the fetus is lying in the spine up position, however, imaging cardiac structures is much more difficult. Turning the mother on one side or the other may improve visualization of cardiac anatomy.

To define the cardiac position and situs, it is essential for the sonographer to be aware of the position of the fetus in the uterus and to identify the right and left sides of the fetus independent of the position of fetal organs.

A complete cardiac evaluation includes scanning the fetal heart in its entirety, right to left, base to apex, including the four-chamber long- and short-axis views (figure 34).

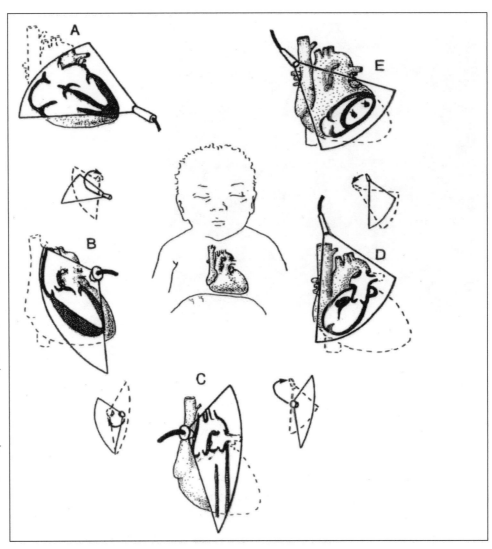

Figure 34.
Sonographic views and approaches to the fetal heart and great vessels. The axis of the fetal heart is more horizontal compared with its postnatal lie in the chest (center). Note that all the views are shown as being obtained from the chest or the abdominal wall; however, it is also possible to achieve all these imaging planes from the back. **A** Four-chamber view showing both atria and the foramen ovale within the atrial septum, both ventricles, and the atrioventricular valves. **B** After slight clockwise rotation and tilt of the transducer toward the fetal left shoulder, the long axis comes into view. **C** Further clockwise rotation and tilt of the transducer results in sagittally oriented planes, which are valuable for depicting the aortic arch and the "ductus arch." **D** Perpendicular to the long axis, the short-axis views are obtained. At the base of the heart, the aorta lies centrally and is surrounded by the structures of the right ventricle and the pulmonary artery, as postnatally. **E** Further toward the apex, the left ventricular structure with two papillary muscles can be seen. Reprinted with permission from Silverman NH, Schmidt KG: Ultrasound evaluation of the fetal heart. In Callen PW (ed): *Ultrasonography in Obstetrics and Gynecology*, 4th edition. Philadelphia, Saunders, 2000, p 380.

Spine

The fetal spine should be imaged in longitudinal and transverse planes throughout its length. Each vertebral segment of the fetal spine normally consists of three ossification centers: the vertebral body and the right and left posterior elements (figure 35). The posterior elements form the lateral and posterior parts of the spinal canal. Real-time imaging of the spine in the transverse plane is essential to exclude a neural tube defect. The sonographer should pay particular attention to the lower lumbar and sacral spine, as defects are most common there.

If imaging is optimal, the spinal cord itself can be visualized by mid-pregnancy. In the longitudinal plane, the spinal cord is hypoechoic, with bright anterior and posterior margins and a bright central line (figure 36). The lower tip of the spinal cord, called the *conus medullaris,* resembles a pencil point.

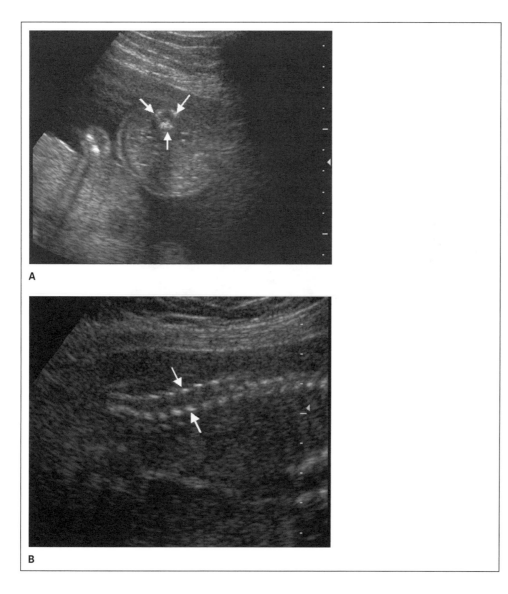

Figure 35.

Fetal spine. **A** Note the three ossification centers (arrows) in this transverse view of the fetal spine. **B** In this coronal view of the fetal spine, both posterior ossification centers (arrows) are visible at each vertebral level in the lumbosacral spine.

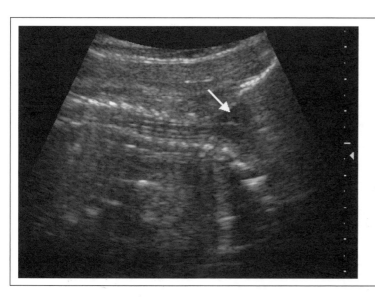

Figure 36A.

Spinal cord. Sagittal sonograms of the fetal spine show the spinal cord. The cervical portion of the cord. Note fluid surrounding the upper portion of the cord and brainstem in the posterior fossa (arrow).

Figure 36B.

Spinal cord. Sagittal sonograms of the fetal spine show the spinal cord. The pointed inferior tip of the spinal cord (conus medullaris) (arrow).

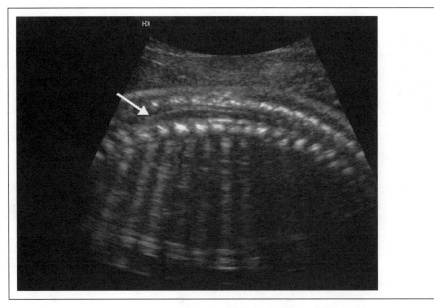

Extremities

The long bones of the upper and lower extremities, as well as the hip and knee joints, can be visualized sonographically beginning in the late first trimester. The simplest way to identify the long bones of the extremity is to begin by scanning the limb transverse to the long axis of the limb. Transverse sonograms through the forearm and calf will show two bones. In the lower leg, the more lateral bone is the fibula, and the medial bone is the tibia.

In the normal fetus, the radius and ulna end at the same level distally, and proximally the ulna is longer than the radius (figure 37). The tibia and fibula end at about the same level proximally, and the fibula is slightly longer distally (figure 38).

Figure 37.

Radius and ulna. Longitudinal view of the radius and ulna. Note that the ulna extends to the elbow proximally.

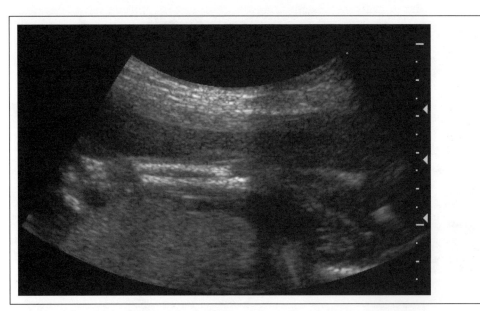

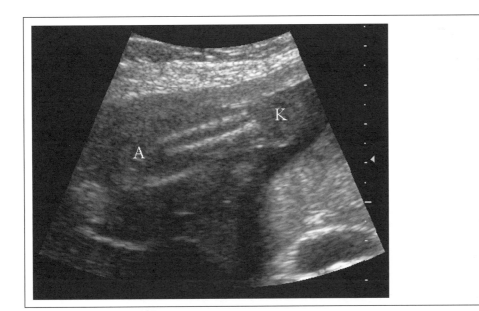

Figure 38.
Tibia and fibula. The fetal knee is to the right in the image. K = knee, A = ankle.

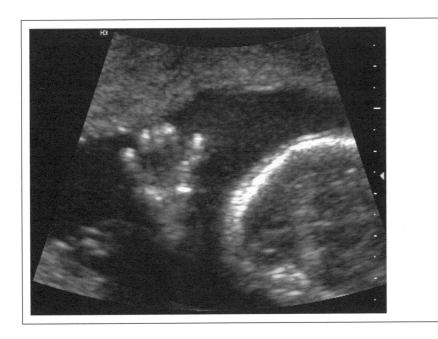

Figure 39.
Fetal hand. All five fingers are visible.

The fingers of the hand may be easier to visualize than the toes of the foot because fingers are longer than toes. With careful scanning, the sonographer can usually discern all four fingers and the thumb in the normal fetus (figure 39). The hand is frequently clenched in a fistlike position, which can hinder visualization. The toes, although smaller, can usually be imaged with current equipment (figure 40).

In the late third trimester, ossification centers appear first in the distal femoral epiphysis (figure 41) and later in the proximal tibial epiphysis. Ossification centers of these epiphyses as seen on x-ray are known to be an indicator of fetal maturity. In normal female fetuses, the distal femoral epiphysis

Figure 40.
Fetal toes.

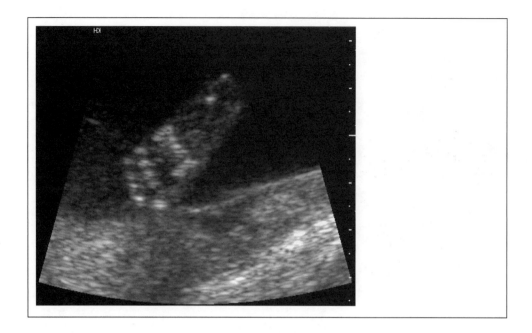

Figure 41.
Distal femoral epiphysis. Sagittal view of the distal femur demonstrating ossification of the distal femoral epiphysis (arrow). The patella (P) is also visualized.

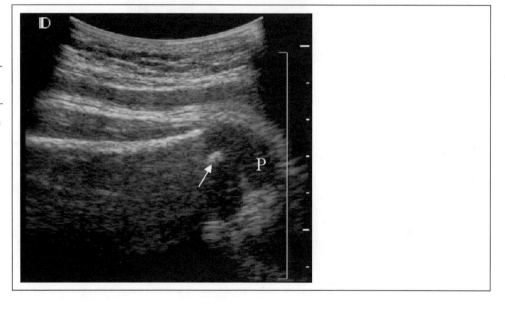

ossifies at about 32 weeks, and the proximal tibial epiphysis ossifies at about 35 weeks. In males, the ossification of these epiphyses occurs about 2 weeks later. The patella can also be visualized, but this bone does not ossify until after birth.

Fetal Abdomen and Pelvis

General

The fetal abdomen is usually viewed primarily in serial transverse planes. The abdomen has a smooth contour, and the inner aspect of the abdominal wall consists of a thin 1 to 3 mm hypoechoic zone of muscle, which should not

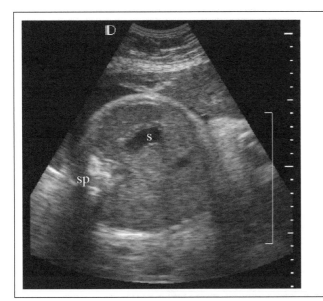

Figure 42.
Fetal stomach. This transverse sonogram demonstrates the fetal stomach (S) and spine (Sp).

be confused with ascites. After the fetal stomach and bladder are identified, the umbilicus and cord insertion can be examined to determine if the cord contains the normal three vessels.

Structures routinely visualized that normally contain fluid include the stomach (figure 42), gallbladder (color plate 1), and urinary bladder. Thus, any fluid-containing small bowel should be viewed with suspicion, although in older fetuses, one may occasionally observe very small amounts of fluid in the small bowel.

Sonograms for measuring the abdominal circumference (AC) are obtained in the transverse plane at the level of the stomach and umbilical vein. Some investigators believe the structure, usually called the *umbilical vein,* should be referred to as the *umbilical portion of the portal vein.* In addition to the liver and stomach, the aorta, inferior vena cava, and adrenal glands are usually visible at this level. The kidneys, colon, and small bowel are visible lower in the abdomen.

The structures usually visible in the fetal pelvis include the iliac bones, sacrum, symphysis pubis, urinary bladder, rectum, and pelvic vessels. By using color Doppler, the two umbilical arteries can be visualized at the level of the urinary bladder. Visualizing the umbilical arteries in the pelvis helps confirm that there are three vessels in the umbilical cord and also helps confirm visualization of the urinary bladder. The iliac and femoral vessels may also be visible with the use of color Doppler. The rectum normally lies directly posterior to the bladder and is similar in echogenicity to the bladder. If the bladder is empty or small, the colon may be confused with the bladder.

Figure 43.
Fetal kidneys. Transverse sonogram of the fetal kidneys and spine (Sp).

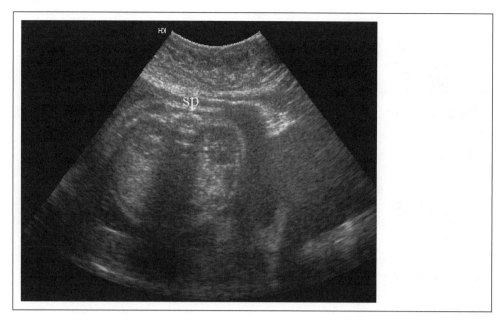

Gastrointestinal

The liver can be consistently imaged from the second trimester onward, although its margins are often indistinct early in the second trimester. The pancreas is not usually visible sonographically, even in the third trimester.

The colon is usually visible by about 22 weeks and becomes progressively more prominent as it fills with meconium. The colon is relatively hypoechoic and should not be mistaken for dilated small bowel. The colon lies near the kidneys, and when a kidney is absent, the colon will often occupy the renal fossa. The average colon diameter is 16–18 mm at term.[15]

Genitourinary

The fetal kidneys lie on either side of the spine in the mid-abdomen and are usually visible by about 14 weeks, but they are optimally visualized later (figure 43). By the end of the second trimester, renal pyramids may be visible. Often, a small amount of urine is present in the collecting system of the kidneys. Color or power Doppler imaging of the renal vessels may help confirm the presence of the kidneys if gray-scale imaging is equivocal. In the normal fetus, the ureters are rarely visible.

Summary

As we have described, many details of fetal anatomy are visible sonographically in the second and third trimester. Thorough knowledge of normal fetal anatomy makes it possible for the sonographer or physician to identify fetal anomalies more confidently.

Placenta

CHAPTER 3

Growth and development (embryology)

Placental size and shape

Abnormalities of placental shape

Intraplacental lesions

Placental grading

Placenta previa

Placental abruption

Marginal and subchorionic hemorrhage

Placenta accreta

Chorioangioma

Placental Doppler

Umbilical cord

. . . .

The placenta is the most important organ for the development of the fetus. It transports oxygen and nutrients to the fetus and carries away carbon dioxide and waste products. The placenta also produces hormones that sustain the pregnancy. As a part of the routine obstetrical sonogram, it is important to note the size, position, and sonographic appearance of the placenta. It is also important to evaluate the retroplacental attachment area, the membranes surrounding the placenta, and the umbilical cord insertion on the placenta.

Growth and Development (Embryology)

Approximately one week after ovulation (3 menstrual weeks), the developing conceptus begins to implant into the uterine wall. The early placental tissue, called the *syncytiotrophoblast,* rapidly burrows into the uterine wall and by approximately 3½ menstrual weeks becomes vascularized by maternal blood vessels. By approximately 4½ menstrual weeks, the gestational sac is visible sonographically and is surrounded by an echogenic rind of tissue. By this time, the growing placental tissue has developed numerous villi surrounding the site of implantation. As growth continues, the villi nearest the endometrial cavity begin to atrophy (decidua capsularis), and the villi adjacent to the myometrium extend into the decidua basalis to form the chorion frondosum. By 10–12 menstrual weeks, the thickened portion of the placenta adjacent to the myometrium is visible sonographically. After 12–13 weeks, blood flow can be observed within the placenta by color and power Doppler.

The mature placenta consists of stem villi bathed in maternal blood (figure 44). The fetal blood circulates within the many-branched villi, surrounded by maternal blood in the intervillus spaces. Exchange of nutrients and waste products between the mother and the fetus takes place here. Many stem villi make up each cotyledon of the placenta.

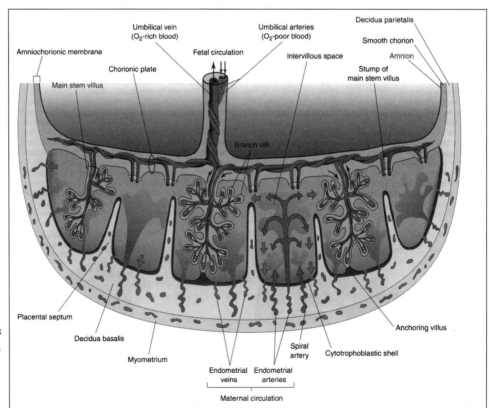

Figure 44.
Full-term placenta. Schematic drawing of a transverse section through a full-term placenta, showing (1) the relation of the villous chorion (fetal part of placenta) to the decidua basalis (maternal part of placenta), (2) the fetal placental circulation, and (3) the maternal placental circulation. Reprinted with permission from Moore KL, Persaud TVN: *Before We Are Born: Essentials of Embryology and Birth Defects,* 6th edition. Philadelphia, Saunders, 2003, p 95.

Placental Size and Shape

The placenta is primarily a fetal organ and thus reflects the health and size of the fetus. In general the thickness of the placenta in millimeters equals the gestational age in weeks plus or minus 10 mm.[16] A full-term placenta should not exceed 4.0 cm in thickness.

A thin placenta may be associated with:

1. Small-for-dates fetus or intrauterine growth restriction (IUGR).
2. Chromosomal abnormalities.
3. Severe intrauterine infection.
4. Severe diabetes mellitus.
5. Hypertension.
6. Toxemia.

A thick placenta may be associated with:

1. Triploidy.
2. Diabetes mellitus.
3. Maternal anemia.
4. Blood group incompatibilities.
5. Placental hemorrhage.
6. Hydrops.
7. Infection.
8. Aneuploidy.

Common pitfalls that may occur when measuring the placenta:

1. An area may appear artifactually enlarged due to oblique section.
2. A contraction may appear as placental thickening.
3. Polyhydramnios may cause the placenta to appear artifactually thin.
4. Oligohydramnios may cause the placenta to seem large.

Abnormalities of Placental Shape

The placenta is normally discoid in shape and attaches to the uterine wall. *Circummarginate placenta* (figure 45) is a condition where the villous (fetal) chorionic membrane does not extend all the way from the center to the edge of the placenta, and the membranous chorion covers the outer placental edge smoothly. A *circumvallate placenta* is similar to a circummarginate one,

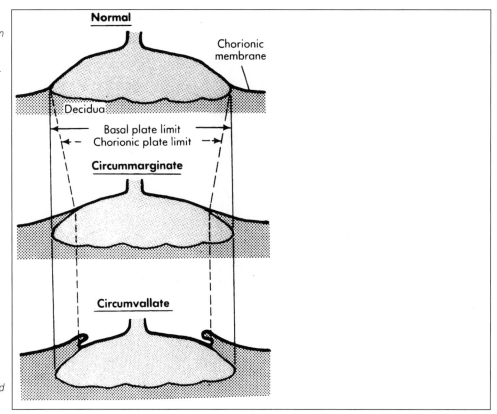

Figure 45.
Diagram in cross section comparing extrachorial to normal placenta. Normally, the membranes extend to the edge of the placenta. With a circummarginate placenta, the transition from villous to membranous chorion occurs at a distance from the edge of the placenta. A circumvallate placenta is similar but has a fold in the membranes at the site of transition. Reprinted with permission from Spirt BA, Kagan EH: Sonography of the placenta. *Semin Ultrasound* 1:293–310, 1980.

but in this case, the villous chorionic membrane is larger than the placenta, and there are folds on the edges (figure 45). Either condition may affect a part of or all of the placental margin. Complete circumvallate placenta is associated with increased risk of placental hemorrhage or infarction, abruption, preterm labor, intrauterine growth restriction, fetal anomalies, and perinatal death. Circummarginate and partial circumvallate placenta are not associated with any fetal problems. Sonographically, a fold of tissue appears to be at the margin of the circumvallate placenta (figure 46). It is important to scan the entire periphery of the placenta to determine if the circumvallate condition is partial or complete. The fold of tissue may be easier to detect before 20 weeks.

Early in pregnancy, the entire surface of the gestational sac is covered with villi; as the pregnancy progresses, the villi usually regress over most of the surface of the sac, and what remains becomes the placenta. If this regression does not occur, the placenta may cover the entire surface of the sac. This condition is called *placenta membranacea.* In this condition, the placenta is thin and is not localized to a specific area. If the regression is patchy, there may be two or more separate areas of placental formation.

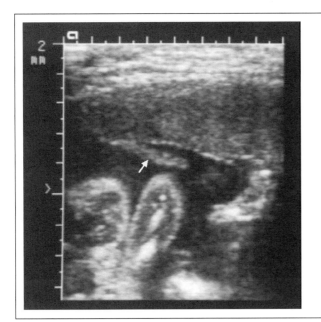

Figure 46.
Circumvallate placenta. Note the fold of tissue at the edge of the placenta (arrow).

A separate portion of placenta is called a *succenturiate* or *accessory lobe* (color plate 2). A succenturiate lobe is connected to the main placenta by a group of vessels running along the uterine wall. It is important to recognize a succenturiate lobe, as it could result in complications such as vasa previa, postdelivery retention of placental fragments, and postpartum hemorrhage.

Intraplacental Lesions

Placental Calcifications

Placental calcification occurs as a result of physiologic processes that take place as pregnancy matures. After 33 weeks, more than 50% of placentas contain some degree of calcification.[17, 18] Calcifications are usually found at the base, septa, and in the subchorionic and perivillous spaces. Calcification is more common in women of lower parity, those who smoke cigarettes, and mothers who have thrombotic disorders and are on heparin or aspirin therapy.

Hypoechoic/Cystic Lesions

Cystic or hypoechoic lesions in the placenta are observed fairly commonly, particularly after 25 weeks' gestation. Most are not clinically significant. From a sonographic point of view, these cystic or hypoechoic lesions can be divided into three general groups:

1. Lesions directly under the fetal surface of the placenta.
2. Lesions in the mid-placenta.
3. Lesions in the deep placenta adjacent to the maternal myometrium.

Subchorionic lesions and cystic or hypoechoic areas immediately under the chorionic membrane adjacent to the fetal surface of the placenta are typically acute or chronic areas of thrombus. Rarely, well-defined subchorionic cysts may be observed. Such cysts do not represent hemorrhagic areas and are insignificant clinically.

1 Mid-Placental Regions

Most hypoechoic or cystic areas in the mid-placenta are due to thrombus in the intervillous space between the fetal and the maternal sides of the placenta. Early in the hemorrhage process, flow may be observed within these hypoechoic areas, and these areas are sometimes termed "maternal lakes." A *septal cyst* is a rare mid-placental cystic structure; it is a cyst that forms between cotyledons of the placenta.

2 Lesions at the Placental Myometrial Interface

Hypoechoic or cystic areas at the placental myometrial interface are more significant. These may represent retroplacental hematomas or areas of abruption. A rare condition called *maternal basal plate infarction* produces massive blood and fibrin deposition in the intervillous space. If blood collections deep to the placenta are large enough, covering 30–40% of the placenta, intrauterine growth restriction or fetal death may occur. In some cases, associated infarction of the deep portion of the placenta may also occur. Placental infarctions are not usually visible sonographically, but occasionally a portion of infarcted placenta may appear echogenic.

Placental Grading

In earlier studies it was thought that fetal lung maturity could be determined on the basis of several parameters including "placental grade." The placenta was graded from 0 to III (figure 47).

- Grade 0—Homogeneous placenta with a smooth chorionic plate.
- Grade I—Scattered echogenic calcifications throughout the placenta.
- Grade II—Scattered echogenic calcifications throughout the placenta and subtle comma-like densities at the chorionic plate.
- Grade III—Scattered echogenic calcifications throughout the placenta and at the base, increased comma-like densities at the chorionic plate, and cystic areas within the placenta.

Placental grading has fallen out of use in obstetrical practice because placental grade does not reliably predict fetal lung maturity. However, grade III placenta occurring earlier in pregnancy than usual may suggest a fetal problem, such as IUGR.

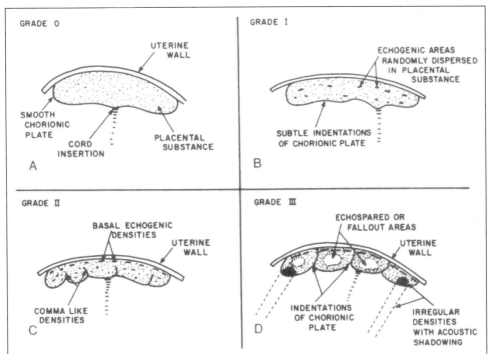

Figure 47.
Maturation of the placenta. Sonographic characteristics used to determine the stage of "maturation" of the placenta. Grade III represents the most mature placenta. Reprinted with permission from Grannum PA, Berkowitz RL, Hobbins JC: The ultrasonic changes in the maturing placenta and their relation to fetal pulmonic maturity. *Am J Obstet Gynecol* 133:915, 1979.

Placenta Previa

Early in pregnancy, the placenta is less localized and often covers the internal os. As the placenta localizes, it usually migrates away from the os. Even if the placental margin covers the os at 15–17 weeks, it is likely to migrate away later as the lower uterine segment elongates. Thus, a diagnosis of placenta previa should not be made before 20 menstrual weeks. The incidence of *placenta previa* is increased in older mothers and in women who have a history of prior abortion, smoking, multiple pregnancy, or previous c-section. In the older or multipara patient, the decidua is thinner, so less is available for implantation. Prior c-section results in scarring at the lower uterine segment; the placenta is unable to migrate. Placenta previa can be misdiagnosed in the mid second trimester because of bladder overfilling or focal myometrial contractions. In that case, the patient can partially void so that more accurate visualization of the internal os can be made. In addition, waiting approximately 20 minutes will allow a contraction to disappear.

1. *Complete previa* occurs when the placenta completely covers the internal cervical os (figure 48).

2. *Marginal/partial previa* occurs when the placenta is at the edge, encroaching, or partially covering, the internal cervical os. Partial previa can be difficult to differentiate on sonogram. Some investigators have chosen the term *incomplete placenta previa.*

Figure 48.

Complete previa. Longitudinal view in the midline pelvis demonstrates the placenta completely covering the os.

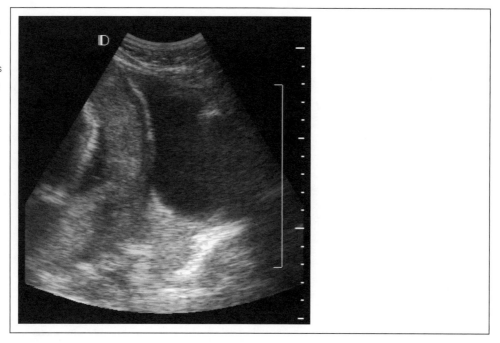

3. *Low-lying placenta* occurs when the placental edge is within 2 cm of the internal cervical os but does not cover any significant portion of it.

Newer techniques such as transvaginal and translabial scanning show the cervix better because the transducer is closer to the area of interest, and higher-frequency sound can be used. The incidence of a placenta previa at term is 5% if the placenta extends more than 15 mm over the internal os at 12–16 weeks; thus, 95% of placentas covering the os in the first trimester will no longer be previa by the third trimester.

Low-lying, or "potential," previa is common in the second trimester. If any doubt exists sonographically, transvaginal sonography is preferable to translabial imaging, especially when the fetal head is low. When the placenta is visualized 2 cm or less from the internal os near term, the patient may require a c-section.

Placental Abruption

Abruption is the premature separation of the normally implanted placenta from the uterus (figure 49). The retroplacental myometrium containing utereteroplacental vessels should not exceed 1–2 mm in thickness unless there is a uterine contraction in the area. Women who have extensive abruption may experience pain, extensive bleeding, and hypovolemic shock. Immediate delivery is usually necessary, and there is no time for a sonogram.

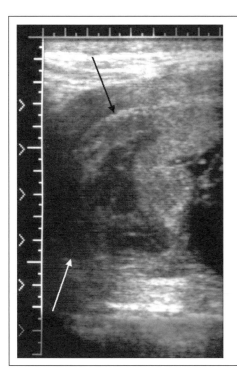

Figure 49.
Placenta abruption. Longitudinal view of the uterus demonstrates echolucent area (arrows) posterior to the placenta.

Typically the hemorrhage from the abruption will appear hyperechoic initially (0–48 hours), and hypoechoic at 1–2 weeks. After 2 weeks, portions of the clot may become anechoic. Generally, an acute abruption will appear to be an ill-defined region in the retroplacental area. Abruption is more likely in patients who have hypertension, have experienced trauma, or use cocaine. Usually placental abruption starts at the edge of the placenta and extends both ways from the margin. If more than 30–40% of the placenta separates, intrauterine growth restriction or fetal demise may often occur.

Marginal and Subchorionic Hemorrhage

If a hemorrhage is located at the edge of the placenta but does not extend posterior to the placenta, it is called a *marginal hemorrhage*. In early pregnancy, hemorrhage outside the amniotic sac but not under the placenta is usually called *subchorionic hemorrhage*.

Placenta Accreta

Accreta is an abnormal adherence of the placenta to the uterine wall (figure 50) with failure to separate after the fetus is delivered. This condition is more common in patients who have had a previous c-section and in patients of advanced maternal age. The underlying cause appears to be a deficiency of the decidua basalis, which is replaced by loose connective tissue.

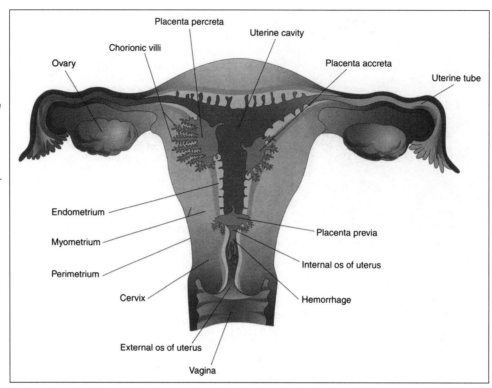

Figure 50.

Placental abnormalities. In *placenta accreta* there is abnormal adherence of the placenta to the myometrium. In *placenta percreta* the placenta has penetrated the full thickness of the myometrium. In *placenta previa* the placenta overlies the internal os of the uterus and blocks the cervical canal. Reprinted with permission from Moore KL, Persaud TVN: *Before We Are Born: Essentials of Embryology and Birth Defects*, 6th edition. Philadelphia, Saunders, 2003, p 104.

The three categories of placenta accreta are:

- *Placenta accreta vera*—the villi extend up to but do not invade the uterine muscle.

- *Placenta increta*—villi invade the muscle.

- *Placenta percreta*—villi penetrate the uterine wall, reaching the serosa. The placenta may invade adjacent organs, such as the bladder or, rarely, the rectum.

Increased risk for placenta accreta exists if the placenta implants over a uterine scar, over a submucous fibroid, in the lower uterine segment, in a rudimentary uterine horn, or in a uterine cornu. Complications that may occur at delivery include retained products of conception, hemorrhage, and uterine rupture. In the past, the maternal mortality rate in this condition was approximately 10–25% but is significantly lower now with better methods of detection, including elevated maternal serum alpha-fetoprotein (MS-AFP), sonography, and magnetic resonance imaging (MRI).

The main sonographic finding in placenta accreta is an area of thinned (<2 mm) or absent retroplacental myometrium (figure 51), and the sonographic interface between the placenta and myometrium is lost. The size of the myometrial defect is important. If the defect is smaller than 2 cm in

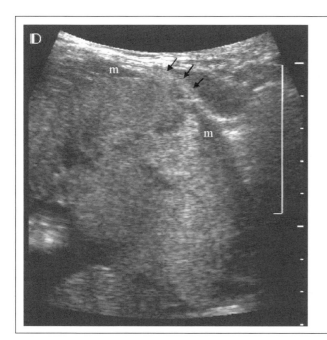

Figure 51.
Placenta accreta. Sagittal view through the lower uterine segment demonstrates an area of loss of retroplacental myometrium (arrows). Note the normal uterine muscle (m) above and below the area of accreta.

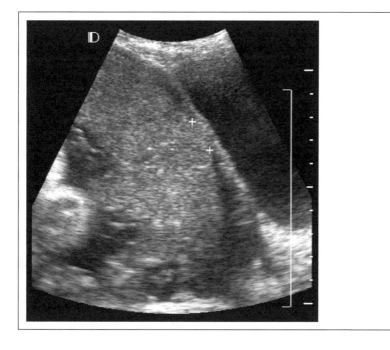

Figure 52.
Placenta accreta. Sagittal view through the placenta. Note the area of myometrial thinning at the calipers. This area of accreta is small enough that it is unlikely to adhere at delivery.

diameter (figure 52), the placenta is unlikely to adhere to the uterine wall at delivery. Another common sonographic finding is the presence of multiple hypoechoic/anechoic spaces in the placenta, sometimes termed "Swiss cheese appearance," but these cystic areas are not usually round or oval, as would be expected in Swiss cheese; they are instead jagged and irregular (figure 53), with fast blood flow within them. Also, there is increased color Doppler flow in the underlying area (color plate 3), especially at the

Figure 53.
Placenta accreta. Longitudinal view of the placenta demonstrates multiple irregular hypoechoic areas ("Swiss cheese appearance").

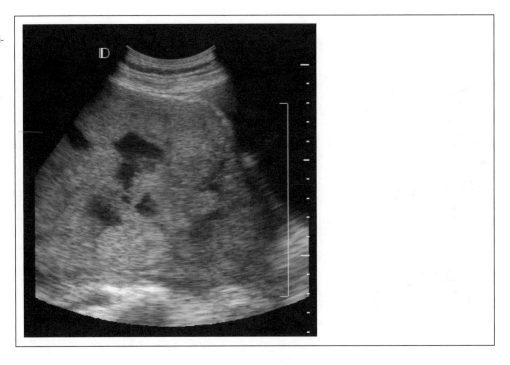

edges of the area of accreta. The sonographer may see placental villous tissue invading the bladder with a nodular thickened bladder wall on transabdominal ultrasound.

Chorioangioma

The most common benign neoplasm of the placenta is chorioangioma, which is a vascular mass arising from chorionic tissue. The majority of chorioangiomas are clinically insignificant. Those larger than 5 cm are associated with a 30% rate of maternal or fetal complications, such as polyhydramnios, intrauterine growth restriction, previa, abruption, congestive heart failure/cardiomegaly, pre-eclampsia, anemia, and congenital anomalies. Arteriovenous shunting may cause fetal cardiac enlargement, which can lead to anemia and eventually high-output congestive failure.

The sonographic appearance of chorioangioma (figure 54) is a well-circumscribed, rounded lesion near the chorionic surface, often near the cord insertion. The sonographer must carefully evaluate the fetus for changes that would indicate fetal hydrops or fluid overload. If the fetus appears normal, serial studies should be performed every 2–3 weeks if the tumor is near the 5 cm size.

Placental Doppler

In the past few years interest has grown in the use of placental Doppler. However, Doppler in the first and second trimester has not generally been clinically useful.

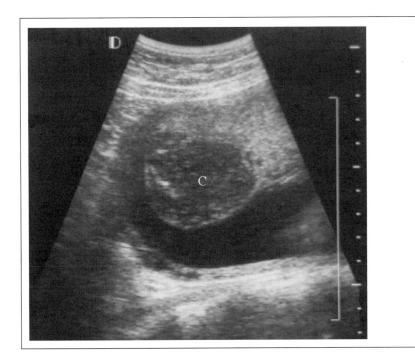

Figure 54.
Chorioangioma. Longitudinal view of the placenta with chorioangioma (C) in the fundal area.

Umbilical Cord

Knowledge of normal umbilical cord development and anatomy is important, and the sonographer should also be aware of cord abnormalities that can be recognized sonographically. Abnormalities of the cord can be associated with fetal anomalies, chromosomal abnormalities, and complications of pregnancy.

Cord Anatomy

The umbilical cord is first visible sonographically at approximately 8 menstrual weeks and appears as a straight, thick structure. The length of the umbilical cord is approximately the same as the crown-rump length (CRL) at that time. The cord diameter during gestation is normally less than 2 cm. The length of the cord depends on the force placed on it by the pull of fetal movement. Adequate amniotic fluid facilitates the fetal activity necessary for normal length and coiling of the cord.

The umbilical cord contains two arteries and one vein. The vein carries oxygenated blood from the placenta and connects to the portal vein in the liver. The umbilical arteries arise from the internal iliac arteries and carry deoxygenated blood from the fetus back to the placenta. The three vessels in the cord can be routinely visualized sonographically. The vessels within the cord are surrounded by Wharton's jelly, a gelatinous connective tissue that protects the umbilical vessels from compression.

The cord is covered by amniotic epithelium, which firmly adheres to the connective tissue. Unlike the placental amnion, which is loosely applied against the chorion, the amnion of the cord cannot be elevated or stripped away.

Cord Abnormalities

1 Vascular Abnormalities

The most common vascular abnormality of the umbilical cord is *single umbilical artery* (SUA), which is seen in approximately 1% of all pregnancies. The cause of single umbilical artery is probably atrophy of a previous normal artery due to thrombosis rather than primary agenesis.[18] Assessment for the presence of a single umbilical artery should be confirmed at the fetal end of the cord because it may represent a normal variant at the placental end, as the umbilical arteries may fuse before entering the placenta.

There is a 20–60% incidence of other fetal anomalies in the presence of a single umbilical artery.[19–21] A single umbilical artery may be associated with malformations of any of the major organ systems and may be seen with chromosomal abnormalities. Even in the absence of associated anomalies, there is an increased risk of intrauterine growth restriction in a fetus that has a single umbilical artery. If a cord has more than two umbilical arteries or more than one umbilical vein, it is called a multivessel cord. Although rare, such cords have been reported in association with congenital anomalies and conjoined twins.[22]

2 Structural Abnormalities

Abnormal Cord Formation

A defective embryonic folding process may result in abnormalities of the fetal abdominal wall and umbilical cord. Generalized and severe malformation of all folds leads to a failure of formation of the umbilical cord, with the fetus directly attached to the placental chorion by a persisting embryonic connecting stalk. The abdominal organs, including the liver, spleen, intestine, and pancreas, lie along the stalk exterior to the fetal body. This abnormality is referred to as *limb-body wall complex, congenital absence of the umbilical cord,* or *body stalk anomaly;* the condition is uniformly lethal. Limb anomalies are often present in such cases.

The sonographic findings in limb-body wall complex include herniation of the liver and viscera from the abdomen without an overlying membrane. The organs extend from the fetal torso to the placenta, and the umbilical cord is not identified. *Amniotic band syndrome,* a similar condition, may show many or all of these findings. (See abdominal wall section.)

Short Cord

A short cord can occur as a primary phenomenon due to failure of embryonic infolding, which leads to limb-body wall defects. Conditions that restrict or reduce fetal movements can also result in a short cord and include:

- Oligohydramnios.
- Twins.
- Tethering of fetus, as in amniotic bands.
- Intrinsic fetal anomalies.
- Musculoskeletal abnormalities.
- CNS abnormalities.

A short cord may predispose to inadequate fetal descent during labor, to fetal heart-rate abnormalities related to cord compression, and to placental abruption.

Long Cord

Problems associated with long cords include:

- Nuchal cord.
- Cord knots.
- Cord prolapse.
- Cord entanglements.

These conditions may lead to cord compression and decreased perfusion due to obstruction of venous return.

Nuchal cords are present in 25% of pregnancies and are of clinical significance when there are two or more loops around the fetal neck.[19, 23] Sonographically they are visualized as two adjacent loops of cord in cross-section posterior to the fetal neck on sagittal images and as loops of cord circumferentially around the neck in the axial plane. A single loop of umbilical cord seen near the fetal neck is most often an incidental finding.

A study by Larson found that pregnancies complicated by multiple nuchal loops were associated with significantly greater likelihood of meconium in the amniotic fluid, abnormal heart rate patterns in advanced labor, operative vaginal delivery, and mild acidosis at birth.[24]

3 Abnormal Twists

Knots of the umbilical cord are classified as *true* and *false knots*. True knots occur in 1% of singleton pregnancies and are a complication of monochorionic twin pregnancy. They are rarely visualized on ultrasound and may result from torsion of the cord, which forms a loop through which the fetus may slip to form a knot.

False knots are actually misnamed, as they simply represent a focal redundancy of the vessels, which appear as vascular protrusions not present in all sonographic planes.

4 Cord Insertion

In early development, the embryo rotates so that the yolk sac and adjacent connecting stalk are positioned opposite the implantation site. This allows the umbilical cord to insert centrally within the placenta. As the placenta develops it may grow toward optimal areas of myometrial perfusion and atrophy in areas of suboptimal blood supply. As a result, the cord may insert eccentrically on the placenta. This process is called *trophotropism.*

The forms of cord insertion are as follows:

- *Battledore placenta:* The cord inserts along the margin of the placenta and is usually of no clinical significance (color plate 4).

- *Velamentous insertion:* The cord inserts beyond the placental edge into the free membranes of the placenta. Velamentous insertion may be complicated by rupture or thrombosis of the umbilical vessels because they are not protected by Wharton's jelly. The fetus may also experience intrauterine growth restriction as a result of the decreased blood flow and nutrition.

- *Vasa previa:* Vasa previa is a rare form of velamentous insertion in which the umbilical vessels cross the cervical os. It may be difficult to detect on routine obstetrical sonography, but color Doppler imaging can demonstrate it (color plate 5). If undetected, the fetus will likely die at delivery from ruptured umbilical cord vessels.

5 Cord Cysts and Masses

Cysts

Umbilical cord cysts (figure 55) may arise from the *omphalomesenteric duct* or *allantois*, distinguishable only by histologic examination. The allantois is an embryologic fluid-filled structure that extends from the developing bladder into the base of the umbilical cord. The omphalomesenteric duct is a connection from the gastrointestinal tract to the yolk sac. These cysts tend to be closer to the fetal end of the cord, and most are small, typically 1–2 cm in diameter. They may be seen in association with anomalies of the gastrointestinal and genitourinary tracts because they are developmentally related.

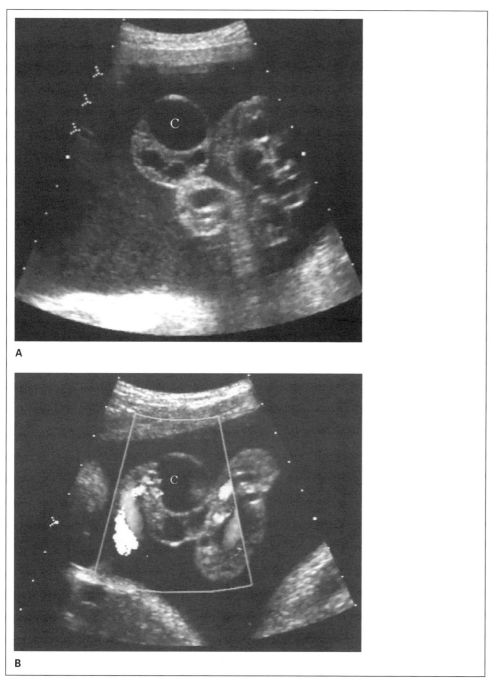

Figure 55.

Umbilical cord. Sonograms **A** and **B** demonstrate cord cysts (C). Note the cystic elements that do not demonstrate evidence of flow.

For instance, allantoic duct cysts (figure 56) have been reported in association with omphalocele, patent urachus, and possibly obstructive uropathy.[25, 26]

Amorphous cystic areas in the umbilical cord may be observed if a small hemangioma exists in the umbilical cord. The condition is sometimes called *mucinous degeneration of the umbilical cord.* The cystic areas are caused by fluid oozing from the hemangioma, and the cysts may enlarge during pregnancy.

Figure 56.

Allantoic cyst. Transverse scan of the fetal cord, demonstrating a large cyst (C) in the cord communicating with the bladder (B). Note the arrows at the periphery of the cyst.

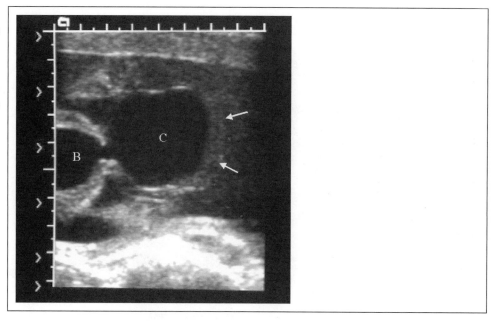

Several studies have shown association of second and third trimester umbilical cord cysts with fetal anomalies and aneuploidy in up to 50% of cases.[27–29] Thus, karyotyping is recommended when an umbilical cyst is detected. Cysts of the umbilical cord detected in first trimester more likely represent normal variants.

Masses

Hemangioma: The most common tumor of the umbilical cord is hemangioma, which may appear as an echogenic mass or multicystic mass located near the placental insertion of the cord.

Varix/aneurysm: Focal dilation of an umbilical artery or vein occasionally occurs. A varix or aneurysm may thrombose and cause fetal death.

Teratoma: A teratoma may have solid or cystic areas and is very rare.

Hematoma: Usually focal, hematomas can be diffuse within the cord. Generally, they are hyperechoic but vary with the age of the bleed. Hematomas are becoming more common as a result of the increased number of invasive procedures being performed, such as cordocentesis. Spontaneous hematomas are usually due to a venous source of bleeding related to umbilical cord knots or torsion. Hematomas are associated with a 50% risk of fetal loss, so if one is suspected, fetal monitoring and possible emergency delivery may be required.[30]

Diffuse Abnormalities: Enlarged cords have been reported with diabetes, hydrops, and diffuse hematoma. Twin-to-twin transfusion can result in diffuse enlargement of the cord of the recipient twin because of the increased flow through the vessels and superimposed edema of Wharton's jelly.

Assessment of Gestational Age

CHAPTER 4

First trimester

Second and third trimester

. . . .

Many clinical problems of pregnancy require accurate assessment of menstrual age before one can proceed with an appropriate management plan. *Menstrual age* refers to the number of weeks' gestation from the first day of the last menstrual period. Obstetricians usually date pregnancies in menstrual weeks but sometimes use the term *gestational age*. In clinical obstetric practice, *menstrual age* and *gestational age* are used interchangeably. In embryology, gestational age is calculated from the time of conception, which occurs approximately two weeks after the beginning of the last menstrual period. In this book we will always refer to menstrual weeks.

Determining accurate menstrual age is important to the obstetrician because it affects clinical management in several important ways.

- The menstrual age is used to schedule such invasive procedures as chorionic villus sampling and genetic amniocentesis. Knowledge of menstrual age is also important when interpreting biochemical tests, such as maternal serum alpha-fetoprotein and triple-screen testing, as the normal range of values changes over time.

- Knowledge of menstrual age allows the obstetrician to anticipate normal spontaneous delivery or to plan elective or cesarean delivery. This knowledge also allows the physician to manage the pregnancy and optimize fetal outcome in case of early or post-term labor.

- In a fetus that has growth restriction, an early sonographic determination of fetal age is vital for evaluating the fetus later in the pregnancy.

- When an anomaly is discovered sonographically, the mother's choices regarding therapy or termination are heavily influenced by menstrual age.

Essentially, all important clinical decisions require knowledge of menstrual age.

Before sonography was available, menstrual age was determined by the patient's menstrual history, which was confirmed during early pregnancy by physical examination of uterine size and later by postdelivery physical examination of the neonate. All three of these parameters alone or in combination are often inaccurate, but menstrual history can be especially misleading for a number of reasons:

- Many women may not accurately recall the first day of their last menstrual period.

- Women may misunderstand the question posed and respond with the last day of the last menstrual period as opposed to the first day.

- For women who do recall the first day of the last period, the date may be unreliable or misleading because of oligomenorrhea, abnormal bleeding events, the use of oral contraceptives, or because the woman became pregnant in the first ovulatory cycle after a delivery. Ovulating early or late may also cause a discrepancy between menstrual age and fetal development.

The most common indication for an obstetric sonogram is related to uncertainty regarding the menstrual age. The use of sonography as a tool for determining menstrual dates has been readily accepted into the practice of clinical obstetrics. Sonographic studies designed to evaluate the duration of pregnancy are based on measurements of the fetus using size as an indirect indicator of menstrual age. The American Institute of Ultrasound in Medicine recommends using crown-rump length (CRL), biparietal diameter (BPD), head circumference (HC), abdominal circumference (AC), and femur length (FL) for estimating menstrual age. See Appendix A on page 345 for AIUM guidelines for the performance of routine obstetrical examinations.

First Trimester

Gestational Sac

The earliest unequivocal sign of pregnancy shown by sonographic evaluation is the demonstration of the "gestational sac." A more precise term may be *chorionic sac,* as it is the developing chorionic villi that create the bright echogenic ring noted near the endometrial cavity. The fluid contained within the sac is nearly all chorionic fluid during very early development. With the use of high-resolution real-time equipment, including transvaginal probes, the gestational sac can usually be seen by 4–5 menstrual weeks.

When measuring the gestational sac diameter, the sonographer should measure across the sac to the interface of the chorionic villi and chorionic fluid.

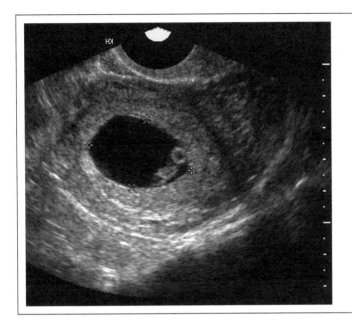

Figure 57.
Mean sac diameter. Sonogram of an early gestational sac demonstrates two of the three usual measurements made (cursors) of the mean sac diameter.

The wall of the sac is not included (figure 57). A mean gestational sac diameter (MSD) is obtained from three dimensions (length, width, and depth) of the gestational sac. The size of the gestational sac when first observed is approximately 2–3 mm MSD. The mean sac diameter increases about 1 mm per day in early gestation.

Data gathered by de Crespigny, Cooper, and McKenna states that the mean sac diameter equals 2–3 mm at 4 weeks and 3–4 days.[31] The gestational sac reaches 5 mm at 5 weeks. A mean sac diameter measurement between 2 and 14 mm (before the embryo can be visualized) represents the earliest possible sonographic measurement. The mean sac diameter becomes progressively less reliable for predicting menstrual age as the first trimester of pregnancy advances.

Up to 8 weeks' gestation, an excellent correlation exists among human chorionic gonadotropin (hCG) levels, menstrual age, and gestational sac size. Concentrations of hCG initially rise exponentially with time, and a range of hCG levels may be observed for any given gestational sac size.

Yolk Sac

The earliest embryonic structure detectable by sonography is the yolk sac. This can be visualized using high-resolution vaginal probes during the 5th menstrual week. The mean sac diameter usually measures 6 to 12 mm when the yolk sac is visible and the embryo has not yet appeared. The yolk sac measures up to 5.6 mm and is located between the amnion and chorion (figure 58).

Figure 58.
Yolk sac. Sonogram of an early intrauterine pregnancy demonstrate the yolk sac (arrow) located between the amnion and chorion.

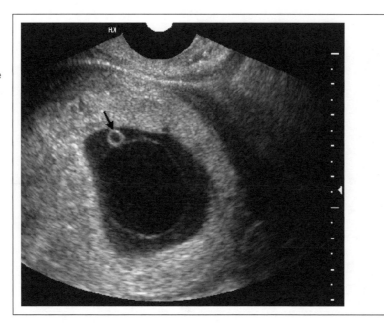

Crown-Rump Length

Once the embryo is visible on ultrasound, the crown-rump length (CRL) becomes the preferred measurement for estimating menstrual age. The developing embryo can be consistently visualized with transvaginal transducers when the crown-rump length reaches 5 mm, although the embryo may be detected when it is as small as 2 mm. If the embryo can be measured, then the mean sac diameter is no longer the most accurate estimation of menstrual age.

By the 5th to 6th menstrual week, one can usually identify the early embryo (figure 59) and cardiac activity. The embryo can be visualized more clearly between 7 and 13 menstrual weeks. When using the crown-rump length to

Figure 59.
Crown-rump length. Sonogram of an early pregnancy. Note the crown-rump length (cursors) adjacent to the yolk sac.

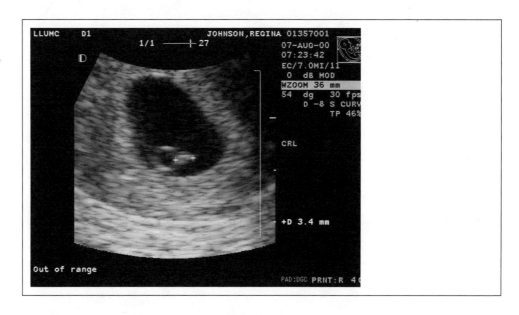

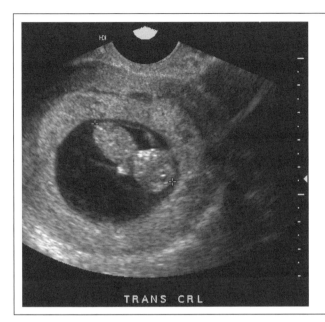

Figure 60.
Crown-rump length. Sonogram during late first trimester demonstrates the crown-rump length (cursors).

predict menstrual age, one should use the average crown-rump length measurement from three good images, always measuring the maximal length (figure 60). The term *embryo* applies up to the end of the 10th menstrual week; the term *fetus* applies thereafter.

Benson and Doubilet recommend the following rules of thumb for visual estimates of early normal first trimester menstrual age[32]:

- If a chorionic sac with no yolk sac or embryo is seen, estimate the age at 5 menstrual weeks.

- If a chorionic sac with a yolk sac but no embryo is seen, estimate the age at 5.5 menstrual weeks.

- If a chorionic sac with a tiny embryo (<5 mm) adjacent to the yolk sac is seen, estimate the age at 6 menstrual weeks.

Although these are simple visual estimates, their accuracy is remarkable.

In summary, the accuracy of first-trimester fetal measurements in predicting menstrual age is well documented; there is very little biologic size variability during this time. It is also well established that once menstrual age has been determined by early mean sac diameter (2–14 mm) or embryonic or fetal crown-rump length in the first trimester of pregnancy, the menstrual age of the pregnancy should never be changed on the basis of biometric measurements made later in pregnancy.

The same can be said of sonographic estimation of menstrual age at any time. An earlier measurement usually supercedes a later measurement, and sonographic estimates of age before 20 weeks' gestation are highly reliable for pregnancy dating. Patients maintaining basal body temperature charts or undergoing assisted conception should use appropriate clinical evidence as the primary method of determining the age of a pregnancy.

When should you perform the first sonogram when dates are uncertain? There are basically two points of view. One is that the earlier measurement is the most accurate because of the biologic variability that increases with gestation. So, if only one sonogram can be performed, the first-trimester sonogram will provide the most accurate dates.

Another viewpoint is to wait until the second trimester to establish dates (15–18 weeks). The dating accuracy may suffer slightly, but 15–18 weeks is an excellent time to make an assessment for most clinical purposes. The value of waiting is that the fetus can be imaged in more detail, and more anomalies will be detectable. Still others believe that both should be performed, which unfortunately many insurance programs will not authorize for payment.

Second and Third Trimester

Gestational Dating

By the second and third trimester of pregnancy, the fetus is more developed, and many anatomic details are visible sonographically. (See the section on "Second/Third Trimester Normal Anatomy.") Multiple structures can be identified and measured during this time. Many sonographic parameters are available for estimating gestational age in the second and third trimester, including biparietal diameter, head circumference, and femur length.

In every case, care must be taken to obtain the best possible images. The sonographer should avoid using measurements from poor images. When making measurements, the sonographer should concentrate on obtaining the best possible images and measuring them, without paying too much attention to what fetal age the measurements correspond to. Otherwise there will be a tendency to repeat or alter measurements to fit the expected age of the pregnancy. It is crucial to obtain each measurement appropriately and accurately.

Biparietal Diameter

A biparietal diameter (BPD) obtained between 14 and 24 weeks menstrual age is comparable in accuracy to the crown-rump length in determining gestational age. The biparietal diameter can be appropriately measured through any plane or section that traverses the ventricle and thalami.

General rules for measuring the biparietal diameter:

- Obtain the correct plane of section through the third ventricle and thalami.
- The calvaria should appear smooth and symmetric.
- Position the cursors in one of the three following ways: outer edge of near calvarial wall to inner edge of the far calvarial wall, inner edge of the near calvarial wall to the outer edge of the far calvarial wall, or middle of the near calvarial wall to the middle of the far calvarial wall.

We prefer the first method. Measuring from the outer edge of the near calvarium to the outer edge of the far wall calvarium is incorrect. To measure the biparietal diameter, the transducer must be perpendicular to the parietal bones and positioned at the correct cephalocaudal position to intersect the third ventricle and thalami. To accurately measure the head circumference, the two criteria for the biparietal diameter must be fulfilled, and the transducer plane must be properly oriented to the skull base. The correct plane of section is through the third ventricle and thalami in the central portion of the brain (as with the biparietal diameter), but the cavum septi pellucidi must be visible in the anterior portion, and the tentorial hiatus must be visible in the posterior portion of the brain. Some refer to this anatomy as an "arrow sign" (figure 61A).

A properly measured biparietal diameter can be obtained on the same image as a properly oriented head circumference measurement. The reverse is not necessarily true. The proper position of the cursors to measure the head circumference is inappropriate for the biparietal diameter. Thus the biparietal

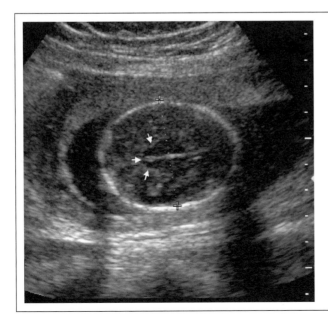

Figure 61A.
Biparietal diameter and head circumference. Sonogram of the fetal cranium (BPD). Note the "arrow sign" (arrows).

diameter can be measured first, then the cursors can be moved for the head circumference. The entire perimeter of the calvaria need not be demonstrated to adequately measure the head circumference. The ellipse adequately estimates the head perimeter even when it is not entirely imaged.

Pitfalls

To obtain an accurate measurement, minimal pressure with a real-time transducer is often sufficient to change an obliquely oriented fetal head to an occiput transverse position. For the head measurements, gain controls should be adjusted so the width of the parietal skull echo is no greater than 5 mm. The measurement error inherent in caliper placement is 1–2 mm.

An abnormal fetal position, such as breech presentation, or a significant reduction in amniotic fluid can affect the shape of the calvarium and thereby reduce the reliability of the biparietal diameter in assessing gestational age. The head circumference, rather than biparietal diameter, should be used for gestational age assessment whenever dolichocephaly or brachycephaly occurs. With oligohydramnios, the fetal head molds to the contour of the uterus. This results in a reduced biparietal diameter and may affect occipitofrontal diameter. Consequently, the biparietal diameter or the head circumference measurements will be more variable in the presence of oligohydramnios than when the amniotic fluid volume is normal.

Head Circumference

Although the biparietal diameter can be obtained in many planes, the head circumference is best obtained through a single plane for consistency. The correct plane of section parallels the base of the skull. Therefore, the plane is more cephalad anteriorly than it is posteriorly. When obtaining a properly measured biparietal diameter, the sonographer must correctly orient the transducer in two planes; measuring the head circumference requires that the transducer be properly oriented in three planes.

The rules for measuring the head circumference are as follows:

- The correct plane of section is through the third ventricle and thalami in the central portion of the brain (as with biparietal diameter), but the cavum septum pellucidi must be visible in the anterior portion of the brain, and the tentorial hiatus must be visible in the posterior portion of the brain.

- Some refer to this anatomy as an "arrow." The cavum septi pellucidi and frontal horns are the feathers.

- The third ventricle and sylvian aqueduct are the "shaft."

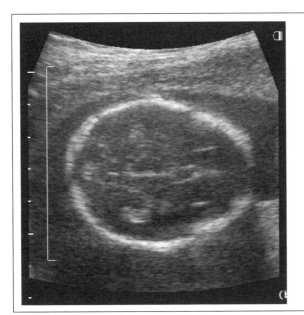

Figure 61B.
Biparietal diameter and head circumference. Sonogram of another fetus demonstrates head circumference measurement.

- The ambient and quadrigeminal cisterns and the tentorial hiatus are the "arrowhead."
- The calvaria must be smooth and symmetric bilaterally.
- After the proper plane of section is obtained, the cursors are positioned at the outer edge of the near calvarial wall and the outer edge of the far calvarial wall.
- Most modern equipment will then allow a computer-generated ellipse to fit the calvarial wall to encompass the cranium and not the outer skin line (figure 61B).

The variability inherent in estimating fetal age from the head circumference is generally greater than with the biparietal diameter. The variability is not constant throughout pregnancy but increases with gestational age. The head circumference is part of several formulas to estimate fetal weight and is also used to monitor growth between examinations. Finally, the head circumference can be compared with other measurements, such as abdominal circumference (AC) and femur length (FL), to assess the possible effects of growth disturbances (e.g. macrosomia and growth restriction) on the fetus.

Cephalic Index

In certain circumstances (e.g. ruptured membranes, breech presentations, and multiple gestations), shape changes in the head may lead to even greater errors than those mentioned previously. To recognize the shape changes, one should always measure the cephalic index of the head to assess head shape.

The cephalic index is calculated from the biparietal diameter and the fronto-occipital diameter (FOD) measured from the outer edge of the calvaria to the outer edge of the calvaria:

$$\text{Cephalic index} = \text{BPD}/\text{FOD} \times 100$$

Technically, equipment manufacturers usually compute a cephalic index from the head circumference ellipse long and short axes. Because the short axis of the head circumference ellipse is not truly a biparietal diameter, a slight and clinically insignificant error is introduced into cephalic indexes computed in this way.

If the cephalic index varies by more than 1 standard deviation (SD) above or below the expected value (<74, >83), the head circumference will give a more accurate estimation of age than the biparietal diameter. Gray et al. found minimal changes in the mean value of cephalic index with advancing age and also concluded that the biparietal diameter should be viewed with suspicion as an age indicator when the cephalic index is more than 1 SD above or below the mean for age.[33]

Doubilet and Greenes recommended an alternative approach to potential head shape variations by routinely calculating a shape-correct biparietal diameter on the basis of an idealized cephalic index of 78:[34]

$$\text{Shape-corrected BPD} = (\text{BPD} \times \text{FOD})/1.265$$

As expected, when this shape correction is performed, the biparietal diameter is equivalent to the head circumference in accuracy of menstrual age prediction because it has been rendered shape-independent.

Abdominal Circumference

The abdominal circumference (AC) is the most difficult of the four measurements. Unfortunately, the abdominal anatomy is not symmetric like the brain anatomy. Also, there is not bright calvarium to check for *perpendicular* accuracy. The abdominal circumference is measured in a location that estimates liver size. The liver is the largest organ in the fetal torso, and its size reflects variations of growth, including growth restriction and macrosomia. Our protocol is to measure the fetal abdominal circumference at the position where the transverse diameter of the liver is the greatest. This can be determined sonographically as the position where the right and left portal veins are continuous with one another. Some refer to this anatomic confluence of the intrahepatic portal veins as "hockey stick" (figure 62).

Important considerations in measuring the fetal abdominal circumference are:

- The correct cephalocaudal plane is the position where the right and left portal veins are continuous with one another.

- The appearance of the lower ribs is symmetric.
- The shortest length of the umbilical segment of the left portal vein is depicted.

After this plane of section is frozen on the screen, the electronic ellipse is fit to the skin edge. Note that this is different from the head circumference where one specifically does not fill the ellipse to the skin edge but rather to the calvarial edge. The rib margin is easily visualized, and one may mistakenly fit the ellipse margin to the rib instead of the skin. This will significantly undermeasure the abdominal circumference. Generally, ultrasound machines are equipped with calculation packages that compute the abdominal circumference from the cursor and elliptical measurements. The circumference can be calculated by using the transverse and anteroposterior diameters of the abdomen (measured from skin edge to skin edge) and the formula (D1 + D2) × 1.57. The menstrual age can then be determined by using a standard reference table.

Many situations will arise when the landmarks for fetal abdominal circumference measurements are less optimally documented. In these cases, the sonographer can rely on the "round" rule. When the anatomic landmarks are difficult to demonstrate, use the circumference estimate where the A-P and transverse measurements are approximately the same, and the results will be reasonable. Excessive pressure with the transducer should be avoided because it distorts the shape of the abdomen.

Of the four basic ultrasound measurements, abdominal circumference is usually the most variable. This is partly because the abdominal circumference is

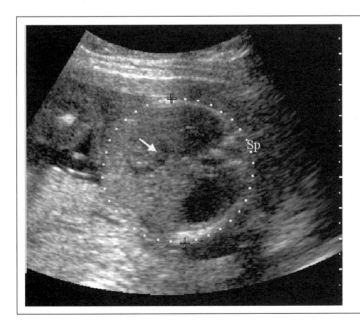

Figure 62.

Abdominal circumference. Sonogram of the fetal abdomen. Note "hockey stick" (arrow). Sp = spine.

more acutely affected by growth disturbances than the other basic parameters. Some believe that the variability is probably due more to measurement error than biological variability. In the study by Benson and Doubilet, the greatest variation between abdominal circumference and the other parameters was observed in the second trimester of pregnancy, a point at which growth variations would be expected to be minimal.[35] The abdomen is not rigid like the head, but soft and flexible, so it is more variable in size and shape.

In early pregnancy and in normally growing fetuses, the abdominal circumference is only slightly less accurate on average than the other basic measurements if one strictly adheres to the rules of measurement. As with all other parameters, however, the variability in predicting menstrual age based on abdominal circumference increases as pregnancy advances.

Femur Length

The femur length (FL) measurement is technically the easiest to obtain of the common biometric measurements, because of the "one-dimensional" nature of the measurement. The transducer should be aligned to the long axis of the bone to obtain the proper plane. No other transducer adjustment is necessary. This does not mean that errors are rare.

Femur length measurement does not actually measure the entire femur. Only the ossified portion of the diaphysis and metaphysis is measured (figure 63). The cartilaginous ends of the femur are excluded. The ossified portion of the femur is more visible sonographically than the nonossified ends. Nonetheless, the cartilaginous ends of the femur are readily demonstrated and, although they are excluded, they are key to accuracy and consistency in femoral length measurements.

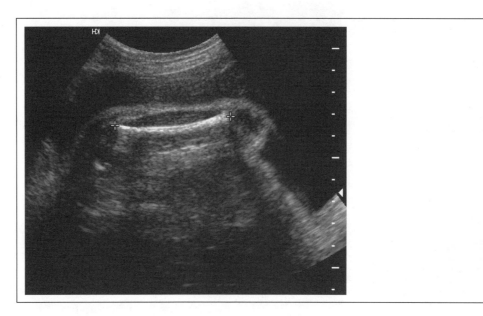

Figure 63.

Femur length. Sagittal sonogram of a fetal femur with cursors for measurements.

Proper alignment of the transducer to the long axis of the femur is ensured by demonstrating both the femoral head or greater trochanter and the femoral condyle simultaneously in the same plane of section. The cursors are positioned at the junction of the bone with the cartilage. A femur imaged vertically can be significantly shorter than one imaged horizontally, with up to a 2.6-week difference in gestational age prediction. Also, the femur closest to the transducer should be measured to minimize the variation associated with measuring at different depths.

Miscellaneous Measurements

Other fetal structures can be imaged and measured with current high-resolution real-time ultrasound equipment. These measurements may rarely be used to estimate gestational age when either fetal head or femur cannot be accurately imaged.

1 Binocular Measurement

When the fetal head is in a direct occiput posterior position, the orbits are easily imaged, and several authors have published normal data for both the binocular distance and the interorbital diameters. Only the outer orbital diameter can be used to estimate fetal age accurately.

2 Transcerebellar Measurement

In some cases, the cerebellum may be visible when a head circumference is difficult to obtain (figure 64). Between 14 and 20 weeks' gestation, the transverse cerebellar diameter in millimeters is roughly equivalent to the gestational age in weeks.

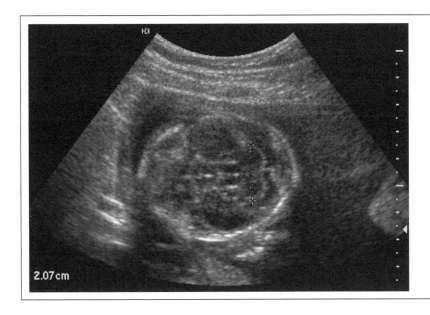

Figure 64.
Transcerebellar measurement. Sonogram showing the correct imaging plane for measuring the cerebellar diameter.

Complications

CHAPTER 5

Intrauterine growth restriction

Multiple gestations

Maternal illness

Fetal therapy

Antepartum/postpartum considerations

• •

Intrauterine Growth Retardation/Restriction

For nearly forty years, it has been recognized that growth-restricted fetuses are more likely to undergo perinatal morbidity or mortality than fetuses of normal size. In 1963, Lubchenco et al. showed that infants with birth weights at or below the 10th percentile were at risk for perinatal morbidity or mortality.[36] In 1966 Scott and Usher showed that the perinatal death rate was 8 times higher for infants with birth weights between the 3rd and 10th percentile and 20 times higher for infants with birth weights below the 3rd percentile.[37] Although the term *intrauterine growth retardation* has been used for years, the phrase *intrauterine growth restriction* is now preferred.

Definition of Intrauterine Growth Restriction

A difference of opinion exists on what criteria should be used to establish the diagnosis of intrauterine growth restriction (IUGR). In general two different definitions of intrauterine growth restriction have been used fairly widely:

1. Fetal weight less than the 10th percentile
2. Fetal weight less than the 5th percentile

Some investigators have proposed a third method of establishing a fetal growth curve from early ultrasound data before approximately 25 weeks and defining intrauterine growth restriction as a fall-off of fetal growth from this Rossavik-calculated growth curve. This third method is still being developed; large studies using this method have yet to be performed.

Fetal Weight Tables

If one is to use a percentile weight definition for intrauterine growth restriction, the first problem that arises is what weight curve to use. Numerous curves have been published correlating fetal weight and percentile weight with fetal age. Many of these early weight distributions were based on data obtained at the time of delivery. One such distribution, published by Williams and others, was based on approximately 2.5 million Caucasian women at sea level in California.[38] The problem with this birth-weight distribution is that fetuses born early tend to weigh less than those born at term. When subsequent medical personnel tried to use this birth-weight distribution to determine which fetuses were less than the 10th percentile or greater than the 90th percentile for weight, they discovered that very few fetuses fell below the 10th percentile or above the 90th percentile on this distribution. Similar problems were observed with other distributions from data acquired at delivery. Subsequent investigators including Hadlock and colleagues have concluded that the most accurate weight percentiles can be calculated on the basis of estimates of fetal weights calculated mathematically from sonographic measurements, taking into account the normal variation of these measurements in sonographic data used to establish fetal age.[39] The resulting fetal weight distributions show much less weight variability than the older weight distributions based on birth-weight data. Because these newer fetal weight distributions are so narrow, it is vital to know precisely the fetal age in order to use these weight percentiles. If the mother is quite certain of menstrual dates, the gestational age based on menstrual dates should be taken seriously, but gestational age based on an early sonogram in the first or early second trimester is generally much more reliable. Gestational age should be established at the time of first sonographic examination of the fetus, and gestational age should not be changed on later sonograms.

Fetal Weight Estimation

Because both the estimated fetal weight and the percentile fetal weight are based on fetal weight estimates made by using sonographic measurements, it is important to understand how fetal weights are calculated from the sonographic measurements. The early equations that were developed to estimate fetal weight used two measurements, either a biparietal diameter (BPD) or head circumference and an abdominal circumference. These equations, such as the Shepard equation, were then compared to birth weights immediately following the fetal weight estimate from sonographic measurements. The difference between birth weight and fetal weight estimate had a standard deviation of 15%. This meant that the actual birth weight was within plus or minus 30% of the predicted weight 95% of the time, resulting in only a rough estimate of the true birth weight. In 1984 Hadlock and Harrist found that adding a third variable to a head and abdomen measurement could improve the fetal weight estimate.[40] The third variable was the femur length. Fetal weight equations were developed using biparietal diameter or head circumference, abdominal circumference, and femoral length. This resulted in fetal weight estimations that were more accurate (table 1). These three variable fetal weight estimations, when compared with subsequent birth weights, had a standard deviation variance of only 7%, meaning that the true fetal weight was within plus or minus 15% of the estimated weight 95% of the time. The reason that these newer fetal weight estimates are more accurate seems to be that the femur length correlates nicely with the overall length of the femurs in most cases. If the femoral length is not an accurate estimate of the overall length of the fetus, as in fetal dwarfism, a three-variant fetal weight will not be accurate.

> ***Scan Techniques to Evaluate Intrauterine Growth Restriction***
>
> 1. Take a complete and comprehensive patient history.
> 2. Assign a gestational age to the fetus via accurate sonographic measurements.
> 3. Estimate the fetal weight and correlate with tables to determine percentiles (table 1).
> 4. Note other sonographic findings that relate to intrauterine growth restriction, head circumference/abdominal circumference (HC/AC), abdominal circumference/femur length (AC/FL), amniotic fluid volume, and umbilical artery and middle cerebral artery and Doppler.

When beginning an examination of a woman who has possible intrauterine growth restriction, the sonographer should obtain a complete maternal history, including:

1. Medications used, including illicit drugs such as cocaine and amphetamines
2. Smoking and alcohol use
3. Maternal disease
   - Vascular disease
   - Diabetes mellitus
   - Chronic hypertension

Table 1.
Percentile values for fetal abdominal circumference.

Menstrual Week	Abdominal Circumference (cm)				
	3rd	10th	50th	90th	97th
14	6.4	6.7	7.3	7.9	8.3
15	7.5	7.9	8.6	9.3	9.7
16	8.6	9.1	9.9	10.7	11.2
17	9.7	10.3	11.2	12.1	12.7
18	10.9	11.5	12.5	13.5	14.1
19	11.9	12.6	13.7	14.8	15.5
20	13.1	13.8	15.0	16.3	17.0
21	14.1	14.9	16.2	17.6	18.3
22	15.1	16.0	17.4	18.8	19.7
23	16.1	17.0	18.5	20.0	20.9
24	17.1	18.1	19.7	21.3	22.3
25	18.1	19.1	20.8	22.5	23.5
26	19.1	20.1	21.9	23.7	24.8
27	20.0	21.1	23.0	24.9	26.0
28	20.9	22.0	24.0	26.0	27.1
29	21.8	23.0	25.1	27.2	28.4
30	27.7	23.9	26.1	28.3	29.5
31	23.6	24.9	27.1	29.4	30.6
32	24.5	25.8	28.1	30.4	31.8
33	25.3	26.7	29.1	31.5	32.9
34	26.1	27.5	30.0	32.5	33.9
35	26.9	28.3	30.9	33.5	34.9
36	27.7	29.2	31.8	34.4	35.9
37	28.5	30.0	32.7	35.4	37.0
38	29.2	30.8	33.6	36.4	38.0
39	29.9	31.6	34.4	37.3	38.9
40	30.7	32.4	35.3	38.2	39.9

Adapted from Hadlock FP, Deter RL, Harrist RB, et al: Estimating fetal age: Computer-assisted analysis of multiple fetal growth parameters. *Radiology* 152:497-501, 1984. Reprinted with permission from Callen PW (ed): *Ultrasonography in Obstetrics and Gynecology,* 4th edition. Philadelphia, Saunders, 2000, p. 1026.

- Renal insufficiency
- Hypercoagulability, antiphospholipid antibody syndrome
- Miscarriages
- Asthma
- Gastrointestinal conditions such as Crohns, ulcerative colitis, GI bypass
- Maternal congenital heart disease
- Infections
    a. Viruses, rubella, cytomegalovirus
    b. Parasites, toxoplasmosis, syphilis, Chagas' disease, malaria
    c. Bacteria, including Listeria

All these conditions have been associated with intrauterine growth restriction.

There are two main types of fetal growth restriction:

1. Restricted fetal growth in the presence of adequate fetal nutrition. This is due to a problem in the fetus that restricts growth. This usually occurs earlier in the second trimester, and the growth reduction is typically symmetric.
2. Inadequate supply of fetal nutrients. This generally occurs in the late second and third trimester, and the fetal growth can be asymmetric.

If the fetus has adequate nutrition and does not grow normally, we must look for fetal anomalies that would suggest fetal syndromes such as trisomy 13 or 18 or possibly trisomy 21. Various other fetal syndromes can also cause intrauterine growth restriction, including triploidy. In many cases, sonographic findings can be detected that suggest the presence of a syndrome. These findings are discussed in the section on syndromes. If the genetic abnormality in the fetus is severe, reduction in fetal growth often occurs earlier in pregnancy and the delay in growth of the different fetal parts is more symmetric.

There are two general classes of intrauterine growth restriction in fetuses that have inadequate nutrition. First, the fetus may have inadequate nutrition because the mother has inadequate nutrition or is ill. Abuse of drugs, alcohol, or cigarettes can lead to intrauterine growth restriction. If the mother has diabetes, hypertension, asthma, vascular disease, heart disease, or gastrointestinal disease, these conditions could lead to inadequate oxygenation or nutrition for both the mother and the fetus. Certain maternal infections including parvovirus, toxoplasmosis, rubella, cytomegalovirus, herpes, and other infections may lead to an intrauterine infection of the fetus with subsequent growth restriction.

Second, if the mother is healthy and has adequate nutrition, intrauterine growth restriction may still occur as a result of abnormalities in the formation of the placenta and its surrounding vasculature.

Fetal intrauterine growth restriction resulting from inadequate nutrition is typically more severe in the middle and latter part of pregnancy when the growth of the fetal abdomen is more rapid than the growth of the fetal head. Intrauterine growth restriction that occurs in this time period is more likely to be asymmetric, with more delay in growth of the abdomen than the head and extremities. However, second and third trimester growth restriction is variable, and asymmetric growth restriction may not occur or may occur only for a short period of time and then may become symmetric.

Compensation will occur if the fetus has inadequate nutrition. The blood flow is redistributed to the heart and the brain, and there is less blood flow through other parts of the body including the liver and kidneys. Because of the redistribution of blood flow, the head may continue to grow normally, with less growth noted in the abdomen, partly because of reduced blood flow and partly because of decreased glycogen storage in the liver from the starving condition. In these fetuses, the head circumference to abdomen circumference ratio may increase. If so, the fetus is considered to have asymmetric intrauterine growth restriction. In this compensation mode, decreased blood flow to the kidneys results in decreased production of fetal urine. Over a period of time, the reduction in fetal urine output will result in oligohydramnios. If Doppler is performed on a fetus in the compensation mode, lower vascular resistance will be noted in the fetal brain. Another finding that can be observed in a fetus that has inadequate nutrition is an increase in the femur length to abdominal circumference ratio. This observation is probably due to relatively normal growth of the femur with reduction of growth in the abdomen. Although this finding may be observed in intrauterine growth restriction, it seems to be variable, and many growth-restricted fetuses do not demonstrate this finding.

In women who have inadequate placental development or extensive vascular disease, intrauterine growth restriction is likely even if the maternal nutrition is adequate. The tissue of the placenta is dependent on oxygenation from the mother for its existence and growth, and if oxygenation is inadequate, placental infarctions may occur during pregnancy. The combination of suboptimal perfusion of the placenta and placental infarction can lead to inadequate fetal nutrition despite adequate maternal nutrition. If the placental infarctions are extensive, there will be an increase in umbilical artery resistance in the placenta. This is usually a fairly late finding. Doppler examination of the umbilical arteries will demonstrate increase in resistance and decrease in diastolic flow.

In general, Doppler measurements are less predictive for intrauterine growth restriction than are non-Doppler criteria. However, if diastolic flow is absent or reversed in the umbilical arteries, the fetus is at great risk for intrauterine demise (color plate 6). Gray scale evaluation of the placenta does not usually demonstrate evidence of placental infarctions, despite severe placental disease. Evaluation of placental calcifications is somewhat helpful, but the degree of calcification in the placenta is not an accurate measure of the degree of placental insufficiency.

As we have discussed, a number of sonographic findings may be observed in intrauterine growth restriction in addition to the low estimated weight percentile. Extensive evaluation of these findings has indicated that no single sonographic finding, with the exception of low estimated fetal weight, can be used by itself to confirm or exclude a diagnosis of intrauterine growth restriction. If the findings are used in combination, however, the diagnosis of intrauterine growth restriction can be more accurately made. Benson and others have indicated that the combination of estimated weight percentile, amniotic fluid volume, and maternal blood pressure can be used to improve the accuracy of diagnosis.[41] They also report that adding femur length, abdominal circumference, or head circumference data to the preceding three parameters did not improve the accuracy. Once the diagnosis of intrauterine growth restriction has been made, the parameters previously described can be used to monitor the growth-restricted fetus and aid in the management of the pregnancy.

In addition to the fetal sonographic parameters previously described, the assessment of fetal well-being can be made as well. This examination, commonly referred to as the biophysical profile, consists of evaluation of fetal breathing movements, number of breaths, fetal movements of the spine and extremities, an assessment of fetal tone and amniotic fluid volume, and assessment of variability of fetal heart rate. The fetal amniotic fluid volume is a chronic marker for fetal distress. As described previously, if perfusion to the kidneys is reduced, the amniotic fluid volume will be reduced over a period of days to weeks. The other four fetal observations are assessments of acute fetal distress; if there is reduction in fetal breathing movements, fetal tone, or in variability of fetal heart rate, these findings indicate fetal distress.

Summary

As we have indicated, there does not seem to be a simple method for diagnosing intrauterine growth restriction. However, if one or more of the following findings are noted, they should raise concern about IUGR:

1. Estimated fetal weight below the 10th percentile. We prefer Hadlock's weight chart.
2. HC/AC ratio above the normal range.
3. Oligohydramnios.
4. Middle cerebral artery resistance equal to or lower than umbilical cord resistance.

Multiple Gestations

Twin Pregnancy

The incidence of twins is approximately 1.1–1.5%, or approximately 1 per 80 live births.[42, 43] The number of multiple births has increased since 1980, most likely because of the increased treatment for infertility and the aging maternal population, both of which are associated with a higher rate of twin pregnancy. Multiple gestations are high-risk pregnancies for both the fetus and the mother.

Twin births account for almost 10% of all perinatal morbidity and mortality.[44] The perinatal mortality rate for twins is approximately 4–6 times as high as for singletons, and the morbidity rate is twice as high.[45] The perinatal death rate for twins is 5–10 times greater than for singletons.[46, 47]

Seventy percent of twins are dizygotic (fraternal), arising from the fertilization of two separate ova, and 30% are monozygotic (identical), resulting from division of a single fertilized ovum. The frequency of monozygotic twinning is relatively constant across populations and is independent of race, age or parity, heredity, use of ovulation-induction agents, and maternal genetics. These factors do influence the frequency of dizygotic twinning.

1 Race

Significant variation exists in the rates of dizygotic twinning among different populations and ethnic groups. The incidence in North America of dizygotic twinning in Caucasians is approximately 7.1 per 1000 live births, whereas the incidence in blacks is approximately 11.1 per 1000. In Nigeria, the incidence is 49 per 1000, and in Japan the incidence is approximately 1.3 per 1000.[43]

2 Maternal Age and Parity

The incidence of twinning increases with advancing maternal age up to 35–40 years old and increases with parity up to seven.

3 Heredity

Maternal family history of dizygotic (DZ) twinning is associated with a higher incidence of twins. This has been attributed to variations in gonadotropin production by the pituitary gland, leading to increased stimulation of the ovaries and multiple ovulations.[48, 49] In a study by White and Wyshak, the incidence of dizygotic twin births in women who themselves were a dizygotic twin was 1 per 58.[50] There is no association with paternal history of dizygotic twinning.

4 Use of Ovulation-Induction Agents

Clomiphene therapy is associated with a 7–9% incidence of twinning, and human menopausal gondadotropin (hMG) is associated with an 18% incidence.[42, 47]

Embryology/Placenta

The placentation type of a twin pregnancy refers to its *chorionicity* (number of placentas) and its *amnionicity* (number of amniotic sacs). Dizygotic twins (fraternal) arise from two separate fertilized ova (zygotes). The two zygotes develop into blastocysts that implant independently, each forming an embryo with its own amnion and chorion and yolk sac, resulting in a dichorionic diamniotic (DC/DA) pregnancy.

The *chorion frondosum* and *decidua basalis* combine to form the placenta. Dichorionic, diamniotic twins have two visibly separate placentas, unless implantation of the two blastocysts is close enough to result in the formation of one apparently fused placenta.

Monozygotic (MZ) twins (identical) arise from the division of a single zygote. The chorionicity and amnionicity of monozygotic twins depends on the stage at which division occurs[43, 51] and may be categorized as follows (figure 65):

1. *Dichorionic diamniotic (DC/DA) twins* arise when the zygote divides between the two-cell stage and morula state, during the first 3 days postconception. This results in the formation of two embryos with two amnions and two chorions. Dichorionic diamniotic twins make up 18–36% of monozygotic twins. As with dizygotic twins, monozygotic dichorionic diamniotic twins have two placentas or one fused placenta (figure 65A and B).

2. *Monochorionic diamniotic (MC/DA)* twinning is the most common form of monozygotic twinning, accounting for approximately 70% of monozygotic twins. Division of the inner cell mass between the 4th and 8th days postconception occurs after the cells destined to become the chorion have already differentiated. Consequently, two embryos, two amnions, and two yolk sacs will be formed within a single chorion. Monochorionic diamniotic twins have a single placenta (figure 65C).

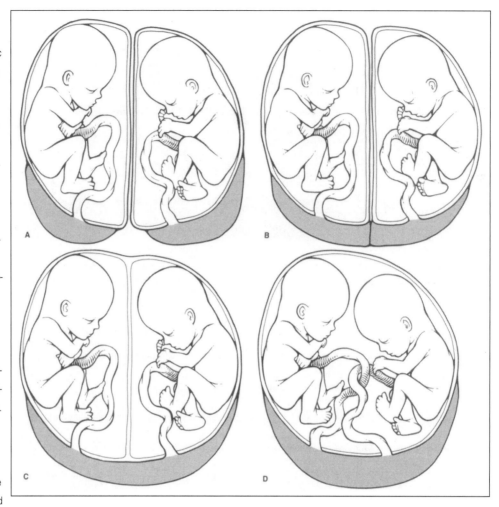

Figure 65.
Placentation types.
A Dichorionic-diamniotic gestation with separate placentas. The membrane separating the twins is thick, with four layers: two chorionic and two amniotic membranes. **B** Dichorionic-diamniotic gestation with fused placentas. The membrane separating the twins is thick, with four layers. **C** Monochorionic-diamniotic gestation. The membrane separating the twins is thin, with two layers of amniotic membrane. **D** Monochorionic-monoamniotic gestation. No membrane separates the twins. The two umbilical cords intermingle in the single amniotic cavity. Reprinted with permission from McGahan JP, Goldberg BB (eds): *Diagnostic Ultrasound: A Logical Approach.* Lippincott Williams & Wilkins, 1998, p 486.

3 *Monochorionic monoamniotic (MC/MA) twins* occur when the embryonic disk divides after day 8 postconception, resulting in the formation of two embryos within a single amnion and a single chorion. The frequency of occurrence is 1% of monozygotic twins (figure 65D).

Sonographic Determination of Chorionicity and Amnionicity

Because of the high perinatal morbidity and mortality in monochorionic compared with dichorionic gestations, all twins should be carefully assessed sonographically to determine the number of chorions and amnions. Chorionicity and amnionicity have important prognostic and diagnostic significance. The placentas in monochorionic diamniotic twin pregnancies usually have vascular anastomoses between the circulations of the two fetuses. These anastomoses may be vein-to-vein, artery-to-artery, or artery-to-vein and may result in *twin transfusion syndrome, twin embolization syndrome,* and the *acardiac parabiotic twin syndrome.*

Sonographically, amnionicity can be assessed by the 6th menstrual week by counting the number of embryonic heartbeats within each gestational sac. If the ratio of embryos to gestational sacs is 1:1, then amnionicity can be assumed to equal chorionicity before visualization of the amnion later in the first trimester. Therefore, identification of two gestational sacs with a single embryo or embryonic heartbeat in each sac confirms the gestation as dichorionic and diamniotic. Identification of a single gestational sac containing two embryos can be a monochorionic diamniotic, or monochorionic monoamniotic pregnancy.

1 First Trimester

Sonographic assessment of chorionicity and amnionicity in multiple gestations is most accurate in the first trimester. Counting the number of gestational sacs is an accurate method for predicting chorionicity from 6 to 10 weeks' gestation. If only one gestational sac is found but two amniotic sacs and embryos are present, the pregnancy is monochorionic diamaniotic (MC/DA). If two embryos lie within one amnion, the pregnancy is monochorionic monoamniotic (MC/MA). Some investigators have noted that the number of yolk sacs is the same as the number of amnions. For instance, a monochorionic monoamniotic pregnancy will have one yolk sac, and a monochorionic diamaniotic pregnancy will have two. As the first trimester progresses, the amniotic cavity enlarges until it obliterates the chorionic cavity at approximately the 10th gestational week. For this reason an early sonogram should be performed in all suspected or known multifetal gestations. Beyond the first trimester, accurate assignment of chorionicity and amnionicity may be more difficult.

2 Second and Third Trimester

The following can be performed sonographically to determine chorionicity and amnionicity:

1. *Identify the presence of a membrane.* The presence of a membrane indicates that the pregnancy is not a monochorionic monoamniotic twin pregnancy. Nonvisualization of a membrane between the fetuses occurs in up to 10% of either dichorionic diamniotic or monochorionic diamniotic twin pregnancies and cannot be used as the sole indicator of a monochorionic monoamniotic pregnancy.

   Visualization of a membrane is useful in determining chorionicity and amnionicity in a twin pregnancy with a single placental mass. Identification of an intervening membrane and evaluation of its thickness and its relationship to both fetuses should be performed in all twin pregnancies.

   The interfetal membrane in a dichorionic twin gestation is composed of two layers of amnion and two layers of chorion, whereas the membrane in a monochorionic gestation is composed of only two layers of amnion with no interposing chorion. This has led to the sonographic assessment of intertwin membrane thickness as a predictor of chorionicity. Prediction of chorionicity based on membrane thickness seems to be more reliable before 26 weeks' gestation, because the membrane thins as pregnancy progresses. Several studies have been done to determine how to define "thick" membrane.[52–54] A thick membrane measures 1–2 mm, and a thin membrane is described as "wispy" and thinner.

2. *Determine fetal sex.* Sonographic evaluation of fetal genitalia is part of the complete examination and can be an indicator of chorionicity and amnionicity. If the examination indicates clearly that one fetus is male and the other female, it can be deduced that the pregnancy is dizygotic and therefore dichorionic diamniotic. If the fetuses are the same sex, then zygosity cannot be inferred. A pregnancy with an apparent single placenta could be either monochorionic or dichorionic.

3. *Assess the sonographic presence of a chorionic "twin peak" or "lambda" sign.* The projection of tissue of similar appearance and echogenicity to the placenta, extending into the intertwin membrane and tapering to a point within this membrane, is called the "twin peak sign."[55] (See figure 66.) According to Finberg, the presence of the chorionic peak sign is due to extension of placental villi into the potential interchorionic space next to the placenta and chorion of its twin. The chorionic peak cannot occur in a monochorionic twin pregnancy because the single chorion serves as a barrier to the growth of

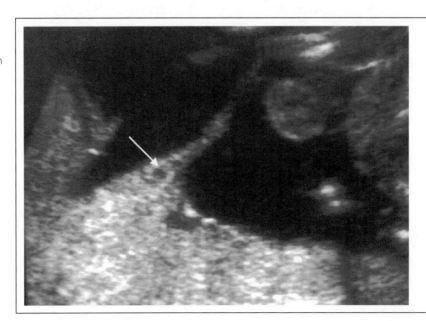

Figure 66.
Twin peak sign. Sonogram demonstrating an extension of placental tissue widening the intertwin septum at its point of contact with the chorionic surface (arrow).

placental villi into the intertwin membrane. The presence of a chorionic peak is diagnostic of a dichorionic diamniotic twin pregnancy. However, nonvisualization of a chorionic peak cannot be used as a predictor of chorionicity.

Growth in Twin Gestations

Although some variation in crown-rump length (CRL) is normal in the first trimester, significant discordance may be ominous. Defining discordance as 5 or more days' difference in estimated gestational age, Weissman and colleagues found that all discordant pairs had major congenital anomalies in the smaller twin.[56]

The growth rate of twins is similar to that of singletons until approximately 28–30 weeks. After this time, twins add weight regularly but more slowly than single fetuses.[57] Discordance in the weights of twins may also be encountered and is potentially of great importance. Twins in dizygotic pregnancies might be expected to differ slightly in size because of their different genetic makeup. Monozygotic fetuses, however, have the same genes and theoretically should have essentially identical parameters at the same time. Discordance, defined as a difference in birth weight of 20% or more, is reported to occur in up to 23% of twin pairs and leads to significantly increased morbidity and mortality compared with twin pairs of nearly equal birth weight.

The causes of discordancy in dizygotic twins are diverse:

1. There may be different genetic growth potential, but this does not usually result in significant discordancy unless there is a significant genetic defect. In either dizygotic or monozygotic gestations, morphologic abnormalities or aneuploidy may affect only one twin and lead to significant growth restriction.
2. Inequality of placentation, in which one twin is supported by an inadequate placenta, may also hinder growth of that fetus relative to its twin.

Complications of Twin Pregnancy

Twin gestations have a higher rate of complications than do singletons, both because some obstetric complications occur more frequently with twins and because certain complications are unique to twins. Multiple gestations are more likely to result in premature delivery than are singletons, and they are at increased risk for neonatal morbidity and mortality associated with prematurity.

Monozygotic twins have an increased incidence of fetal anomalies, including anencephaly, hydrocephalus, holoprosencephaly, sirenomelia, and sacrococcygeal teratoma. These anomalies are often discordant, affecting only one twin, even though both twins arise from a single fertilized egg.

Complications specific to twins depend on placentation type.[58] Monochorionic twins may develop complications resulting from vascular anastomoses through the common placenta. Monoamniotic twins are also at high risk for umbilical cord entanglement and cord accidents within their common amniotic cavity.

1 *Twin-twin transfusion syndrome* is a complication of monochorionic twins that results from unbalanced exchange of blood from one fetus (donor twin) to the other (recipient twin) across artery-to-vein anastomoses in their common placenta. The sonographic features of twin-twin transfusion syndrome include discrepant amniotic fluid volumes and discordant fetal sizes. Discordance is significant when the difference in the estimated fetal weights between the twins is greater than 25% of the weight of the larger twin.[59, 60] The anemic donor twin is smaller and has oligohydramnios. The oligohydramnios may be so severe that the donor twin is compressed against the uterine wall by the diamniotic membrane. When this occurs, the affected fetus is called a "stuck twin" (figure 67). The polycythemic recipient twin usually is appropriate in size, has polyhydramnios, and may be hydropic. Both the donor and the recipient twin carry a poor prognosis, with a mortality rate (intrauterine and perinatal) of approximately 70%. The prognosis is especially poor in the presence of a stuck twin.

Figure 67A.
Stuck twin. Transverse view of the stuck twin.

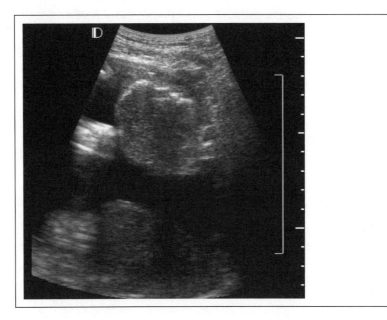

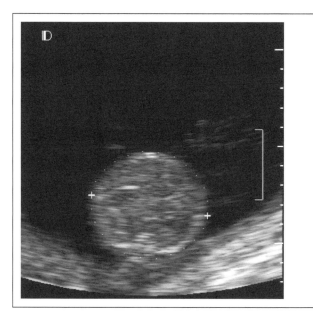

Figure 67B.
Stuck twin. Transverse view of the other twin demonstrating polyhydramnios.

2 *Twin embolization syndrome.* With the demise of one twin in dichorionic diamniotic pregnancies, the surviving twin is not at significant risk.[61, 62] If co-twin demise occurs in the second trimester, as the surviving twin grows, the water content and most of the soft tissue of the dead fetus may be reabsorbed, resulting in a small flattened fetus surrounded by minimal or no amniotic fluid, referred to as *fetus papyraceus*.[43]

In monochorionic twins, demise of the co-twin may result in renal, hepatic, and cerebral damage in the surviving twin.[63–65] (See figure 68.) Benirschke originally postulated that demise of the co-twin may result in

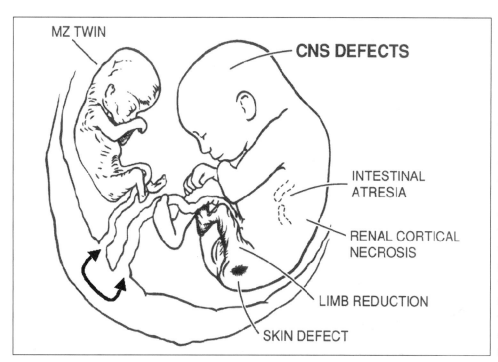

Figure 68.
Twin embolization. Depiction of the abnormalities that may occur in twin embolization syndrome. The living twin may pump blood into the dying twin and experience hypotension and hypoxia. Emboli may move from the dying twin to the living twin. In Gray P, Rouse G, DeLange M: Sonographic evaluation of twin embolization syndrome, a report of three cases and review of the literature. *JDMS* 9:3–10, 1993.

Figure 69.

Porencephalic cyst. Postnatal coronal sonogram from living twin shows a porencephalic cyst (C) caused by twin embolization syndrome.

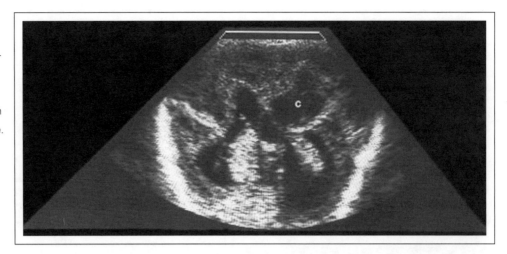

transfusion of thromboplastin-rich blood or embolization of clot and debris across the placental vascular anastomoses to the surviving twin. More recently, Benirschke has suggested that the damage to the surviving twin is caused by the living twin pumping its blood into the dying twin. The living twin then becomes hypoxic. Common intracranial manifestations of the twin embolization syndrome (TES) include ventriculomegaly, porencephalic cysts (figure 69), diffuse cerebral atrophy, and microcephaly.[64] Gastrointestinal manifestations include hepatic and splenic infarcts and gut atresias.[64] Other anomalies, including renal cortical necrosis, pulmonary infarcts, facial anomalies, aplasia cutis, and terminal limb defects, may also occur (figure 68).

■ 3 *Acardiac twin (TRAP sequence).* The acardiac anomaly is a rare complication of monochorionic twins that results from large artery-to-artery and vein-to-vein anastomoses in their common placenta. In such cases, one twin becomes the "pump" twin, with its heart supplying blood both to

Figure 70A.

Twin reversed arterial perfusion. Sagittal view of the malformed hydropic twin.

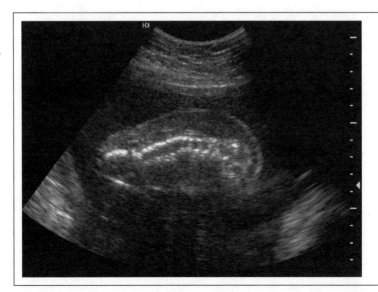

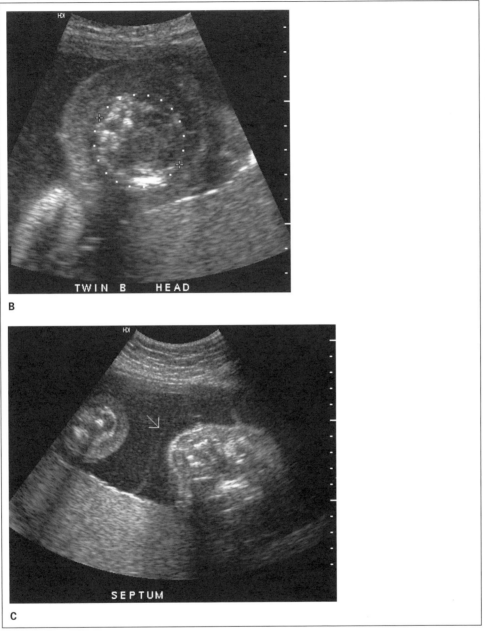

Figure 70.

Twin reversed arterial perfusion. **B** Transverse view demonstrates hydrops of the abdomen. **C** Septum (arrow) between the abnormal twin on the left and pump twin on the right.

itself and to the acardiac co-twin (figure 70). The direction of blood flow in the co-twin is reversed, with blood entering this twin through its umbilical artery and exiting through its umbilical vein. This phenomenon is called *twin reversed arterial perfusion* (TRAP) sequence (color plate 7).

Because the acardiac twin receives poorly oxygenated blood through the umbilical artery, structures supplied by the iliac arteries and distal abdominal aorta are relatively well perfused, whereas the upper body and head receive essentially no oxygenated blood. As a result, the acardiac twin has limited development of the upper half of the body, characterized by anencephaly or a small rudimentary head with holoprosencephaly, absent or hypoplastic upper torso and limbs, and absent or anomalous two-chambered heart.[66–68] A multiloculated dorsal cystic hygroma is usually present. The acardiac twin usually has a two-vessel umbilical cord. The reversed direction of blood flow in the acardiac twin's umbilical vessel can be documented with Doppler.[69–71]

4 *Cord entanglement.* Monoamniotic twins and their umbilical cords reside in a common amniotic sac, leading to potential intertwining of the two cords that may cut off blood flow to one or both fetuses. This complication occurs frequently in monoamniotic twins and contributes to the high mortality rate in such twins.[72]

5 *Conjoined twins.* Conjoined twins are rare, occurring in approximately 1 in 50,000 births. They are classified according to the location of conjoining (figure 71), with the most common sites being anterior thoracic and

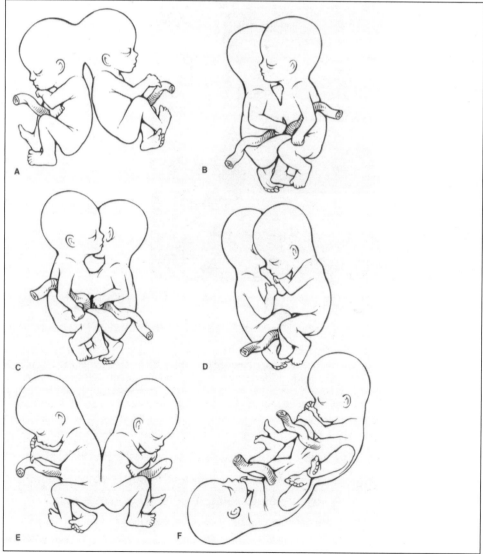

Figure 71.
Types of conjoined twins. Incomplete division of the fertilized ovum leads to conjoined twins with shared organs. **A** Craniopagus twins are joined at the head. **B** Xiphopagus twins are joined at the xiphoid. **C** Thoracopagus twins are joined at the thorax. **D** Omphalopagus twins are joined across the anterior abdomen. **E** Pygopagus twins are joined at the pelvis, facing away. **F** Ischiopagus twins are joined at the pelvis, opposed. Modified with permission from Mariona FG: Anomalies specific to multiple gestations. In Chervenak FA, Isaacson VS, Campbell S (eds): *Ultrasound in Obstetrics and Gynecology.* Boston, Little, Brown, 1993, p 1051.

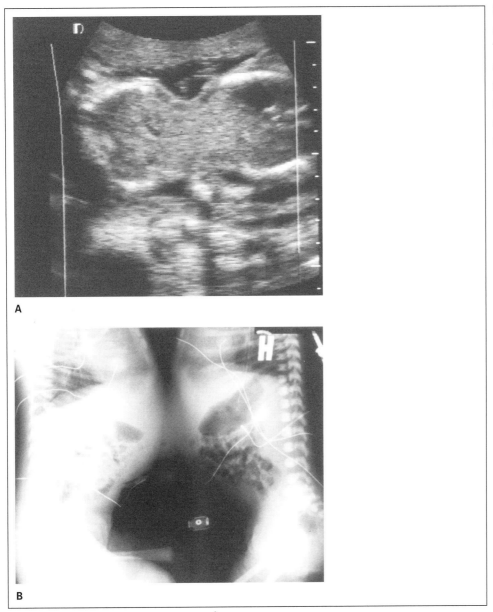

Figure 72.
Conjoined twins. **A** Transverse sonogram showing conjoined twins with shared liver (omphalopagus). **B** Radiograph of the same twins.

abdominal walls. Conjoined twins are easily identified by ultrasound. Sonography is particularly useful for determining the location of conjoining and the extent of organ sharing (figure 72). This technique allows assessment of prognosis, surgical planning, and parental counseling before delivery.

Maternal Illness

Many maternal diseases may affect pregnancy. The result may be early pregnancy loss, late fetal demise, or major malformations. Maternal conditions that can affect pregnancy include diabetes mellitus, maternal hypertension, and Rh incompatibility. Although the placenta acts as a filter between the mother and the fetus, many infectious agents, drugs, and antibodies can move across the placental barrier and affect the fetus.

Diabetes Mellitus

Two types of diabetes can affect the developing fetus. In the first type, the mother has *pre-existing diabetes mellitus* and is insulin-dependent. In the second type, the mother has *gestational diabetes,* which develops during pregnancy. Women who have pre-existing diabetes may develop hypoglycemia in the first trimester, during organogenesis. If that occurs, the developing embryo may exhibit a variety of abnormalities. In gestational diabetes, the fetus is not at risk for major structural anomalies because the blood sugar variation occurs after embryogenesis.

Anomalies associated with pre-existing diabetes mellitus include:

- Cardiac anomalies specifically include:

    Ventricular septal defect (VSD).

    Great vessels anomalies.

    Coarctation of the aorta.

    Pulmonary atresia.

    Truncus arteriosus.

    Transposition of great vessels.

- CNS malformations:

    Anencephaly.

    Holoprosencephaly.

    Encephalocele.

    Spina bifida.

    Caudal regression.

    Sirenomelia.

- Renal and urologic anomalies specifically:

    Ureteral duplication.

    Hydronephrosis.

    Multicystic dysplastic kidney.

    Renal agenesis.

- Gastrointestinal anomalies:

    Situs inversus.

    Duodenal atresia.

    Imperforate anus.

These anomalies are discussed in detail in the section on fetal abnormalities.

Absence of the sacrum (caudal regression) is strongly associated with diabetes mellitus, but other neural tube defects may also occur. In our experience, encephaloceles observed in diabetic pregnancies contain only the cerebellum. This type of encephalocele is rarely observed in nondiabetic pregnancies. Cardiac anomalies are the most common anomalies associated with diabetic pregnancy. In diabetic pregnancy, renal anomalies and renal agenesis are associated with fusion of the lower extremities (*sirenomelia*). Table 2 shows the relative risk for fetal anomalies in women with pre-existing diabetes compared with other pregnant women.

A mother who has diabetes mellitus exposes her fetus to varying levels of glucose throughout the pregnancy, and the fetus often produces excess insulin. This can lead to overgrowth of the fetal trunk and abdominal organs in late pregnancy, while the cranium and brain grow at a more normal rate. The result is a larger abdomen in the fetus of a diabetic mother.

Macrosomia is usually defined as fetal weight greater than 4000 grams or a birth weight above the 90th percentile for gestational age. Macrosomia can result in a stillbirth or intrapartum trauma. In addition to macrosomia, large placenta, polyhydramnios, excessive anasarca, and organomegaly may be observed in the diabetic pregnancy. The detection of macrosomia in the third trimester is helpful for clinical management and for planning the delivery. In pre-existing diabetes, IUGR may be observed because of vascular disease.

Anomalies	Relative Risk*
Cardiac	4:1
Anencephaly	3:1
Holoprosencephaly	40:1
Caudal regression	200–600:1

Table 2. Relative risk for fetal anomalies in women with pre-existing diabetes compared with other pregnant women.

*The relative risk ratio indicates how much more likely it is that a diabetic woman will have a fetus with one of these anomalies. In the case of cardiac anomalies, for example, a woman with preexisting diabetes is 4 times more likely to have an afflicted fetus.

Data from: Congenital malformations in diabetes. In Gabbe SG, Oh W (eds): *Infants of Diabetic Mother: Report of the 93rd Ross Conference on Pediatric Research*. Columbus, Ohio: Ross Laboratories, 1987, pp 12–19.

When performing a sonogram on a diabetic mother, a sonographer should:

- Take a complete maternal history.
- Establish if the mother has gestational diabetes or pre-existing diabetes mellitus.
- Scan carefully to rule out the anomalies mentioned above, paying particular attention to the fetal brain, spinal column, sacrum, and heart.

Maternal Hypertension

Toxemia of pregnancy occurs in the third trimester and is characterized by maternal edema, hypertension, proteinuria, and CNS irritability. This disease can be classified in two stages, *pre-eclampsia* and *eclampsia.* Findings in pre-eclampsia are hypertension and proteinuria, edema, or both. In the eclamptic stage, one or more convulsions occur, which significantly increases the risk of maternal and fetal mortality. When the convulsions occur, the mother usually experiences vasospasm, which can lead to stroke, hepatic hemorrhage, or both.

Maternal hypertension occurs most commonly in young primigravidas and older multiparas. The cause remains unclear, but immunologic, hormonal, and nutritional factors may be responsible. Some investigators suggest the decrease in prostaglandin synthesis observed in pre-eclamptic patients promotes placental vascular disease and decreased uteroplacental blood flow. Placental abruption, low birth weight, and fetal distress are associated with toxemia.[73]

Sonography plays a role in monitoring pre-eclamptic pregnancies. A variety of sonographic findings may be observed in these patients, including:

- Oligohydramnios
- Intrauterine growth restriction (IUGR)
- Decreased placental volume
- Accelerated placental maturation
- Fetal demise
- Increased placental resistance. Doppler can be performed serially to monitor placental vascular resistance.

Maternal Isoimmunization (Rh Incompatibility)

The major blood types, A and B, are actually antigens on the surface of red cells. In addition to A and B there are other antigens, such as D (rhesus or Rh), M, and Kell. If a fetus has a red cell antigen that the mother lacks, the mother may develop antibodies against that antigen. This process is called *alloimmunization* or *isoimmunization*. Usually, the mother is exposed to the fetal antigen at delivery. If the mother subsequently has another fetus with the same antigen, and a transplacental hemorrhage occurs, she will begin making antibodies, which will cross the placenta and attack the red cells of the affected fetus.

Why does alloimmunization cause hydrops? When the fetus has red cell antigens that the mother does not have and transplacental hemorrhage occurs, the mother produces antibodies that cross the placenta and attack the fetal red cells, hemolyzing them. As the fetal red cells are destroyed, the fetus must circulate the blood faster in order to keep itself oxygenated. Eventually the fetus will go into high-output failure, and hydrops develops.

Sonographic findings (figure 73) associated with hydrops include:

- Polyhydramnios (one pocket greater than 8 cm or four quadrants greater than 20–24 cm).
- Placental edema, 4–6 cm.
- Changes in the umbilical vessels. Umbilical artery Doppler demonstrates decreased pulsatility with blunted systolic peak and increased diastolic flow.
- Peritoneal, pleural, or pericardial effusions.
- Skin thickening (anasarca) edema greater than 5 mm, usually seen first around the calvaria.

The most common cause of maternal isoimmunization is maternal sensitization to the Rh antigen. At the time of delivery of her first pregnancy, an Rh-negative woman is usually given Rhogam. Rhogam contains immunoglobulins collected from women who are sensitized to the Rh antigen. The Rhogam will attach to the Rh antigens on fetal red cells that have entered the maternal bloodstream and "cover them up" so the mother does not begin to make antibodies.

The number of cases of immune hydrops has decreased. Factors contributing to declining incidence of fetal immune hemolytic disease include:

1. Postpartum prophylaxis (Rhogam).
2. Antepartum prophylaxis (Rhogam) in some women, specifically in women who experience spontaneous transplacental hemorrhage (TPH) in utero or who undergo invasive procedures during pregnancy.
3. Therapeutic immunoglobulin G (IgG) for massive exposure.

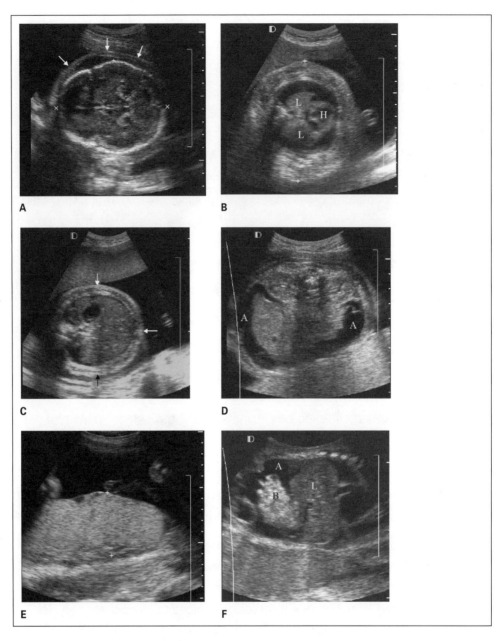

Figure 73.

Hydrops. **A** Fetal cranium. Note edema (arrows). **B** Transverse of the fetal chest. Note pleural effusion surrounding the lung (L) and heart (H), as well as chest wall edema. **C** Transverse fetal abdomen. Note wall thickening (arrows). **D** Transverse fetal abdomen. Note ascites (A). **E** Thickened placenta (cursors). **F** Sagittal of fetal abdomen. Note ascites (A) and fluid surrounding liver (L) and bowel (B).

Alloimmunization occurs when the fetal blood crosses to the maternal circulation or by transplacental hemorrhage. About 75% occur at delivery, but 10% occur before 28 weeks, as a result of abruption or subchorionic hemorrhage.

Invasive obstetrical procedures that are likely to cause transplacental hemorrhage include:

- Genetic amniocentesis.
- Chorionic villus sampling (CVS).
- Percutaneous umbilical blood sampling (PUBS).
- External version.

The use of ultrasound guidance for these procedures can decrease the chance of transplacental hemorrhage by:

- Identifying the origin of the cord at the placenta.
- Visualizing the position of the cord.
- Localizing the placenta.
- Detecting anomalies including placenta succenturiate lobe and vasa previa.

If transplacental hemorrhage is strongly suspected, a maternal Kleihauer test can be performed, which samples maternal blood to assess whether blood cells from the fetus are present.

Management of the Anemic Fetus

When fetal anemia is suspected, several procedures can be performed:

- Amniocentesis.
- Cordocentesis.
- Evaluation of the middle cerebral artery (MCA) peak systolic velocity (a newer technique).

A study done by Mari demonstrated that the following criteria must be met to use the middle cerebral artery evaluation successfully:

- The fetus should be at risk for anemia.
- The incidence angle between the ultrasound beam and the MCA should be close to 0 degrees.
- The highest peak velocity should be recorded.[74]

If the peak systolic velocity of the middle cerebral arterial bloodflow is below the normal 50th percentile, the fetus is considered nonanemic (see figure 74) and cordocentesis may be delayed. Because the highest velocities are associated with the most severe cases of anemia, the middle cerebral artery peak systolic velocity has the potential to estimate the degree of anemia. This approach may reduce the number of invasive procedures required to manage affected fetuses.

Amniocentesis can assist with evaluation of amniotic bilirubin, but this is valuable only in certain types of alloimmunization, such as Rh but not Kell or M. In patients who have Rh immunization, amniocentesis is performed to evaluate the level of bilirubin in the amniotic fluid. Amniocentesis is repeated to recheck the bilirubin level. If the bilirubin level in the amniotic fluid rises enough, fetal anemia is presumed to be present. When fetal anemia is established, then a fetal transfusion can be performed.

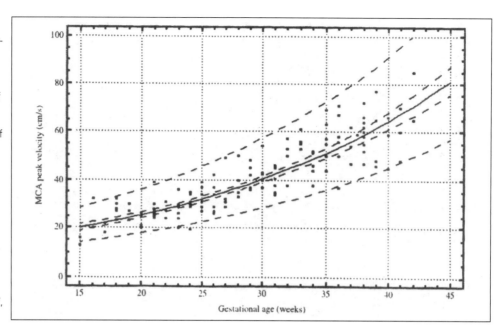

Figure 74.
MCA peak velocity. Normal range of middle cerebral artery peak velocity as a function of gestational age, constructed from a study of 135 normal fetuses. Inner dashed lines represent 95% confidence intervals and outer dashed lines represent 95% prediction interval. Reprinted with permission from Mari G, Adrigno A, Abuhamad Z, et al: Diagnosis of fetal anemia with Doppler ultrasound in the pregnancy complicated by blood group immunization. *Ultrasound Obstet Gynecol* 5:400–405, 1995.

Fetal Therapy

Although intrauterine fetal diagnosis and therapy is an emerging field, several forms of therapy have been developed for various fetal conditions.

Fetal Blood Sampling/Transfusion

Cordocentesis

Cordocentesis is a procedure that is performed when a fetal blood sample is required for any reason. In cases of immune or nonimmune fetal anemia, the procedure may be performed to establish the degree of fetal anemia. Cordocentesis may also be performed if blood tests on the fetus are desired to determine if the fetus has a genetic disease or congenital infection or possibly to establish fetal blood type in anticipation of neonatal transplantation.

If the placenta is located anteriorly, a needle is advanced through the anterior uterine wall and through the placenta and is directed to puncture the umbilical vein at the insertion of the umbilical cord on the placenta. Puncturing the cord at the placental insertion stabilizes the vein so that it does not move or roll significantly during the puncture. After puncture of the vein, a blood sample is aspirated from the umbilical cord. If there is uncertainty as to whether the blood is fetal or maternal blood, a portion of the sample can be tested to establish the presence of fetal hemoglobin. In some cases, the needle may be kept in the vein after the aspiration if additional procedures such as fetal transfusion are anticipated.

If the placenta is located posteriorly, cordocentesis is more difficult, as the fetus may move between the anterior abdominal wall and the cord insertion point. An initial sonogram will usually establish whether or not the umbilical cord insertion on the placenta is accessible from an anterior approach. If it is accessible, placental cord insertion is still the preferred cordocentesis site. Before cordocentesis can be performed, however, the fetus must be immobilized. Usually a muscle relaxant is injected into the fetal buttock or thigh. After a wait of a few minutes to observe the affects of the medicine, additional injections may be administered to paralyze the fetus. Once the fetus is paralyzed, the needle is advanced through the anterior uterine wall into the amniotic fluid and into the umbilical vein at the placental cord insertion. Blood is then aspirated for testing.

If the placenta is located posteriorly and the cord insertion is not accessible, puncturing a loose loop of umbilical cord may be attempted. This can be rather difficult, as the cord tends to move away from the needle during the puncture. Another possible cordocentesis site is the fetal cord insertion. If either a loose loop of cord or a fetal cord insertion puncture is attempted, it is advisable to paralyze the fetus before the procedure.

Intravascular Fetal Transfusion

Intravascular fetal transfusion is performed by using the same technique described above in the section on cordocentesis. Once the needle is inserted into the umbilical cord, a sample of blood is aspirated. Usually some clinical estimate of the degree of fetal anemia, based on middle cerebral artery velocity or amniotic bilirubin levels, is available, and the fetal transfusion is begun while the fetal blood sample is being evaluated. It is important to proceed promptly with the transfusion, for the transfusion needle may be dislodged at any time and would require a lengthy repositioning. Typically, a 20-gauge needle is used for a cordocentesis and fetal transfusion. Packed red blood cells travel slowly through the needle; therefore, 15–25 minutes of transfusion time may be required. During the transfusion, the position of the needle tip and the umbilical vein and the adjacent umbilical cord are observed sonographically. In most cases, bright speckles can be observed within the umbilical vein during the transfusion. These speckles are observed during injection but not between injections. Once the fetal blood sample has been analyzed for hematocrit, a calculation is made to determine how much blood should be transfused into the fetus, and the transfusion is completed. If the transfusing needle has not been dislodged, a post-transfusion blood sample may be taken to establish post-transfusion hematocrit. After withdrawing the needle, the physician should observe the puncture site on the umbilical vein for several minutes to establish whether blood is leaking into the amniotic fluid from the site. If so, it usually will cease within 1–2 minutes. In the unlikely event of severe hemorrhage after transfusion or cordocentesis, a few investigators have reported using direct intracardiac transfusion with the needle.

Intraperitoneal Fetal Transfusion

Before intravascular fetal transfusion techniques were perfected, another procedure was used for fetal transfusion. The physician advanced a needle directly into the fetal peritoneal cavity, taking care to avoid major organs in the abdomen such as the liver, spleen, and kidneys, and blood was transfused directly into the peritoneal cavity of the fetus. This technique is rarely used today. Intraperitoneal fetal transfusion usually was not successful if the fetus had ascites or subcutaneous edema.

Other Therapy

Diaphragmatic Hernia Repair

For several years, a few centers in the United States have been performing diaphragmatic hernia repair on an experimental basis in human fetuses.

1 Initially, primary repair of the diaphragmatic defect was attempted, but this approach did not yield good results, for there was a high rate of miscarriage after the procedure. Untreated, fetal mortality for antenatally diagnosed diaphragmatic hernia ranges from 60 to 75%. This high mortality is the primary reason that diaphragmatic hernia repairs were attempted.

2 More recently, a different surgical approach has been used.[75] In fetuses selected for diaphragmatic hernia repair, a laparoscopic procedure is performed. A clip is surgically placed across the trachea, clamping it shut below the larynx. As the fetus continues to produce fluid within the lungs, the lungs gradually expand, increasing their volume and displacing herniated abdominal contents back into the abdomen. This surgical approach has been more successful than the earlier attempts, for there is a gradual change in the fetal lung and abdominal volumes, and a gradual reduction into the abdomen of the hernia contents. In the earlier diaphragmatic operations, compression of intra-abdominal contents with subsequent ischemia of bowel and other abdominal organs probably contributed to the miscarriage rate. The newer approach still carries a significant risk of miscarriage and is therefore used only for fetuses that have the lowest likelihood of survival without treatment.

3 Before diaphragmatic hernia surgery is performed on a fetus, careful sonographic examination is performed to:

- Make sure there are no other fetal anomalies.
- Discover how severe the herniation of abdominal contents is.
- Establish whether portions of the liver are herniated into the chest.

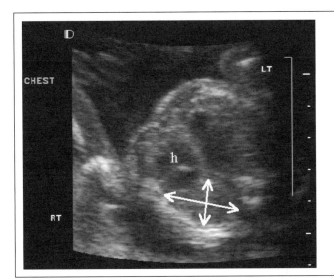

Figure 75.

Congenital diaphragmatic hernia. Lung measurement in congenital diaphragmatic hernia. The lung position in relation to the heart is measured on two perpendicular axes.

4 One semiquantitative way of estimating the degree of herniation is to measure the fetal lung-head ratio (LHR). In this assessment, the size of the remaining lung posterior to the heart is imaged and measured. The largest amount of lung posterior to the fetal heart is measured in two perpendicular axes (figure 75). The measurements along the two axes are multiplied together and divided by the head circumference. If the lung-head ratio is greater than 1.4, the prognosis for survival without surgery is considered relatively good and surgery is not performed.[76] Recently, the fetal lung–head ratio has been called into question as a reliable predictor of fetal outcome.

Fetal Bladder Decompression

If the fetus has bilateral hydronephrosis, oligohydramnios, and a prominent urinary bladder, bladder outlet obstruction is likely and fetal bladder decompression may be beneficial. Before bladder decompression is attempted, a careful sonographic survey of the fetus should be performed to evaluate for possible potentially lethal anomalies. In addition, the kidneys should be carefully examined to evaluate for possible cystic dysplasia that may develop from continuous bladder outlet obstruction. Finally, a fetal urine sample from the bladder can be tested for the urine sodium level and for fetal urinary β_2-microglobulin. In the normal fetus, the amount of sodium in the urine should be lower than in normal saline. If the kidneys are damaged, the urine will become isotonic.

Various methods of urinary bladder decompression have been used. Most commonly, a double pigtail catheter is placed from the fetal bladder to the amniotic fluid space. This procedure is usually performed in the mid-second trimester of pregnancy. Disadvantages of this procedure include possible obstruction of the urinary catheter and possible removal of the urinary catheter from the bladder by the fetus. Another procedure that has been used in some cases is open fetal surgery, with placement of fetal vesicostomy from the skin to the bladder. Although this is a more definitive treatment of bladder obstruction, it has been performed only rarely.

Other fetal conditions and anomalies have been treated surgically or surgical treatment is being considered. These include myelomeningocele, sacrococcygeal teratoma, placental vascular anomalies, twin reversed arterial perfusion (TRAP) sequence, and fluid aspiration from the thorax or abdomen.

Selective Reduction of Multifetal Pregnancy

It is well established that the risk of pregnancy complications for twins is higher generally than for singleton pregnancy. The risk of fetal morbidity and mortality increases rapidly with triplets, quadruplets, and pregnancies of higher fetal number; therefore, selective fetal reduction is offered in large centers. In this procedure, the number of viable fetuses is reduced by selective termination of some of the fetuses in the multiple pregnancies. Before fetal termination in multifetal pregnancy is attempted, it is important to establish that the fetus to be terminated has a separate placenta from the other fetuses. If fetal termination is attempted in a monochorionic pregnancy, both fetuses will likely die. Usually the fetuses that are easiest to reach are the ones selected for termination. Fetal reduction procedures are usually performed in the late first or early second trimester. The procedure involves injecting potassium chloride into the heart of the fetus to be terminated.

If a fetal reduction is performed primarily for an abnormal fetus, the term *selective fetal reduction* is used rather than *multifetal pregnancy reduction*.

Antepartum/Postpartum Considerations

Preterm Delivery

Preterm delivery is defined as spontaneous delivery regardless of birth weight that occurs before 37 weeks. This diagnosis is made when regular uterine contractions are accompanied by changes in the cervix or rupture of the amniotic membranes. The frequency of preterm labor and preterm birth has not changed in the past 30 years. Reasons for this appear to be:

1. The mechanism of preterm labor is not really understood but could possibly be due to infection or uterine distention.
2. High-risk patients are not easy to identify.
3. The diagnosis is often made at a late stage.
4. Current therapy (betaminetric drugs, $MgSO_4$) does not significantly prolong pregnancy and does not improve neonatal outcome.

Clinical factors associated with preterm delivery are:

1. Maternal habits, including smoking, stress, nutrition, and drug use.
2. Socioeconomic status (education, marital status).
3. Medical conditions (uterine or cervical anomalies, infection, and history of preterm labor).
4. Complications of pregnancy, including multiple gestation, vaginal bleeding, and poor fetal growth.

Methods used to assess those at risk for preterm delivery include:

1. Visual cervical examination. When the cervical plug begins to loosen, fetal fibronectin is present in the cervicovaginal secretions.
2. Monitoring uterine activity measured by portable tocodynamometer.
3. Salivary estriols.
4. Sonographic evaluation of cervical length.

In general, if the cervical length is less than 3 cm in the latter part of pregnancy, the woman is at risk for preterm delivery. When a patient presents in labor and has a cervical length less than 3 cm, she is even more likely to deliver prematurely.

Ultrasound Determination of Risk for Preterm Delivery

Sonography can assist in detecting incompetent cervix. Sonographic criteria include shortening of the cervical length to less than 3 cm and the presence of funneling and dilatation of the cervical canal. These sonographic findings visualized before 12 weeks usually indicate inevitable abortion. When seen in the second trimester in the absence of uterine contractions or spontaneous rupture of membranes, the findings indicate cervical incompetence. In the third trimester, a dilated cervix indicates premature delivery is likely. A patient whose cervix is shorter than 2.5–3 cm is more likely to deliver prematurely

1 Transabdominal Approach

The patient must have a full bladder for the transabdominal sonogram. It is important to determine that the bladder is not overdistended, as this could result in an inaccurate assessment of the cervical length (figure 76). Scanning is performed in the midline to assess the true cervical length. The scans are obtained parallel to the long axis of the cervix so that the endocervical canal can be visualized. Because measurement of the cervix is more difficult during late gestation, placing the patient in the Trendelenburg position may be useful.

It may be beneficial to have the patient stand for several minutes or to apply transfundal pressure while the sonographer images the cervix. In general,

Figure 76.

Dilated cervix and bladder distention. **A** Longitudinal sonogram of the lower uterine segment and cervix with full bladder. Some cervical dilatation is visible. **B** With partial bladder emptying, the cervical dilatation is more evident. Note the "hourglass" appearance.

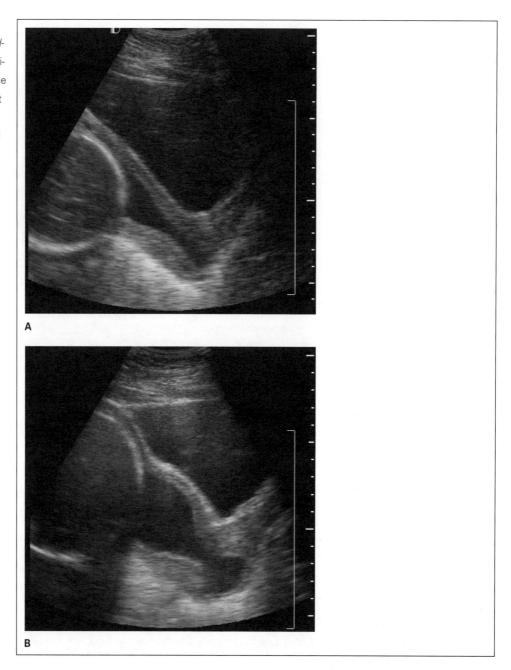

transabdominal sonography through a full bladder cannot exclude cervical shortening because the lower uterine segment may close by pressure from the filled urinary bladder.

2 Transperineal (Translabial) Approach

In the transperineal approach, sonography is performed on a patient who has an empty bladder. The patient is in the supine position with hips abducted and transducer placed between the labia minora at the vaginal introitus. Posi-

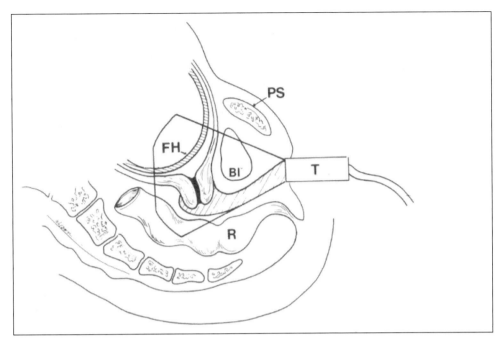

Figure 77.

Transperineal approach. Sagittal diagram of the female pelvis with transducer (T) positioned at the vaginal introitus shows typical scanning plane during transperineal sonography. PS = pubic symphysis, BI = bladder, R = rectum, FH = fetal head. Reprinted with permission from Mahoney BS, Nyberg DA, Luthy DA, et al: Translabial ultrasound of the third-trimester uterine cervix: Correlation with digital examinations. *J Ultrasound Med* 9:717–723, 1990.

tion the transducer in the sagittal plane and direct the beam along the vagina (figure 77). The cervix is usually oriented at a right angle to the vagina. This approach is particularly effective during the third trimester and in patients who have ruptured membranes. Patient acceptance is usually good.

3 Transvaginal Approach

In the transvaginal approach, sonography is performed on a patient who has an empty bladder. The patient is in the supine position with hips abducted. The transducer is introduced through the vagina, and longitudinal and transverse views can be obtained. Several reports suggest that the transvaginal approach is superior to the transabdominal and transperineal approaches.[77] Complications include:

- Increased risk of amniotitis after rupture of membranes
- Stimulation of contractions with preterm labor
- Induction of vaginal bleeding

4 Normal Cervix

The cervical length is obtained by measuring the length of the endocervical canal (figure 78) from internal to external os. The transvaginal approach generally produces less distortion.

If the internal cervical os dilates more than 5 mm before 30 weeks, the risk of preterm delivery rises from 3.5 to 33%, compared with an undilated internal os.[78] Cervical dilatation is the most significant predictor of preterm delivery. If

Figure 78.

Sagittal sonogram of the cervix. Note the measurement is taken from internal os (I) to external os (E).

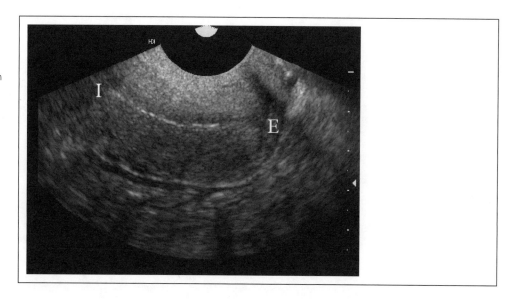

Figure 79.

Measurements of the cervix with funneling. Reprinted with permission from Berghella V, Kuhlman K, Weiner S, et al: Cervical funneling: Sonographic criteria predictive of preterm delivery. *Ultrasound Obstet Gynecol* 10: 161, 1997.

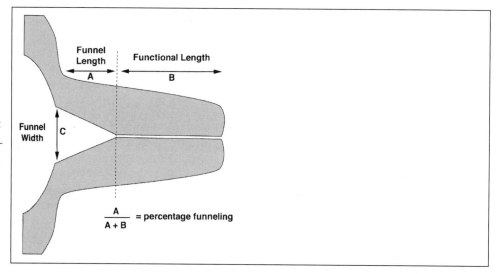

the internal cervical os dilates slightly, and the cervical walls are still concave, the configuration is called *funneling* (figure 79). If the cervical canal dilates more, the walls of the cervix become convex. Eventually the external os dilates, and the membranes bulge through the open os (figure 80). As the cervical degree of dilatation increases, the probability of premature delivery increases.

5 Clinical Aspects of Cervical Incompetence

1. Causes can be congenital or acquired, including traumatic injury, laceration, amputation, conization, and excessive cervical dilatation before diagnostic curettage or therapeutic abortion.

2. The incidence of cervical incompetence is reported to be 0.05 to 1% of all pregnancies[79] and accounts for up to 16% of second trimester losses.[80]

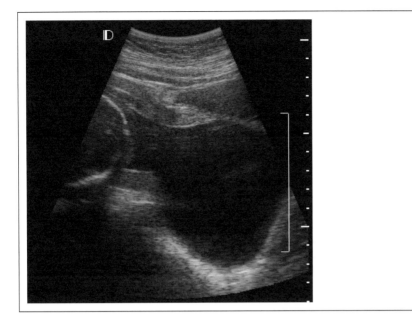

Figure 80.
Bulging membranes. Longitudinal sonogram of the lower uterine segment demonstrates "bulging membranes."

3. Congenital cervical incompetence has been reported in women prenatally exposed to diethylstilbestrol (DES) with associated uterine malformations.[81]

4. The classic presentation is painless cervical dilatation and recurrent second trimester loss.

6 Cervical Cerclage

Cervical cerclage is a surgical procedure in which a purse-string suture is applied to the cervix by using one of two techniques. In a patient who has documented history of incompetent cervix, a suture is usually inserted electively at 13–16 weeks. Use of cervical cerclage has been associated with risk of puerperal fever.

Postpartum Bleeding

Hemorrhage is one of the most significant causes of maternal morbidity after childbirth. Postpartum hemorrhage (PPH) can be subclassified according to the timing of the hemorrhage.

1 Primary Postpartum Hemorrhage

Primary postpartum hemorrhage is bleeding that occurs during the first 24 hours after delivery as a result of acute clinical problems such as:

- Coagulopathies.
- Chorioamnionitis.
- Abnormal placental implantation such as previa or accreta.

- Uterine relaxation due to such agents as halothane or magnesium sulfate.
- Retained placenta.

The clinical presentation at delivery usually indicates diagnosis and guides management.

2 Secondary Postpartum Hemorrhage

Secondary postpartum hemorrhage is bleeding that occurs after 24 hours postdelivery; it occurs in 1% of all patients. The cause is usually retained placental tissue. Sonographically it is difficult to differentiate hemorrhage from retained products of conception. Doppler assessment has not proven to be successful. It is very important to assess the appearance of the endometrial stripe.[82]

1. If the endometrial stripe appears thin or there is a small amount of endometrial fluid in the cavity, it is likely within normal limits.

2. If echogenic masses are present in the endometrial cavity and the A-P measurement is greater than 1.5 cm, it likely represents products of conception.

3. If small hyperechoic foci are present in the cavity but no mass is noted and the endometrial cavity is less than 1.5 cm wide, retained products are unlikely. This pattern is seen after instrumentation of the uterus.

4. If a heterogeneous mass is present and the endometrium is more than 1.5 cm wide, it likely represents retained products.

Postpartum Infection

Puerperal infections occur after 3–4% of vaginal births and after 10–15% of c-sections; higher rates are noted in certain populations at risk.[83] Endomyometritis is a clinical diagnosis associated with fever, uterine tenderness, and elevated WBC; it usually presents at 3–4 days. Primarily it is a clinical diagnosis, but sonography may show an irregular endometrial cavity containing fluid and, sometimes, shadowing. Retained products of conception predispose the uterus to infection.

Cesarean Section

C-sections are one of the most common surgical procedures performed during pregnancy. In this procedure, an incision is made into the uterus, typically a transverse incision in the lower uterine segment, and the fetus is delivered through this incision rather than through the cervix. This surgical procedure is widely used to improve fetal outcome.

1. A typical indication for c-section is fetal macrosomia; in this condition there is concern that vaginal delivery may result in injury to the shoulders of the fetus or the brachial nerves. Usually, c-section for macrosomia is considered in fetuses with estimated fetal weight exceeding 4500 grams in nondiabetic women and exceeding 4000 grams in diabetic woman.

2. Another indication for c-section may be fetal malposition. If a baby is in breech presentation, c-section is often performed to improve the likelihood of a smooth delivery and optimal fetal outcome.

3. If the mother has genital herpes, a c-section may be performed to prevent infection of the fetus.

In the nonpregnant woman, a previous c-section may be suspected if an echogenic line is noted through the anterior lower uterine segment on sagittal view. In women who have had previous c-sections performed, there is increased risk of a condition called *placenta accreta*. In this condition, the placenta attaches to or invades through the surgical scar in the muscular wall of the lower uterine segment. The sonographic findings observed in placenta accreta are reviewed in Chapter 3. Identifying women who have placenta accreta is important because profuse bleeding may occur during delivery if placenta accreta is present but unsuspected.

CHAPTER 6: Amniotic Fluid

Amniotic fluid volume

Fetal pulmonic maturity studies

. . . .

Amniotic Fluid Volume

The volume of fluid surrounding the fetus can be affected by fluid inflow from maternal circulation across amniotic membranes, fluid inflow from the placental surface, and fluid inflow from the fetal lungs and bladder. Fluid may also flow out of the amniotic cavity across the same membranes if conditions are right. Fluid may also be removed from the cavity by the fetus swallowing. The volume of amniotic fluid present in the amniotic cavity at any particular time during pregnancy can be thought of as the net result of all fluid flowing into and out of the space.

Before 15–20 weeks' gestation, most of the fluid in the amniotic space comes from the maternal circulation and flows across the membranes into the cavity. After about 15–20 weeks, the fetal contribution to the amniotic fluid increases rapidly; most of the fluid is contributed as fetal urine. A much smaller amount of fluid is contributed from the fetal respiratory tract as a result of fetal breathing.

The main cause of fluid removal from the amniotic volume is swallowing of amniotic fluid by the fetus. If the amniotic membranes rupture, fluid may leak through the ruptured membranes.

Normally during pregnancy the volume of amniotic fluid surrounding the fetus gradually increases through early pregnancy and reaches a maximum of approximately 800 ml at about 33 weeks, decreasing gradually thereafter. The amniotic fluid volume increases during the second trimester primarily because of increased urine output and decreases in the latter part of pregnancy because of increased swallowing and decreased urine output.

Amniotic Fluid Volume Estimation

Many different methods have been described to qualitatively estimate the amount of amniotic fluid present within the uterus. The oldest and still one of the most accurate methods is to visually evaluate the amniotic fluid volume while scanning the fetus. A disadvantage of the visual assessment method is that it is difficult to communicate a volume amount from the examiner to other health care givers. Some have proposed subjective assessment of amniotic fluid on a 5-point scale with 1 indicating no amniotic fluid and 5 severe polyhydramnios.

A widely used method of estimating amniotic fluid volume in a semiquantitative way is the *amniotic fluid index* (AFI). The largest vertical pocket of fluid is measured in each quadrant of the uterus and the sum of the measurements is recorded as the amniotic fluid index. Generally, an amniotic fluid index of less than 5–7 cm is considered to indicate oligohydramnios, and an amniotic fluid index exceeding 20–24 cm is considered to indicate polyhydramnios.

Oligohydramnios

A number of different definitions of *oligohydramnios* have been proposed, including total amniotic fluid volume less than 300–500 ml, a minimum vertical pocket less than 1–2 cm, or an amniotic fluid index less than 5 cm. As discussed previously, common causes of oligohydramnios include conditions with low production of fetal urine, including fetal renal dysplasia, fetal urinary obstruction, and intrauterine growth restriction. Rupture of amniotic membranes may also cause oligohydramnios.

Polyhydramnios

The most common definition of *polyhydramnios* is an amniotic fluid index (AFI) greater than 20–24 cm. Causes of polyhydramnios may be divided into two general groups:

1. Conditions that result in increased urinary or respiratory fluid production.
2. Conditions that result in decreased swallowing of fluid into the gastrointestinal tract.

Maternal diabetes may cause increased fetal blood sugar levels and cause fetal polyuria. In cardiac disease, high output failure can cause polyhydramnios.

Reduced gastrointestinal swallowing of fluid may be due to a mechanical obstruction of the proximal gastrointestinal tract such as absent mouth, esophageal atresia, duodenal atresia, jejunal atresia, or other obstruction of the gastrointestinal tract. In diaphragmatic hernia, gastroschisis, or omphalocele, the gastrointestinal tract is intact but kinked. Reduced swallowing may also be due to a central nervous system defect that results in decreased or absent swallowing, such as anencephaly, hydrocephaly, hydranencephaly, or other severe CNS abnormalities. Or it may be due to muscular abnormalities such as myotonic dystrophy or arthrogryposis. In these conditions the end organ muscles cannot contract normally, and swallowing does not take place.

Fetal Pulmonic Maturity Studies

For years many studies have been done to try to establish a sonographic way of diagnosing fetal lung maturity, but no successful imaging method has been discovered. The standard method of establishing fetal lung maturity is through the use of biochemical tests, which measure materials in the amniotic fluid that are produced by the fetal lung. The *lecithin/sphingomyelin* (L/S) ratio has been in use for 30 years. If the lecithin/sphingomyelin ratio is 2.0 or greater, the fetus is unlikely to develop respiratory distress syndrome after delivery. A newer test that measures *phosphatidylglycerol* (PG) in the amniotic fluid is also helpful. If phosphatidylglycerol is identified in the amniotic fluid, it is unlikely that the fetus will develop respiratory distress after delivery. However, neither of these tests is very effective, for many fetuses with immature lecithin/sphingomyelin ratio or phosphatidylglycerol level will *not* develop respiratory distress.

CHAPTER 7
Genetic Studies

Diseases arising from a single gene

Maternal serum testing

Chorionic villus sampling

. . . .

Diseases Arising from a Single Gene

Medical conditions arising from a single gene occur in about 1% of newborn infants. Approximately 10,000 single-gene diseases are known; about half are autosomal dominant, about a third are autosomal recessive, and the remainder are X-linked.

An *autosomal recessive disorder* is a condition in which a defective copy of the gene is contributed by each parent. If each parent carries one copy of the defective gene, the likelihood of the child contracting the disease is 25%. Every person in the population carries five or six recessive genes for significant diseases, and if the parents of the child are closely related, it is more likely the child will contract a recessive disease. An affected child will inherit two copies of the defective gene, one from each parent. People who have one normal copy and one defective copy of a gene will often have some decrease in enzymatic activity of defective protein, but in recessive conditions, that person is clinically normal.

In *autosomal dominant conditions,* only one defective gene is required to cause the associated disease. A person who has an autosomal dominant disease usually possesses one copy of the defective gene and a normal copy of the gene. Assuming the other parent has normal copies of that particular gene, the risk of their child having the disease is 50%, for the child could receive either a defective copy or the normal copy of the gene from the affected parent. In many autosomal dominant diseases, the severity of the disease varies from individual to individual, and it may be difficult to predict the severity of the disease in a given case.

Autosomal dominant diseases are more likely to appear as new mutations, because only one copy of the defective gene is needed to get the disease. Many autosomal dominant diseases are more severe if both copies of the gene are affected.

Most *X-linked diseases* are recessive. This means that a female who has one defective X chromosome and one normal X chromosome will be a carrier but will not manifest the disease. Because males possess only one copy of the X chromosome instead of two, a woman who has one normal and one abnormal copy of an X chromosome gene will transmit the abnormal gene to 50% of her offspring. If that offspring is male, he has a 100% chance of contracting the disease because the child will have only one X chromosome. In order to contract an X-linked disease from the father, the father must be affected by the disease, as he carries only one X chromosome.

Maternal Serum Testing

It has been recognized for many years that older women are at higher risk for developing certain fetal anomalies, including such chromosomal anomalies as trisomy 13, 18, and 21. Genetic testing has been performed for many years to detect these chromosomal abnormalities. In recent years, additional testing has been offered to detect structural anomalies in the fetus. Many states now offer screening programs to detect neural tube defects, abdominal wall defects, and chromosomal anomalies. One of the least invasive forms of screening uses maternal serum to detect abnormal levels of certain chemicals within the mother's blood. A number of components of maternal blood may be tested. The most common blood component that is tested for is *alpha-fetoprotein.* Other substances that are tested for include *acetylcholinesterase, unconjugated estriol,* and *human chorionic gonadotropin.*

Alpha-Fetoprotein

Alpha-fetoprotein (AFP) is a protein produced by the fetal liver and yolk sac. It is the main protein that circulates in the fetal serum in early fetal life. The level of this protein in the fetal blood is 2 million units per liter. Normally the amount in the amniotic fluid is 20,000 units per liter and the amount in the maternal serum is 20 units per liter. In fetal anomalies in which the skin is not intact, such as open spina bifida, omphalocele, gastroschisis, and aplasia cutis, the result is high levels of alpha-fetoprotein in the amniotic fluid (AF-AFP) and in the maternal serum (MS-AFP). The standard way of reporting maternal serum alpha-fetoprotein results is in multiples of the median (MOM). The maternal serum alpha-fetoprotein result is divided by the median value from a group of women at the same gestational age. Typically, patients who have maternal serum alpha-fetoprotein results greater than 2 or 2½ multiples of the median are referred for additional testing. Each screening program determines the cutoff that will be used in that particular screening program. The highest cutoff typically used is 2.5 multiples of the median.

In analyzing the maternal serum alpha-fetoprotein results comparing unaffected fetuses and fetuses with a neural tube defect, it can be shown that there is significant overlap between the normal and abnormal distributions. The cutoff used by a particular screening program is selected to try to optimize the results and minimize the number of false-positive and false-negative tests.

In addition to open neural tube defects and aplasia cutis, other abnormalities may be detected with the use of maternal serum alpha-fetoprotein screening. Anencephaly fetuses have higher levels of maternal serum alpha-fetoprotein than those with spina bifida. Open abdominal wall defects, including omphalocele and gastroschisis, may also elevate maternal serum alpha-fetoprotein. Conditions in which the fetus is spilling protein into the amniotic fluid will also result in an abnormal test. Conditions that may or may not give rise to an elevated maternal serum alpha-fetoprotein include encephalocele, triploidy, autosomal recessive polycystic kidney disease, sacrococcygeal teratoma, cystic adenomatoid malformation of the lung, and bilateral renal agenesis. In the case of renal agenesis, there is much less amniotic fluid than normal, and the maternal serum alpha-fetoprotein is concentrated in the scant volume of amniotic fluid.

Elevated maternal serum alpha-fetoprotein levels may also be observed in patients who do not show fetal anomaly. If the assumed fetal age is incorrect, maternal serum alpha-fetoprotein levels may be either higher or lower than expected. If the fetal age is less than expected, the maternal serum alpha-fetoprotein may be lower. If the fetal age is greater than expected, the maternal serum alpha-fetoprotein results may be high. Many screening programs will not change the presumed fetal age unless the sonographic measurement of fetal size differs from the fetal age determined by last menstrual period by more than two weeks.

Another cause of elevated maternal serum alpha-fetoprotein is multiple gestation. Twins will have a maternal serum alpha-fetoprotein approximately twice as high as a singleton pregnancy. Other causes of maternal serum alpha-fetoprotein elevation without fetal anomaly include transplacental fetal maternal hemorrhage. Maternal ovarian or liver tumors, which may secrete alpha-fetoprotein, are other possible causes of elevated maternal serum alpha-fetoprotein.

Acetylcholinesterase

Acetylcholinesterase (ACHE) is another protein that can be evaluated. This protein is more specific for neural tissue and is usually tested by performing amniocentesis in patients who have elevated maternal serum alpha-fetoprotein. Although acetylcholinesterase is more specific for neural abnormalities, it is also elevated in omphalocele, gastroschisis, cystic hygroma, hydrops, and maternal fetal hemorrhage.

Chromosomal Abnormality

It has been observed that maternal serum alpha-fetoprotein is slightly lower in chromosomally abnormal pregnancies than in normal pregnancies. The typical value in Down syndrome is 0.74 multiples of the median. The maternal serum alpha-fetoprotein is corrected for age, race, weight, and diabetic status, and a risk of Down syndrome is calculated. If the risk for Down syndrome is one in 350 or less, amniocentesis is offered to evaluate for chromosomal abnormality.

Triple Screen

Because maternal serum alpha-fetoprotein screening is relatively insensitive for Down syndrome and other chromosomal abnormalities, a combination of maternal serum tests for unconjugated estriol (UE3) and human chorionic gonadotropin (hCG) are also tested on the maternal serum and the results compared with the alpha-fetoprotein. Unconjugated estriol is 25–30% lower in Down syndrome than in normal pregnancies, and hCG is about twice as high in Down syndrome pregnancies as in normal controls. With this combined testing, the improved sensitivity for detection of possible Down syndrome fetuses can be realized. Triple-screen testing may detect between 58 and 91% of Down syndrome fetuses with a 5–6% false positive rate. Trisomy 13 may also be detected on the basis of triple-screen testing. In trisomy 18, all three markers will be lower than normal.[84]

Chorionic Villus Sampling

History

Chorionic villus sampling (CVS) had its beginnings in the 1960s, when the method primarily used endoscopic techniques that had high complication and failure rates.[85, 86] In the 1970s a study from China described successful chorionic villus sampling using a blind catheter-aspiration technique.[86] The chorionic villus sampling technique developed more rapidly after 1982 when a report by Kazy et al. described its benefits for genetic diagnosis and emphasized ultrasound's role for guidance in successful chorionic villus sampling.[87]

Concept/Indications

Chorionic villus sampling is a method of prenatal assessment that permits the diagnosis of many genetic disorders in the first trimester. Genetically the placenta is a fetal organ. Cytogenetic DNA and biochemical studies of chorionic villi, therefore, reflect fetal genetic composition. The villi along the site of implantation proliferate rapidly, creating an area of increased echogenicity that can be visualized sonographically. This structure is known as the *chorion frondosum*, which eventually becomes the placenta. The chorion frondosum is the optimal site for obtaining a chorionic villus sample. The chorionic villi opposite the site of implantation degenerate and become the *chorion levae*.

Indications for chorionic villus sampling include:

- Maternal age 35 or greater at delivery
- Previous child with nondisjunctional chromosome abnormality
- Parent carrier of balanced translocation or other chromosome disorder
- Both parents carriers of autosomal recessive biochemical disease
- Women who are carriers of an X-linked disease

Two Technical Approaches for Chorionic Villus Sampling

1 Transcervical Approach

The transcervical approach is performed between 10 and 12½ weeks. Before the procedure is begun, sonography is performed to establish fetal viability and locate the placenta. The patient is then placed in the lithotomy position, a speculum is inserted, and the vagina is cleaned with an antibiotic solution. Under direct ultrasound visualization, a biopsy catheter is inserted into the developing chorion frondosum of the placenta, a syringe is attached to the catheter, and the catheter tip is moved to and fro in the sample site

Figure 81.

Sonographically guided transcervical chorionic villus sampling. Diagram illustrates the technique.

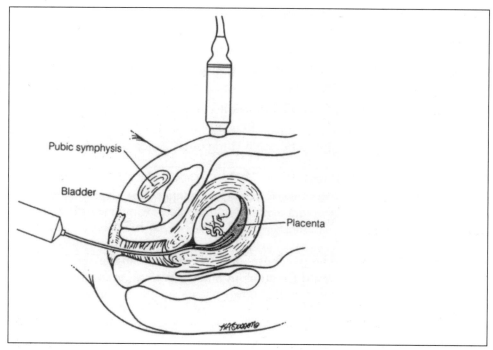

while suction is applied (figure 81). After the procedure, the catheter is withdrawn and the sample material is visualized under a microscope. Additional passes may be performed, and the fetal heart rate and placenta appearance are evaluated after each pass.

Potential risks of the transcervical approach include:

- Spontaneous abortion
- Maternal sepsis
- Perforation of the amniotic sac
- Unexplained midtrimester oligohydramnios

The fetal loss rate associated with transcervical chorionic villus sampling has been evaluated in several large studies, and 1–2% above the background risk has been quoted.[88, 89]

2 Transabdominal Chorionic Villus Sampling Technique

Chorionic villus sampling can also be performed transabdominally, especially in cases of an anterior placenta. Before the procedure is begun, a sonogram is performed to establish the position of the placenta and the viability of the

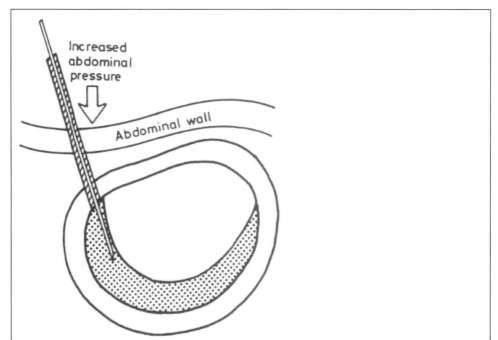

Figure 82.
Transabdominal chorionic villous sampling approach.

fetus. Under direct ultrasound visualization the physician inserts an 18- to 20-gauge needle into the placenta under aseptic conditions (figure 82). A syringe is attached to the needle and suction is applied to the needle while the needle is moved to and fro within the placenta. This technique can be performed at any time in pregnancy for an anterior placenta.

The fetal loss rate associated with transabdominal chorionic villus sampling is not significantly different from transcervical chorionic villus sampling. Early studies suggested that if chorionic villus sampling was performed before 9 weeks, there was risk of limb-reduction defects in the fetus. Subsequent studies in larger groups have suggested that if chorionic villus sampling is performed after 10 weeks, limb-reduction defects are less common. Also, the fetal loss rate is lower if chorionic villus sampling is performed later.

Fetal Demise

The primary method for establishing fetal death is to demonstrate lack of heartbeat in the fetus. Additional findings may be observed, including subcutaneous edema, indistinct abdominal organs, overlapping skull bones (Spaulding sign), and cystic changes in the degenerating placenta.

Fetal Abnormalities

CHAPTER 8

Abnormalities of the fetal head and face

Embryology of the fetal face

Fetal brain and cranium

Abnormalities of the fetal neck

Neural tube defects

Abdominal wall abnormalities

Thoracic abnormalities

Genitourinary abnormalities

Gastrointestinal abnormalities

Skeletal abnormalities

Cardiac abnormalities

Syndromes

. . . .

Abnormalities of the Fetal Head and Face

Although AIUM guidelines do not include imaging of the face in the basic fetal examination, examination of the fetal face has become a standard part of the examination in many obstetrical sonography practices. If fetal anomalies are suspected, the fetal face should always be carefully examined. A complete examination of the fetal face would include axial views of the forehead, orbits, nasal bridge, maxilla, lips, tongue, mandible, neck, and oral pharynx. The coronal view should include the nose and lips, anterior and mid–hard palate, tongue, and mandible. The soft tissues of the neck including the oropharynx can also be examined in this plane. If possible, profiles of the facial soft tissues and facial bones including the mandible should be viewed as well. This may not be possible in every fetus, but three-dimensional imaging may help to obtain profile views if the fetus is facing to the side. Views of the fetal ears and neck may be important in some cases as well. Visualization of the fetal face will be difficult if the fetus is facing posteriorly, if there is oligohydramnios, or if the mother is obese.

Embryology of the Fetal Face

At 6–7 menstrual weeks, the basic structures of the maxilla, mandible, and later the eyes, orbits, and nose develop. The eyes first develop on the lateral side of the face. As the face develops, the orbits and eyes migrate medially in the face, and the nasal structures migrate from a supralateral position inframedially. The nostril, lip, and anterior palate form from a projection of tissue that folds together from lateral and medial prominences and fuse under the nostril to form the anterior lip. If this process does not proceed normally, unilateral or bilateral cleft lip will develop.

The maxilla and mandible begin to ossify at about 8–9 menstrual weeks, and the bony structures of the face should be visible sonographically by 11–12 menstrual weeks, although the structures are better formed and easier to examine in a detailed way by 14–16 menstrual weeks.

Subjective assessment of the orbits should show orbits of reasonable size, with the intraorbital distance approximately equal to the orbital diameter. Orbital measurement tables have been established.[90] Outer orbital diameters and interorbital diameters can be measured if necessary. The orbits should be imaged in the axial plane slightly below the plane used for the biparietal diameter (BPD) and head circumference (HC). During scanning, the sonographer should attempt to show the maximum diameter of each orbit, and the orbits should normally be equal in size. The lens of the eye, the eyelid, and sometimes the hyaloid artery can be visualized sonographically.

Hypotelorism

The term *hypotelorism* means reduced intraorbital distance. In fetuses that have hypotelorism (figure 83), the interorbital diameter will typically be below the 5th percentile, and the outer orbital diameter may be reduced as well.

The most common condition associated with hypotelorism is *holoprosencephaly.* Holoprosencephaly is a complex malformation sequence involving the brain and the face. The brain does not divide into hemispheres normally, and the face is not normally formed, as the brain and face form simultane-

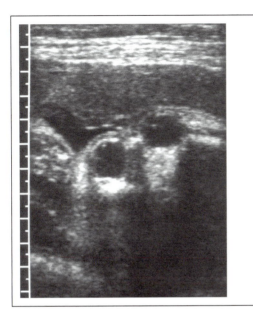

Figure 83.

Hypotelorism. Axial sonogram demonstrates hypotelorism. Note that the orbits are closer together than normal.

ously. A more detailed description of the malformation of the brain and holoprosencephaly may be found later in this chapter under "Fetal Brain and Cranium." A wide spectrum of facial anomalies is associated with holoprosencephaly. The most severe facial anomalies are usually associated with the more severe brain abnormalities, but severe brain malformations may be present even if the facial abnormalities are absent or minor. The most severe form of facial malformation observed in holoprosencephaly is *cyclopia*. In cyclopia a single orbit exists in the middle of the upper face (figure 84). One or two globes may be present within this orbit. Often, the mid-facial structures, including the maxillary bone, are not well ossified. The mass of tissue that should have made the nose produces a "bump," or proboscis, in the center of the forehead above the single orbit. The upper lip in these fetuses is smooth and flat.

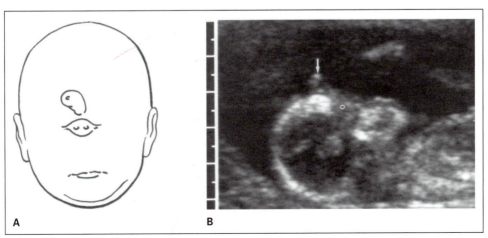

Figure 84.

Holoprosencephaly with cyclopia. **A** Drawing of fetal face with cyclopia. Note the proboscis above the single orbit. **B** Sonogram of a fetus with cyclopia. Note the proboscis (arrow) above the orbit (O). Reprinted with permission from Bernal R, Rouse G, DeLange M: Sonographic evaluation of holoprosencephaly. *JDMS* 8:256–261, 1992.

Figure 85.

Ethmocephaly. Drawing of fetal face with ethmocephaly. Note the proboscus above the hypotelar orbits. Reprinted with permission from Bernal R, Rouse G, DeLange M: Sonographic evaluation of holoprosencephaly. *JDMS* 8:256–261, 1992.

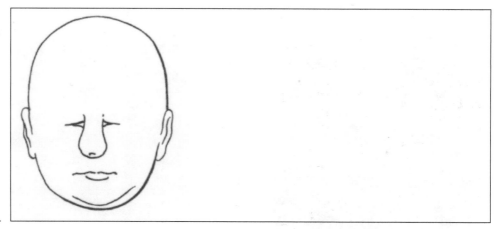

A slightly less severe form of facial malformation associated with holoprosencephaly is *ethmocephaly* (figure 85). In this facial malformation, separate orbits form but hypotelorism exists and, again, a midline proboscis extends from above the orbits anteriorly.

A milder form of facial malformation is *cebocephaly*. In this condition, there is hypotelorism of the orbits, but a better-formed nasal bridge is present. There is, however, a single depression in the end of the nose instead of two normal nostrils. Cyclopia, ethmocephaly, and cebocephaly are typically lethal malformations, as no well-formed nostrils are present and the neonate is unable to breathe through its nose. Another mild form of facial anomaly associated with holoprosencephaly is a midline cleft. In this condition, the anterior bony palate does not form (premaxillary agenesis) and a Y-shaped cleft appears in the midline, which extends into the nostrils bilaterally (figure 86). The midface may be quite flat and there is typically hypotelorism.

Holoprosencephaly can be associated with many chromosomal anomalies, most commonly trisomy 13, and with nonchromosomal syndromes, including diabetic embryopathy.

Figure 86.

Premaxillary agenesis. **A** Drawing of a face of a fetus with premaxillary agenesis. **B** Sonogram of fetal lip in a patient with premaxillary agenesis. Note the oblique clefts (arrows) above the lower lip (LL). Reprinted with permission from Bernal R, Rouse G, DeLange M: Sonographic evaluation of holoprosencephaly. *JDMS* 8:256–261, 1992.

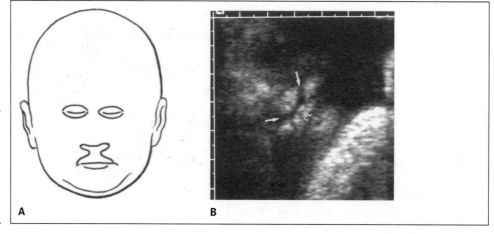

Microphthalmia

If the orbit itself is smaller in diameter than normal, the condition is termed *microphthalmia*. This condition, which may be unilateral or bilateral, has been observed in many syndromes. When microphthalmia is observed, fetal karyotyping may be helpful.

Hypertelorism

In *hypertelorism,* the orbits are farther apart than usual, with the interorbital distance visually larger than an orbital diameter. Two conditions are typically associated with marked hypertelorism, and many other syndromes have also been reported with milder hypertelorism. One such condition is midline facial cleft syndrome in which the face retains its early embryologic appearance with its eyes on the side of the head and the nostrils widely separated one from another. A midline cleft lip is often observed in this condition as well. The other relatively common condition associated with hypertelorism is a frontal encephalocele. In this condition, there is an anterior bony defect in the skull and protrusion of brain tissue and meninges; subcutaneous tissue is noted between the orbits and in the low forehead. Anterior encephaloceles are uncommon in the United States but are apparently more common in far eastern countries. Anterior encephaloceles are less commonly associated with severe mental retardation than are occipital encephaloceles.

Lips and Mouth

As described briefly in the embryology section of this chapter, the nostrils, lips, and hard palate form simultaneously. Each nostril forms from a fold of tissue with a medial and lateral prominence. The portion of the lip directly inferior to the nostril forms by fusion of this fold of tissue (figure 87). A cleft

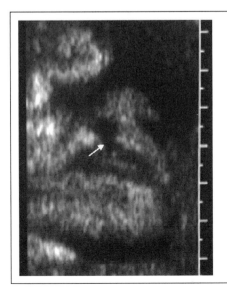

Figure 87.

Cleft lip. Coronal sonogram demonstrating a unilateral cleft lip.

Figure 88.

Bilateral cleft lip and palate. **A** Coronal sonogram of the face in a fetus with bilateral cleft lip and palate. The mid portion of the lip and palate (arrows) are displaced anteriorly. n, nose. **B** Coronal sonogram of fetus with bilateral cleft lip and palate. This view is posterior to Part A and shows the hard palate, which is bilaterally clefted (arrows).

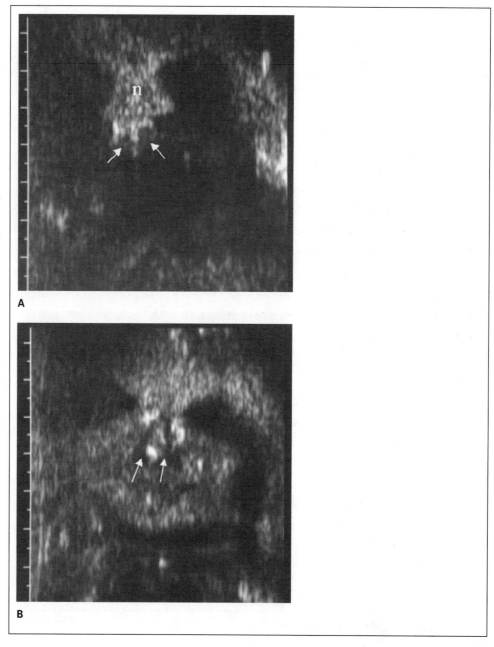

lip (color plate 8) may form as a defect of the lip only or as a defect of both the lip and palate unilaterally. Bilateral cleft lip and palate results from lack of fusion of the inferior fold of the nostril bilaterally. In this case, the lip and anterior palate both are typically affected. In bilateral cleft lip and palate (figure 88), the middle portion of the bony maxilla is not fused to the lateral portion and is therefore weakly supported by underlying bone. Movement of the fetal tongue can displace the middle portion of the maxillary ridge anteriorly. Therefore, the central part of the lip and palate is typically observed in the coronal plane to lie anterior to the remainder of the face. The posterior part of the hard palate may be clefted alone or with the lip and anterior palate.

Cleft lip and palate are usually due to multiple factors, but cleft lip, palate, or both, are also observed in many syndromes.

Micrognathia

An abnormally small mandible is called *micrognathia*. Micrognathia may occur as part of many syndromes and, if severe, may compromise respiration. Although charts have been developed for mandibular length, micrognathia is typically diagnosed as a subjective observation of the midline profile of the fetal face when the fetal chin is noticeably small and receding (figures 89 and 90).

Macroglossia

Macroglossia is a tongue that is too large. On routine sonography of the fetal face, the tongue may be observed moving in the mouth, but if the tongue extends beyond the fetal lips repeatedly or persistently, the diagnosis of macroglossia should be considered. The most common syndrome with

Small mandible

Macroglossia - tongue is to big, commonly assoc. w/ Beckwith Weidman
- also seen in BW, oophalocele, big intra abd. organs & asymetry of fetal limbs

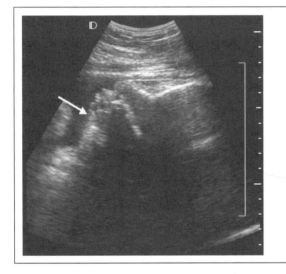

Figure 89.

Micrognathia. Sagittal midline face demonstrating markedly receding chin (arrow).

Macroglossia usually seen in late preg. & observed w/ 20+ syndromes

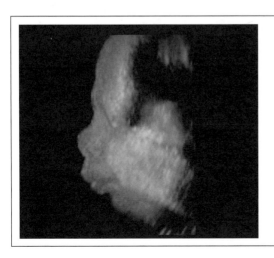

Figure 90.

Micrognathia. Three-dimensional sonogram of another fetus with micrognathia.

macroglossia is *Beckwith-Wiedemann syndrome.* In Beckwith-Wiedemann syndrome, omphalocele, enlargement of intra-abdominal organs, and asymmetry of the fetal limbs may also be observed. Macroglossia is typically visualized late in pregnancy. At least 20 other syndromes have been observed with macroglossia.

Fetal Brain and Cranium

To detect malformations of the fetal brain and spinal cord is one of the most common reasons for performing fetal sonography. Neural tube screening programs have increased the number of patients being examined for central nervous system anomalies.

Embryology of the Fetal Brain and Cranium

The fetal central nervous system begins to develop at approximately the 5th menstrual week. The neural tube begins to form by fusion in the middle of the embryonic spine cephalad and caudad. The fetal ventricles are initially quite large and should be well visualized and filled with choroid plexus by 13 menstrual weeks. From approximately 14 to 40 weeks, the fetal ventricles do not change significantly in transverse diameter. Instead, the brain grows and enlarges around the ventricle. The transverse diameter of the fetal ventricle in the region of the atrium is normally approximately 7 mm with a standard deviation of 1 mm. Therefore, the 3 standard deviation limit for ventricular diameter is 10 mm. As the fetus enlarges, the choroid plexus, which initially fills the entire ventricle anteroposteriorly, begins to predominate in the posterior aspect of the ventricle. By 12 weeks, the corpus callosum begins to develop and completes development by approximately 20 menstrual weeks. By 18–20 menstrual weeks the cavi septi pellucidi is also visible inferior to the corpus callosum. The vermis of the cerebellum develops superiorly to inferiorly, and the inferior portion of the vermis should be present by about 18 weeks. The fetal calvarium begins to ossify at about 8 menstrual weeks and should be largely visible by 10–11 weeks and well ossified by 15 weeks.

Ventriculomegaly and Hydrocephaly

Congenital enlargement of the ventricles occurs in 0.03–1.5 per 1000 births.[91] Two findings suggest ventricular enlargement, hydrocephaly, or both. One is enlargement of the lateral ventricle to more than 10 mm in transverse diameter (figure 91). Another is to observe whether or not the choroid plexus fills the lateral ventricle. If the choroid plexus does not fill the ventricle from side to side in the trigone region, hydrocephaly should be suspected. Mahony and associates observed that a 3 mm or greater separation between the

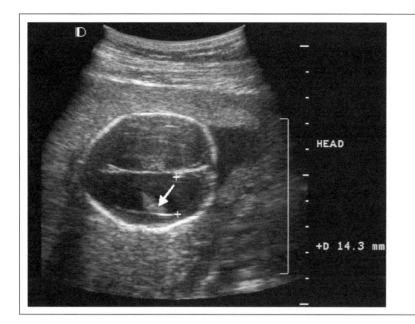

Figure 91.
Hydrocephaly. Axial sonogram of fetal head demonstrates markedly enlarged lateral ventricle. Note the small dependent choroid plexus (arrow).

choroid plexus and the lateral ventricular wall in the dependent ventricle is abnormal.[92] Hertzberg et al. found that while 20% of these individuals had abnormalities, 80% were normal.[93] If the ventricle is much larger than the choroid plexus, the likelihood of brain abnormality and hydrocephaly increases. When the choroid plexus is small relative to the size of the lateral ventricle, the choroid may be observed to be dangling in the dependent ventricle. This is another sonographic sign that suggests hydrocephaly.

Not all ventricular enlargement is due to intracranial pressure. In some cases, there may be brain destruction or lack of brain development, as may be observed in congenital infections of the brain or periventricular infarction. Late in pregnancy, enlargement of the ventricle may be observed if the brain cortex is not developing normally. If cortical gyri do not develop in late pregnancy, the condition is called *lissencephaly*.

Mild Lateral Cerebral Ventriculomegaly

If the ventricles are only mildly dilated, with a lateral atrial dimension of 10–15 mm, most affected fetuses will have no significant sequelae, but this finding may be observed in a variety of conditions, including subtle forms of agenesis of the corpus callosum. Enlargement of the lateral ventricle to more than 15 mm is more commonly associated with obvious CNS malformations. Aqueductal stenosis is one of the common causes of in-utero hydrocephalus. In this condition, the lateral and sometimes the third ventricle are enlarged and the fourth ventricle is spared. In some cases, an X-linked gene defect has been implicated in males that have aqueductal stenosis and hydrocephaly.

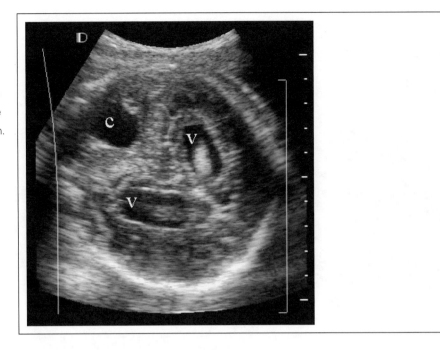

Figure 92.
Dandy-Walker malformation. Coronal sonogram of the posterior fossa demonstrating a cystic defect (C) in the vermis and cerebellum. V = lateral ventricle.

Dandy-Walker Malformation

Dandy-Walker malformation (DWM) consists of absent or incomplete development of the cerebellar vermis associated with cystic dilatation of the posterior fossa (figure 92). The lateral ventricles may be enlarged with Dandy-Walker malformation, but this is a variable finding.

In the most severe form, Dandy-Walker malformation shows marked hypoplasia of the cerebellar hemispheres and a large posterior fossa cyst. If the posterior fossa cyst is smaller and the cerebellar hemispheres are larger, the condition is sometimes called *Dandy-Walker variant*. If some vermian tissue is still present, the prognosis is improved.

Because the vermis does not form inferiorly until 18 weeks, the diagnosis of Dandy-Walker variant should not be made early in the second trimester.

The appropriate plane of examination of the cerebellum should show the cavum septum pellucidum anteriorly and the cerebellum posteriorly. If a more coronal plane is used, the posterior fossa will appear enlarged and the inferior vermis may not be well visualized. Also, the soft tissue outside the skull may be inappropriately interpreted as being abnormally thickened.

In the normal plane, which runs through the cerebellum and the cavum septi pellucidi, the cisterna magna normally should measure 5–10 mm in depth.

Dandy-Walker variant is estimated to occur in approximately 1 of 30,000 births. Dandy-Walker malformation or Dandy-Walker variant is associated with other intracranial and extracranial malformations, most commonly agenesis of the corpus callosum.

The differential diagnosis for Dandy-Walker malformation is posterior fossa arachnoid cyst. Dandy-Walker malformation can be differentiated from a posterior fossa arachnoid cyst; an arachnoid cyst will not communicate with the fourth ventricle. Arachnoid cysts do not have an association with other congenital malformations.

Agenesis Corpus Callosum

The corpus callosum is a midline structure above the cavum septi pellucidi, which represents white matter tracts extending from one hemisphere to the other. The corpus callosum develops between 12 and 18 weeks, and the cavum septi pellucidi develops inferior to the corpus callosum. With normal development of the corpus callosum, the cingulate gyrus forms above the corpus callosum.

In the absence of corpus callosum formation, a number of anomalies are noted within the brain.

1. The cingulate gyrus does not form. Because corpus callosum is absent, the sulci and gyri form on the interhemispheric surface of the brain in an irregular somewhat random pattern. Often the sulci form a radial pattern, sometimes called the "rising sun" configuration.

2. The lateral ventricles of the brain have a different configuration than normal. The lateral ventricles migrate farther into the central portion of each hemisphere and are therefore farther from one another.

3. The tissue that should have formed the corpus callosum lies immediately medial to each lateral ventricle in each hemisphere and moves the ventricle into a more vertical alignment in the coronal view. Also, the ventricle is oriented in a linear fashion anteroposteriorly rather than curving inward toward the midline.

4. In many cases, the transverse diameter of the posterior aspect of the lateral ventricle is larger than the anterior horn. In agenesis corpus callosum, there is sometimes an interhemispheric cyst (figure 93) between the ventricles or an extension of the third ventricle superiorly above the usual position of the corpus callosum.

There is a high frequency of associated malformations with agenesis corpus callosum, most commonly Dandy-Walker malformation. Agenesis corpus callosum is sometimes observed in trisomy 18.

Holoprosencephaly

If the brain does not normally divide into two hemispheres, the condition is called *holoprosencephaly*. A wide range of malformations is referred to as holoprosencephaly.

Figure 93.

Agenesis corpus callosum. Coronal (**A**) and axial (**B**) sonograms of a fetus with agenesis corpus callosum. Note the midline cyst (C) separating the lateral ventricles.

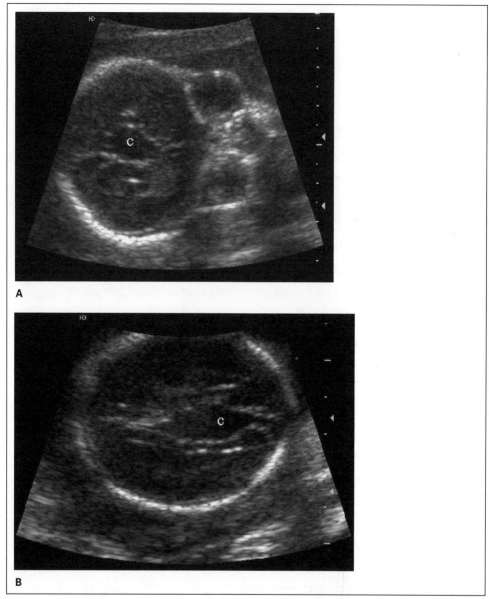

1. *Alobar holoprosencephaly* is a condition in which the hemispheres fail completely to divide; a single horseshoe-shaped ventricle in the midline of the brain arches over a fused thalami (figure 94).

2. *Semilobar holoprosencephaly* is partial separation of the brain and hemispheres, with a partial formation of the midline interhemispheric fissure, but the brain cortex continues across the midline above an undivided ventricle (figure 95). These cases typically have a little more separation of the thalami and a little better formation of the third ventricle in the midline.

3. *Lobar holoprosencephaly* is the condition in which the brain divides into hemispheres, but there is open communication across the midline between the lateral ventricles and the third ventricle.

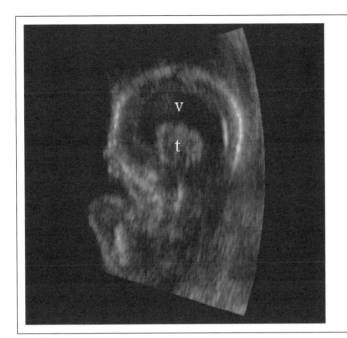

Figure 94.

Alobar holoprosencephaly. Note the monoventricle (V) arching over the fused thalami (t) in this coronal sonogram.

Alobar, semilobar, and lobar holoprosencephaly are all associated with severe mental retardation.

In cases of lobar holoprosencephaly a falx may be present and is often asymmetric, with one occipital horn much larger than the other. If there is nearly complete separation of the brain into hemispheres, with fusion only of the frontal horns of the lateral ventricles and of the inferior aspect of the frontal lobe of the brain (figure 96), the condition is sometimes referred to as *septo-optic dysplasia*. Many authors consider this to be the mildest variation of holoprosencephaly.

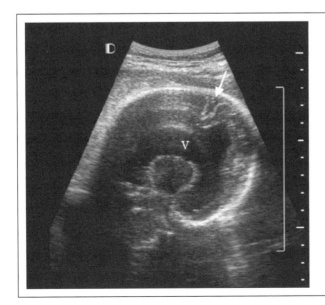

Figure 95.

Semilobar holoprosencephaly. Note the partially formed interhemispheric fissure (arrow) above the monoventricle (V) in this coronal sonogram.

Figure 96.

Septo-optic dysplasia. Coronal sonogram of a neonate with septo-optic dysplasia. Note the fused frontal horns (Fh). cn = caudate nucleus.

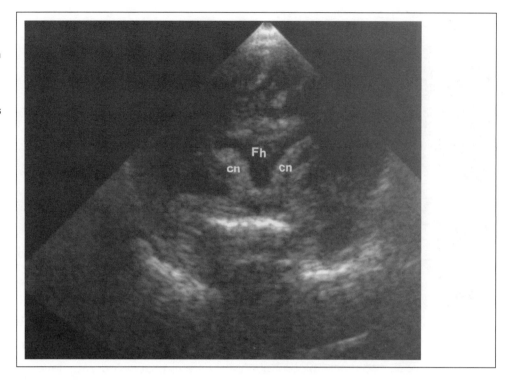

Facial Anomalies

As described previously, a range of facial anomalies is associated with holoprosencephaly. Because the brain and the face develop simultaneously, the degree of malformation of the face and degree of malformation of the brain will correlate to a certain degree.

Holoprosencephaly with Dorsal Cyst

In some patients who have holoprosencephaly, a large cyst may develop posterior to the cerebral hemispheres and above the tentorium. A dorsal cyst often encompasses much of the space inside the skull, with displacement of the cerebral hemispheres anteriorly into the frontal fossa (figure 97). A dorsal cyst may occur with any degree of severity of holoprosencephaly. In a case of lobar holoprosencephaly, the dorsal cyst may occur on one side of the falx only.

Differential Diagnosis

Conditions that may be confused with holoprosencephaly include hydranencephaly and severe hydrocephaly. In both hydranencephaly and severe hydrocephaly, a well-formed falx is typically present in the midline. In holoprosencephaly with dorsal cyst, there is always brain tissue in the anterior fossa. In hydranencephaly there may be no detectable cortical tissue, and in severe hydrocephaly, careful examination will show a thin layer of cortical parenchyma in the periphery of the cranium adjacent to the skull.

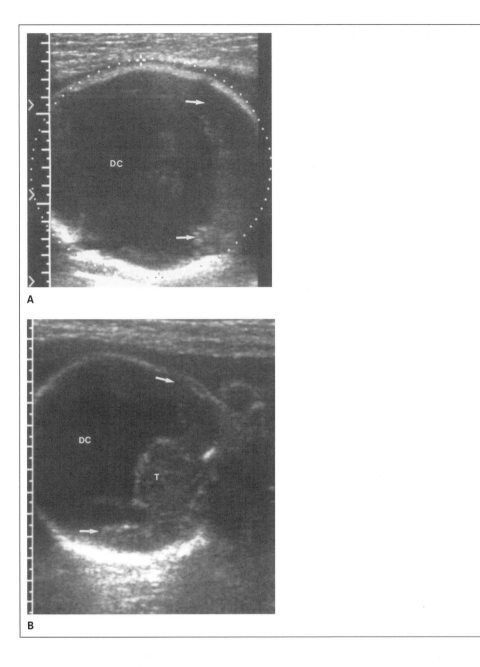

Figure 97.

Holoprosencephaly and dorsal cyst. Axial (**A**) and coronal (**B**) of fetus with holoprosencephaly and dorsal cyst. Note the cerebrum lies in the frontal fossa and extends only part way up laterally in the mid-head (arrows). The remainder of the head is filled with the dorsal cyst (DC). The thalami are fused (T).

Neural Proliferation Differentiation

1 *Hydranencephaly.* In hydranencephaly the meninges and falx are normally formed, but cerebral tissue above the tentorium is nearly totally absent. The conventional explanation for this condition is occlusion of the supraclinoid carotid arteries. Other conditions, such as infection, may give rise to a similar presentation. Some brain tissue may be present in the occipital lobe above the tentorium in some cases. Head size is variable, and the prognosis is quite poor, because the cerebral cortex is almost completely destroyed. Hydranencephaly can be differentiated from severe hydrocephaly if careful examination of the periphery of the head shows no evidence of thinned cortex.

2 *Porencephaly.* Porencephaly is defined as a cystic cavity that communicates with the ventricle, subarachnoid space, or both. Porencephalic cysts are typically lined by white matter, not gray matter. If a large porencephalic area is present in the middle cerebral artery distribution, a fluid-filled cavity may extend from the ventricle to the skull. This represents a smaller area of brain infarction than hydranencephaly.

3 *Schizencephaly.* Schizencephaly is a rare condition in which clefts are noted to extend from the skull through the brain tissue into the lateral ventricles either unilaterally or bilaterally (figure 98). Schizencephaly differs from porencephaly in that the clefts are lined by cortical brain. Some authors believe that this is a fundamental error of neuronal migration, but most consider this a destructive vascular infarct, which occurs early in brain development, before 20 menstrual weeks, with subsequent cortical overgrowth extending into the defect.

4 *Microcephaly.* Microcephaly is defined as an abnormally small head, with a head circumference more than 2 or 3 standard deviations below the mean for age. Typically microcephaly is associated with abnormal brain development such as holoprosencephaly or lissencephaly (no sulci or gyri), or brain injury, such as porencephaly. In microcephaly, the head size is small relative to abdominal circumference and femoral length. Although diagnosis of microcephaly may be made in some cases as early as 15 ½ weeks, most cases of microcephaly will develop later in pregnancy.

5 *Intracranial calcifications.* Fetal intracranial calcifications are rarely reported in the ultrasound literature. There are two general groups of causes of these calcifications. Congenital infections such as cytomegalovirus (CMV) or toxoplasmosis may result in scattered or periventricular calcifications.

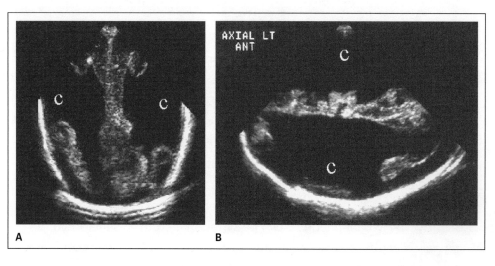

Figure 98.
Schizencephaly. Coronal (**A**) and axial (**B**) sonograms demonstrating schizencephaly. Note clefts (C).

Typically these occur late in pregnancy and may be associated with ventricular dilation. Noninfectious causes of calcifications include teratoma, tuberous sclerosis, sagittal sinus thrombosis, and Sturge-Weber syndrome.

Abnormalities of the Fetal Neck

Various abnormalities may affect the fetal neck, including cystic hygromas, occipital or suboccipital encephalocele, cervical meningomyelocele, and diffuse thickening of tissue in the posterior neck. Abnormalities of the anterior neck include enlargement of the thyroid gland, hemangioma, teratoma, branchial cleft cysts, and thyroglossal duct cyst.

Neural Tube Defects

Embryology

At approximately 4½ menstrual weeks, the neural plate develops. Early in the 6th menstrual week, the neural groove begins to fold into the neural tube. The neural tube forms from the middle and extends cephalad and caudad. By the end of the 6th week, the tube is closed and the brain is beginning to develop. Neural tube defects can be organized according to the type of failure in neural tube closure that gives rise to them.

Anencephaly

Anencephaly is the most common open neural tube defect and occurs because the cranial end of the neural tube fails to close. The diagnosis of anencephaly is difficult to make before 10–11 weeks, in part because the cranium does not calcify until that time. During the second trimester, sonographic findings suggesting anencephaly include absence of the cranial vault and absence of an organized brain above the skull base. Sonographically the face is typically visualized, with identification of orbits, mouth, and nose, and with no cranium or organized brain tissue visualized above the skull base (figure 99).

Associated anomalies observed with anencephaly include spina bifida, cleft lip and palate, clubfoot, and omphalocele. Polyhydramnios is commonly observed with anencephaly, presumably as a result of brain dysfunction and lack of fetal swallowing. Conditions that may resemble anencephaly include some cases of amniotic band syndrome with disruption of the fetal calvarium and some large encephaloceles.

Exencephaly/Acrania

Acrania is an abnormality similar to anencephaly in that the cranial vault is absent, but it differs from anencephaly in that the brain is fairly well developed and hemispheres of the brain may be observed.

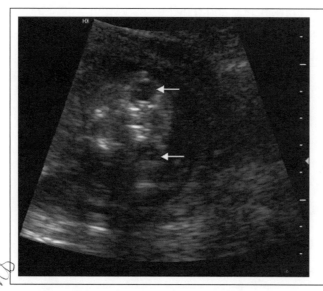

Figure 99.
Anencephaly. Coronal sonogram of fetal face demonstrating orbits (arrows). Note that there is no cranium above the level of the orbits.

Cephaloceles/Encephalocele

A *cephalocele* is a defect in the skull such that intracranial contents herniate through the defect. If brain tissue is herniated, the lesion is an *encephalocele*, a subset of cephaloceles. In the United States, the most common type of encephalocele is an occipital encephalocele in the midline above the tentorium. Posterior encephaloceles may herniate above or below the tentorium (figure 100). In some cases the skull defect may be large, and both occipital lobes and cerebellum will be herniated. Large occipital encephaloceles are associated with profound mental retardation. Frontal encephaloceles are rare in the United States and more common in the Far East; they are not as likely to be associated with mental retardation.

Because cephaloceles are often associated with other fetal anomalies, careful review of the remainder of the fetus is indicated if cephalocele is observed. Many syndromes include cephaloceles as a part of their presentation. One of the most common is Meckel-Gruber syndrome, which is an autosomal recessive condition manifesting with occipital encephalocele, marked cystic renal dysplasia, and often polydactyly. Because of the severe cystic renal dysplasia, Meckel-Gruber syndrome is lethal.

A cranial meningocele differs from an encephalocele in that no brain tissue extends into the cystic herniation. In general, normal intelligence is more common with meningoceles than with encephaloceles. If a mass is observed on the posterior aspect of the fetal head or neck, careful examination of the posterior skull can help differentiate between cystic hygromas and other posterior neck masses such as cranial meningoceles or encephaloceles. A bony defect must be present and brain tissue must be herniated into the extracranial space in order for the lesion to be an encephalocele.

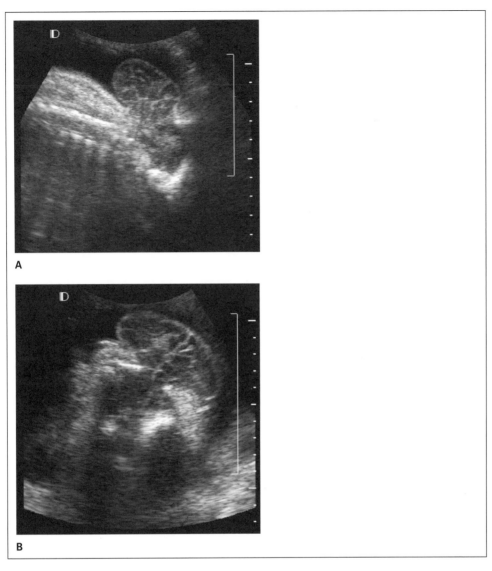

Figure 100.
Encephalocele with brain herniation. Sagittal (**A**) and axial (**B**) sonograms demonstrating a large posterior encephalocele with brain herniation.

Spina Bifida

Spina bifida is a defect in formation of the bony spinal column. *Spina bifida operta* refers to a defect in the skin, subcutaneous tissues, and posterior neural arches of the spinal canal. The defect is typically covered by a thin meningeal membrane. This membrane may be flat or may bulge, forming a sac extending posteriorly from the spinal canal. If the sac contains neural tissue, it is referred to as a *myelomeningocele*. Virtually all cases of spina bifida operta represent myelomeningoceles. The size and location of the defect is variable. The most common location is in the lumbosacral spine.

Open spina bifida, or *spina bifida operta*, is often associated with *ventriculomegaly*, "lemon sign" (frontal scalloping or indentation of the frontal bones), and "banana sign" (obliteration of the cisterna magna around the cerebellum in the posterior fossa) (figure 101). Ventriculomegaly often does not occur until late in pregnancy.

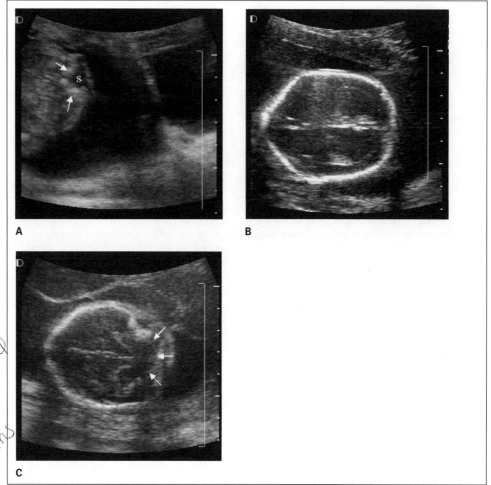

Figure 101.
Spina bifida. **A** Lower lumbar spine demonstrates spina bifida. Note the splaying of the posterior neural arches (arrows) and fluid-filled sac (S). **B** Axial sonogram demonstrating hydrocephaly and "lemon sign." Note the "beaking" of the frontal bones. **C** Axial sonogram demonstrates compressed cerebellum "banana sign" (arrows).

A milder form of spina bifida, usually called *spina bifida occulta,* is characterized by a defect in the bony posterior neural arch of the spinal canal, with preservation of tissue and skin overlying it. These cases are much more difficult to detect sonographically and often have associated pigmented lesions on the skin or subcutaneous lipomas overlying the neural tube defect. The incidence of spina bifida varies throughout the world. In the United States the incidence varies from approximately 0.5 to 1.5 per 1000 births. Elsewhere in the world the incidence varies from 0.3 to 4 per 1000 births.

A severe rare form of spina bifida is *rachischisis.* In this condition, the entire spinal canal is open posteriorly from the neck to the sacrum. Typically, this is associated with either anencephaly or acrania.

Miscellaneous

1 Choroid Plexus Cysts

Choroid plexus cysts are sometimes observed in the fetal brain. These are cystic structures within the choroid plexus, which, in turn, is within the ventricle (figure 102). Choroid plexus cysts are observed in 1–2% of mid-trimester

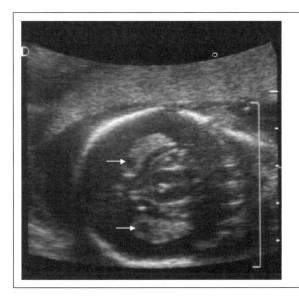

Figure 102.
Choroid plexus cysts. Coronal sonogram demonstrates small bilateral choroid plexus cysts (arrows).

fetuses. If a choroid plexus cyst is observed in a fetus, detailed evaluation of the fetal heart, brain, abdomen, and extremities is indicated, because if additional anomalies are observed, the incidence of chromosomal trisomy 18 is much higher. An association between choroid plexus cyst and other chromosomal abnormalities has not been convincingly demonstrated. Although some authors have suggested that larger choroid plexus cysts or bilateral choroid plexus cysts may be associated with increased risk for trisomy 18, this data is controversial, and others find no association between size and bilaterality of cysts and trisomy 18.

Choroid plexus cysts in most fetuses will resolve by approximately 26 weeks. Resolution of a choroid plexus cyst does not increase or decrease the likelihood that the fetus has trisomy 18.

2 Vein of Galen Aneurysm

When a cystic structure is noted in the midline posteriorly in the fetal head, the possibility of vein of Galen aneurysm should be considered. The dilated vein of Galen is typically due to increased blood flow from an arterial venous malformation in the fetal head that is often not well demonstrated sonographically. Doppler can demonstrate blood flow within the cystic structure. At birth, the shunting may be severe enough from arterial venous malformation that heart failure may develop. Hydrops may be a presenting symptom. Detection of vein of Galen aneurysm usually occurs late in pregnancy. No cases have been reported before 32 weeks' gestation.

3 Fetal Intracranial Tumors

Intracranial tumors in the fetus are rare. Most intracranial tumors detected in utero are supratentorial and 50% are teratomas. Other tumors noted include glioblastomas, craniopharyngioma, sarcomas, and oligodendrogliomas. In general, intracranial tumors in utero or in the neonate have a poor prognosis.

4 Intracranial Hemorrhage in Utero

Intracranial hemorrhage in utero is rare. The usual causes of fetal intracranial hemorrhage include severe maternal hypoxia, severe trauma, or the presence of maternal platelet antibodies.

5 Intracranial Calcifications

Intracranial calcifications observed in the fetal brain are quite rare. Usually the calcifications are due to intrauterine infection and are apparent only late in pregnancy. Typical infections include cytomegalovirus and toxoplasmosis. In addition, intracranial calcifications can be rarely observed in noninfectious conditions such as intracranial teratomas, tuberous sclerosis, or Sturge-Weber syndrome. When the calcifications are due to intrauterine infection, they typically occur in areas of cell necrosis and may be observed adjacent to ventricles. Microcephaly, ventriculomegaly, and porencephalic cysts may also be observed in these patients.

Abdominal Wall Abnormalities

In the past 10 years, there has been improvement in the detection rate of abdominal wall defects, primarily due to a widespread use of alpha-fetoprotein screening and increasing use of the AIUM guidelines for prenatal obstetrical sonography, which include standard views of the cord insertion.

Embryology of the Abdominal Wall

The anterior abdominal wall forms as a part of a complex process early in the embryonic phase. In the latter part of the 6th menstrual week, the embryo forms from the flat neural plate. In the process, there is a folding of tissue from the head end and the tail ends of the embryo. In the central portion of the embryo lateral folds develop. Simultaneously, the tissue surrounding the yolk sac and the allantois fuses to form the umbilical cord. By about 10 menstrual weeks, the embryo becomes recognizably human in appearance.

At the beginning of the 8th menstrual week, the gastrointestinal tract elongates. The mass of small bowel becomes too large to be contained in the developing peritoneal cavity and herniates into the proximal umbilical cord. As the midgut herniates, the bowel rotates 90 degrees counterclockwise around the superior mesenteric artery (figure 103). By about 12 menstrual weeks, the peritoneal cavity enlarges, and the mass of bowel returns to the peritoneal cavity. As it does so, it rotates an additional 180 degrees counterclockwise for a total bowel rotation of 270 degrees. According to one observation,[94] a

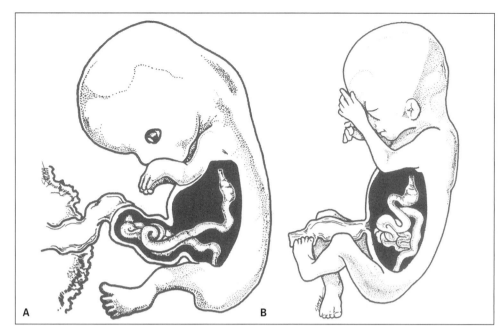

Figure 103.
Physiological herniation. **A** Drawing of a fetus at 9 menstrual weeks demonstrating normal herniation of bowel into the cord. **B** Drawing of a fetus at 14 menstrual weeks showing return of bowel into the abdominal cavity. Reprinted with permission from Cyr DR, Mack LA, Schoenecker SA, et al: Bowel migration in normal fetus: US detection. *Radiology* 161:119–121, 1986.

small persistent bulge at the base of the umbilical cord at 12 weeks exists in approximately 20% of patients. Most investigators recommend not making a diagnosis of omphalocele until after 13–14 menstrual weeks.

Gastroschisis

Gastroschisis has been reported to occur in 1.75–2.5 per 1000 live births. Most cases are sporadic, but a few familial cases have occurred. Other names used to describe gastroschisis are *paraomphalocele, laparoschisis,* and *abdominoschisis*. Various theories have been proposed to explain the production of gastroschisis, including abnormal involution of the right umbilical vein, disruption of the omphalomesenteric artery with subsequent ischemia, and early rupture of omphalocele during the embryonic period.[95–97]

Proposed Explanation for Gastroschisis

1. Abnormal involution of the right umbilical vein
2. Disruption of the omphalomesenteric artery with subsequent ischemia
3. Early rupture of omphalocele during embryonic period

In most cases of gastroschisis the small bowel is herniated (color plate 9), but rarely the stomach and other organs including the liver may be herniated. Typically the herniated bowel is nonrotated and there is no covering membrane. The abdominal wall defect almost always lies to the right of the umbilical cord insertion on the fetus.

Associated Anomalies

In 7–30% of cases, associated anomalies can be observed with gastroschisis. These anomalies can be classified in two groups:

1. Anomalies associated with bowel herniation, including bowel rotation, absent secondary fixation of the bowel to the dorsal abdominal wall, ischemia, and atresia in multiple areas due to chemical irritation and hypoperistalsis.

2. Other anomalies not related specifically to bowel herniation, including anencephaly, cleft lip and palate, atrial septal defect (ASD), ectopia cordis, diaphragmatic hernia, scoliosis, syndactyly, and amniotic bands. However, the non-bowel anomalies are more commonly associated with omphaloceles than gastroschisis.

Fetal karyotyping is not usually recommended because chromosomal abnormalities do not occur at a greater rate among fetuses with gastroschisis than among the general population.

With aggressive neonatal management, survival is typically 90% or greater. If there is associated bowel wall thickening or bowel distention, or other organs are herniated, the prognosis is less favorable. Fetuses with gastroschisis may develop intrauterine growth restriction (IUGR) and may deliver early. Serial sonograms may be helpful to evaluate the fetal well-being, but diagnosis of intrauterine growth restriction may be difficult to establish sonographically, as the abdominal circumference will be smaller as a result of the herniated bowel. Some examiners have begun to evaluate blood flow to the bowel in fetuses that have gastroschisis to monitor fetal well-being.

Omphalocele

Omphalocele is defined as a midline defect of the abdominal wall, with extrusion of the abdominal contents into the base of the umbilical cord. The herniated mass is typically covered by parietal peritoneum and amnion. The incidence of omphaloceles is similar to that of gastroschisis, approximately 2.5 per 10,000 births. There is a higher associated incidence of anomalies in omphalocele than is observed in gastroschisis, primarily because of an association between omphalocele and chromosomal anomalies. The incidence of associated anomalies with omphalocele has been reported to be as high as 50–88%, with chromosomal anomalies reported in 40–60%.

The most common chromosomal anomalies observed with omphalocele include trisomy 18, 13, and 21 and, less commonly, Turner's, Klinefelter, and triploidy. In 50% of fetuses that have omphalocele, an associated cardiac defect exists. Ventricular septal defect, atrial septal defect, tetralogy of Fallot, pulmonary artery stenosis, double outlet right ventricle, coarctation of the aorta, bicuspid aortic valve, and transposition of great vessels have all been reported in association with omphalocele. In addition to chromosomal anomalies, omphaloceles are also associated with Beckwith-Wiedemann syndrome, pentalogy of Cantrell, and cloacal exstrophy. These syndromes will be described later.

Diagnosis of Omphalocele

Elevated maternal serum alpha-fetoprotein (MS-AFP) has become a common reason for referral of fetuses that have omphalocele. Positive acetylcholinesterase increases the suspicion further. Typically an omphalocele will present sonographically as a mass in the base of the umbilical cord. It is important to establish that the umbilical cord inserts on the apex of the mass and to determine what organs are noted within the mass (figure 104). Rarely the membrane covering the herniated material will rupture, complicating the diagnosis. The prognosis depends primarily on the associated anomalies. Polyhydramnios and oligohydramnios are associated with omphalocele. Polyhydramnios is typically due to associated atresias or obstruction of bowel by kinking. The presence of either polyhydramnios or oligohydramnios suggests a somewhat poorer prognosis. The size of the omphalocele affects morbidity and surgical management but does not directly correlate with incidence of fetal death. A small omphalocele containing only bowel increases the risk of chromosomal anomaly.

Pentalogy of Cantrell

Pentalogy of Cantrell was first described by Cantrell in 1958.[98] The components of pentalogy include a midline supraumbilical anterior wall defect, a deficit in the lower sternum, a deficiency of the anterior diaphragm, a deficit in the diaphragmatic pericardium, and congenital intracardiac defects.

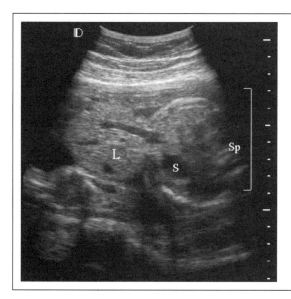

Figure 104.
Omphalocele. Transverse sonogram of a fetus with an omphalocele. Note liver (L) extending into the omphalocele. Sp = spine, S = stomach.

> **Pentalogy of Cantrell Components**
>
> 1. A midline supraumbilical anterior wall defect
> 2. A deficit in the lower sternum
> 3. A deficiency of the anterior diaphragm
> 4. Deficit in the diaphragmatic pericardium
> 5. Congenital intracardiac defects

From a practical point of view, the usual abnormalities observed sonographically are ectopia cordis and omphalocele. Pentalogy of Cantrell is caused by abnormal folding of the lateral mesoderm at the end of the 6th menstrual week and early in the 7th menstrual week. The lateral mesoderm gives rise to the anterior abdominal wall, the sternum, and portions of the diaphragm. Associated anomalies include atrial septal defect (50%), ventricular septal defect (20%), and tetralogy of Fallot (10%). Noncardiac anomalies include cleft lip, microphthalmia, low-set ears, kyphoscoliosis, vertebral anomalies, clinodactyly, two-vessel cord, and ascites. An association between pentalogy of Cantrell and trisomy 13 and 18 has been observed. This group of anomalies has also been observed in monozygotic twins. The degree of protrusion of the heart from the chest and the size of the omphalocele in pentalogy of Cantrell is highly variable. The extension through the abdominal wall may be minimal. Pleural or pericardial effusion may be present.

Beckwith-Wiedemann Syndrome

Beckwith-Wiedemann syndrome is characterized by omphalocele, macroglossia, and visceromegaly, including the liver and kidneys, and asymmetry of the fetal limbs. Cardiac anomalies, diaphragmatic hernia, or diaphragmatic eventration may also be observed. In later life there is a known risk for tumors, including nephroblastoma, sarcoma, and adrenal tumors. The syndrome appears to be related to a defect in the insulinlike growth factor 2 gene. This defect leads to increased levels of growth hormone and insulinlike growth factor, which gives rise to the malformation. The diagnosis may be suspected prenatally on the basis of omphalocele and large fetal size but is typically not established until after birth.

Limb-Body Wall Complex

Limb-body wall complex (LBWC) is characterized by a number of disruptive abnormalities of the anterior abdominal wall, including extensive deficiency of the anterior abdominal wall, short umbilical cord, scoliosis, limb defects, and facial and cranial anomalies. Typically, the umbilical cord is attached to the lateral abdominal wall region in a sheet of amnion. This condition is also known as *body stalk anomaly* (figure 105).

The incidence of limb-body wall complex is approximately 1 in 7500 to 1 in 42,000 births in Great Britain. The prevalence in the United States is unknown. The most widely held view of the cause of limb-body wall complex is alteration of blood flow leading to disruption and incomplete development of various parts of the embryo at 4–6 menstrual weeks. Another proposed cause is early amniotic rupture. A third possibility is faulty folding of the head, tail, and lateral folds of the abdomen during formation of the abdominal wall. Associated anomalies include scoliosis and limb anomalies including clubfeet, oligodactyly, arthrogryposis, absent limbs, split hand, and radial and ulnar hypoplasia. Facial clefts, cephalocele, and exencephaly have been observed. Absent diaphragm is common, and bowel atresia and renal abnormalities have also been observed.

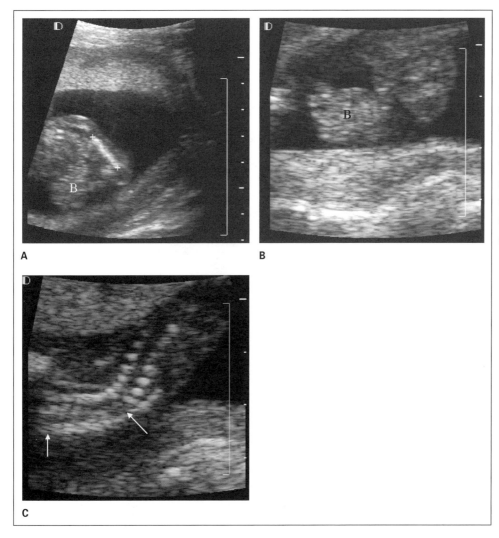

Figure 105.

Limb-body wall syndrome. **A** Transverse sonogram showing bowel (B) outside the abdomen. The bowel is adjacent to the femur (cursors). **B** Another view of bowel (B) anterior to the abdomen. **C** Sagittal sonogram showing marked scoliosis of the spine (arrows).

Amniotic bands are observed in 40% of cases, but these bands may be due to a vascular disruption rather than classical amniotic bands. Limb-body wall complex is always fatal but is unlikely to recur in later pregnancies. Sonographically, a grotesque mass of tissue and marked scoliosis of the spine are typical findings. Internal organs may be difficult to identify. The limbs may be difficult to locate if scoliosis is severe.

Amniotic Band Syndrome

In fetuses that have *amniotic band syndrome,* multiple and bizarre anomalies are noted, with limb amputations, constricting bands of tissue, deformities of the face, facial clefts, rib clefts, scoliosis, abdominal wall defects, ambiguous genitalia, lymph edema, syndactyly, and clubfoot (figure 106). Cases with major abdominal wall defects are usually characterized as limb-body wall complex.

The cause of amniotic band syndrome is unknown, but there are two prominent theories. One is rupture of amniotic membrane with intact chorionic membranes and subsequent entanglement of the fetus in the amniotic membranes. The second theory is that the defects are due to vasospasm or arterial disruption. Experimental studies using vasoactive drugs in rats have demonstrated defects quite similar to those observed in amniotic band syndrome.[99, 100] Prognosis is variable, depending on the degree of malformations. There is no evidence of significant risk of recurrence.

An amniotic sheet may be confused with amniotic bands. An *amniotic sheet* develops when a pregnancy occurs in a uterus with an adhesion

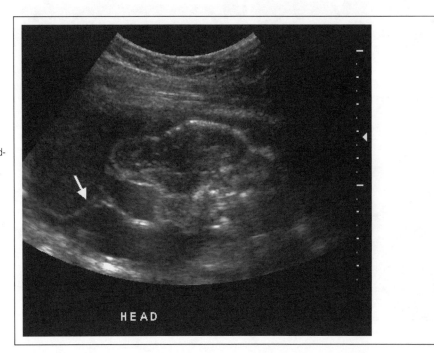

Figure 106.
Amniotic band syndrome. Sagittal sonogram of a fetus with amniotic bands. Note the marked irregularity of the fetal head and the band (arrow) extending from the fetal head.

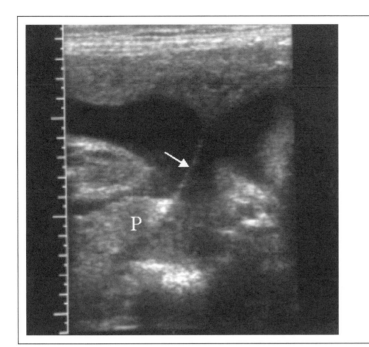

Figure 107.
Amniotic sheet. Sonogram of an intrauterine pregnancy demonstrating an amniotic sheet (arrow) attached at the edge of the placenta.

between the anterior and posterior walls of the uterus. When this happens, the amniotic membranes fold around the adhesion, forming a sheet of amniotic membrane extending from the wall of the uterus to the adhesion site (figure 107). This finding is not associated with fetal anomalies or fetal morbidity.

Cloacal Exstrophy

Cloacal exstrophy is a rare association of anomalies involving omphalocele, exstrophy of the bladder, imperforate anus, and spina bifida. The incidence is approximately 1 per 200,000 births. Isolated bladder exstrophy occurs in approximately 1 in 30,000 births.

The *cloaca* is an early embryologic structure, which subsequently develops into the rectum and bladder. The cloaca divides in a vertical fashion, and the rectum forms posteriorly, the bladder anteriorly. If the lower abdominal wall fails to develop, an unusual anomaly of the bladder area is observed, with portions of the bladder mucosa exposed on the skin surface and a central protruding bowel loop connecting to the colon. Numerous other anomalies of the genitourinary tract may be observed, including multicystic dysplastic kidney, hydronephrosis, and undescended testes. Anomalies of the diaphragm, CNS, and spinal column are also observed. An association with trisomy 21 has been reported.[101]

Maternal serum alpha-fetoprotein is markedly elevated in many of these cases. Sonographically, a mass of tissue is noted inferior to the umbilicus in the region of the abdominal wall. In some cases a large fluid-filled structure may be identified in the pelvis, which represents the cloaca rather than the urinary bladder. The anterior bones of the pelvis are either deficient or absent.

> ***Sonographic Approach to Evaluating Abdominal Wall Defects***
>
> 1. What is the relationship of the abdominal wall defect to the umbilical cord?
> 2. Is there a membrane covering the herniated structures?
> 3. What organs are herniated?
> 4. Is the herniated bowel dilated or strictured?
> 5. What other anomalies are present in this fetus?
>
> ***Potential Pitfalls That May Lead to Incorrect Diagnosis:***
>
> 1. Normal small bowel herniation into the umbilical cord between 8 and 14 menstrual weeks
> 2. Distorted anterior abdominal wall (i.e., in oligohydramnios), which leads to a suspicion of an abdominal wall defect
> 3. Scars or adhesions within the uterus, giving rise to amniotic sheets within the uterine cavity, which may be confused with amniotic bands
> 4. Cord masses, including omphalomesenteric duct cyst or allantoic cyst that may resemble an omphalocele.

Thoracic Abnormalities

Embryology

The lung buds begin to develop early in the 5th menstrual week, and by 16–20 menstrual weeks the normal number of bronchi are formed. Between 16 and 24 menstrual weeks and continuing thereafter, more and more air spaces and alveoli develop in the fetus. The surfactant in the lungs, which allows normal breathing with maintenance of air pressure in the alveoli during expiration, is not present in normal quantities until approximately 35 menstrual weeks. Four factors are required for normal lung development, including:

1. Adequate thoracic space
2. Normal fetal breathing movements
3. Fluid production in the lungs
4. Adequate amniotic fluid volume

Intrathoracic masses and pleural effusions do not decrease the intrathoracic space but decrease the effective intrathoracic volume available for lung development. Neuromuscular conditions may decrease fetal respiratory movements, and any condition that causes longstanding oligohydramnios will also affect the development of the lung. The precise mechanism of pulmonary hypoplasia caused by oligohydramnios is somewhat unclear; however, extrinsic compression of the lungs and the fetal chest may be a contributing factor.

Sonography of the Normal Lung

In the normal chest, the fetal heart should occupy approximately one-third of the thoracic volume on transverse images. Typically, the right lung is slightly larger than the left because of the left-sided cardiac apex. Normally, the right atrium and a portion of the left atrium lie to the right of midline. In the sagittal plane, the diaphragm can be visualized, with adjacent stomach, spleen, and liver below the diaphragm. The echogenicity of the lungs should be homogeneous and of medium level. Typically, the echogenicity of the lungs is slightly greater than the liver. The higher frequency probe will demonstrate brighter lungs.

Pulmonary Hypoplasia

In the absence of an intrathoracic pulmonary mass or pleural effusion, pulmonary hypoplasia is usually due to one of two causes:

1. Oligohydramnios
2. Small thoracic cage

In general a fetus that has a thoracic circumference smaller than the 5th percentile is likely to experience respiratory distress, which could be fatal. By using subjective criteria, if the chest is visibly small compared with the abdomen and if there is a sharp change in diameter in the A-P dimension from the chest to the abdomen, the possibility of pulmonary hypoplasia should be considered.

Causes of oligohydramnios that lead to pulmonary hypoplasia in the fetus include:

1. Longstanding rupture of membranes beginning before 24 menstrual weeks
2. Absence of the fetal kidneys or severe renal dysplasia in which little urine is output
3. Severe intrauterine growth restriction

Pleural Effusion

Fetal hydrothorax is estimated to occur in approximately 1 in 15,000 pregnancies. Pleural effusion may be on a primary basis (primary chylothorax) or may be secondary to various causes of fetal hydrops. Pleural effusions may be unilateral or bilateral. Secondary pleural effusions may be due to many causes, but most will arise as a result of lymphatic dysplasia, high output failure in the fetus, or low osmotic pressure within the vascular system. In some cases, shunting with a double pigtail catheter has been performed to manage pleural effusions.

Chest Masses

Unilateral fetal chest masses are summarized in table 3.

One of the more common pulmonary masses that may be observed in the fetus is the *cystic adenomatoid malformation* (CAM) of the lung. Three types have been described (figure 108): Type I, with large cysts (2–10 cm, or macrocystic) of variable sizes (figure 109); Type II, with smaller cysts (<2 cm); and Type III, with very small cysts (<0.5 cm, or microcystic), which are not visible sonographically. Some have suggested that bronchial atresia is the primary abnormality in these patients, and the lung distends distal to the atresia.

Table 3. Unilateral fetal chest masses.

Sonographic Appearance	Mass
Cystic	CAM* I
	Bronchogenic cyst
	Congenital diaphragmatic hernia
	Enteric cyst
	Mediastinal meningocele
	Esophageal duplication cyst
Cystic and solid	CAM II
	Enteric cyst
	Teratoma (pericardial)
	Congenital diaphragmatic hernia
	Mixed CAM III and sequestration
	Pulmonary sequestration (predominantly solid)
	Thoracic neuroblastoma
Solid	CAM III
	Pulmonary sequestration
	Tracheal atresia
	Congenital diaphragmatic hernia (bowel or liver)

*CAM = cystic adenomatoid malformation.

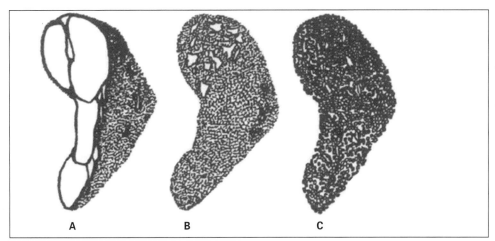

Figure 108.
Types of cystic adenomatoid malformations. The three types of congenital cystic adenomatoid malformation of the lung as described by Stocker et al. **A** Type I lesions have large cysts of variable sizes. **B** Type II lesions have smaller cysts. **C** Type III lesions appear solid owing to reflections from numerous adenomatoid structures, along with scattered, thin-walled structures similar to bronchioles. Reprinted with permission from Stocker JT, Madewell JE, Drake RM: Congenital cystic adenomatoid malformation of the lung: Classification and morphologic spectrum. *Hum Pathol* 8:155, 1977.

Although early work suggested that there is a difference in prognosis between the different types of cystic adenomatoid malformation, more recent investigation suggests that the size of the lesion is more important than its internal characteristics.

Mediastinal shift by a cystic adenomatoid malformation mass is associated with an increased likelihood of fetal demise. It is well established that many cystic adenomatoid malformation lesions become relatively smaller when compared with total lung volume as the pregnancy progresses. After delivery, cystic adenomatoid malformation lesions are typically resected, because if left in place, they may result in later infection and abscess. The policy in many centers is to avoid intervention during pregnancy in fetuses that do not have hydrops.

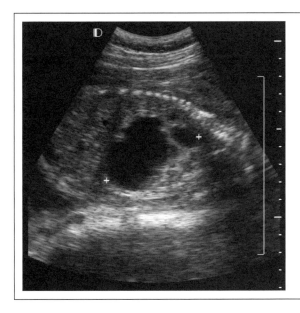

Figure 109.
Cystic adenomatoid malformation (CAM). Sagittal sonogram of a fetus with CAM. Note the large cysts filling most of the chest.

Pulmonary Sequestration

Pulmonary sequestration is an abnormality of the lung in which lung tissue develops that is not connected to the normal tracheal bronchial tree. Two categories of pulmonary sequestration are described, *extralobar sequestration* (ELS) and *intralobar sequestration* (ILS). Intralobar sequestration is more commonly seen in adults, and extralobar sequestration is more commonly seen in fetuses, neonates, and young children. It has been proposed that in adults intralobar sequestrations are acquired lesions in which the tracheal tree obstructs as a result of inflammation and fibrosis. Extralobar sequestrations typically demonstrate a blood supply arising directly from the abdominal aorta rather than from the pulmonary artery. Extralobar sequestrations account for approximately 0.5–6% of all congenital lesions of the thorax.[102] Color and spectral Doppler are extremely helpful in establishing a diagnosis of extralobar sequestration by identifying a separate vessel arising from the aorta and supplying the echogenic mass of tissue (color plate 10).

Associated abnormalities may occur with extralobar sequestration, including congenital diaphragmatic hernia (CDH), diaphragmatic eventration, or paralysis. Recent investigations suggest that most fetuses that have pulmonary sequestration survive. Occasionally fetal hydrops may develop with pulmonary sequestration.

Rarely, "pulmonary" sequestrations are found in the abdomen rather than the chest; approximately 10–15% of extralobar sequestrations are found below the diaphragm and appear as brightly echogenic masses within the abdomen.

Tracheal Atresia

Tracheal atresia is a rare pulmonary anomaly. Sonographically the lungs show diffuse hyperechogenicity bilaterally. The lungs are enlarged, and the heart appears relatively small and is compressed in the midline (figure 110).

The lungs become echogenic because very small fluid-filled spaces dilate within the lungs. The level of tracheal obstruction is typically at the larynx. Other anomalies are commonly observed in fetuses that have laryngeal obstruction, including renal anomalies, CNS malformations, and tracheal-esophageal atresia.

A surgical procedure performed while the fetus is still attached to the placenta at the time of delivery is necessary to establish a patent airway in these individuals.

Bronchogenic Cysts

Bronchogenic cyst is a rare cystic lesion that arises within the lung, probably as a result of abnormal development of bronchi between the 26th and 40th

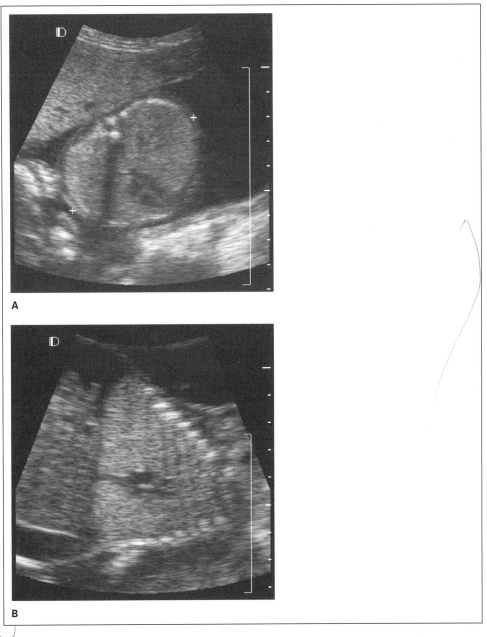

Figure 110.
Tracheal atresia.
A Transverse sonogram.
B Sagittal sonogram showing enlarged markedly echogenic lungs. Note the small compressed heart.

day of life. Bronchogenic cysts are not usually associated with other congenital anomalies. The cysts may be uni- or multilocular.

Congenital Diaphragmatic Hernia

Congenital diaphragmatic hernia (CDH) is a result of incomplete fusion of the diaphragmatic structures at 6–10 weeks. The diaphragmatic defect may be either right or left sided, but left-sided diaphragmatic hernias are more commonly observed because of herniation of stomach, intestines, and spleen to the chest in left-sided hernia. Right-sided diaphragmatic defects are typically obstructed by the liver, although if large enough, may result in diaphragmatic hernia.

Figure 111.
Congenital diaphragmatic hernia. **A** Transverse sonogram of a chest in a fetus that has congenital diaphragmatic hernia. Note the displacement of the heart to the right with the apex angled to the left. **B** An additional transverse sonogram of the same fetus showing bowel and stomach (arrows) in the left chest.

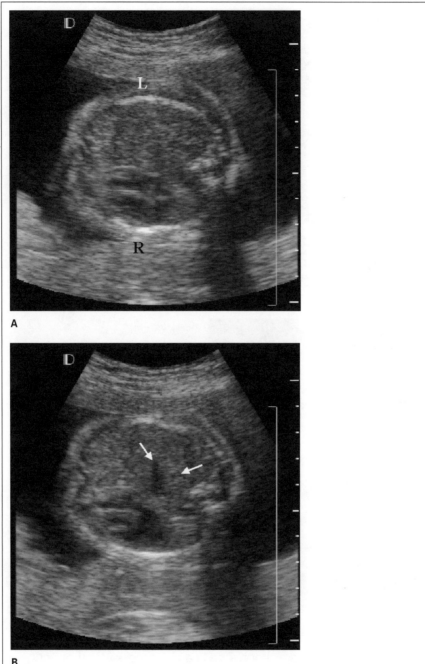

Sonographically, the most notable intrathoracic abnormality in congenital diaphragmatic hernia is displacement of the fetal heart toward the right chest wall (figure 111). Typically, the cardiac apex will be angled to the left. More careful examination usually suggests either bowel or stomach in the left hemithorax. A diaphragmatic hernia can be differentiated from an intrathoracic mass by failure to visualize the diaphragm on the affected side. Typically in patients that have pulmonary sequestration or cystic adenomatoid malformation, the diaphragm will be visible below the lesion.

Diaphragmatic hernias are associated with various other anomalies and syndromes; the most commonly associated syndrome is trisomy 18.

Recently, experimental surgical procedures have been developed to repair congenital diaphragmatic hernia. The procedure is described elsewhere (see "Fetal Therapy" in Chapter 5), but patients are selected for surgery if the diaphragmatic hernia is severe, that is, little remaining lung is noted posterior to the heart on the right and the liver extends into the hernia. Detection of liver extension into the hernia may be made easier by the use of Doppler and color flow to evaluate the intrahepatic vessels.

Other Intrathoracic Masses

Mediastinal masses, including teratomas, enteric cysts, and thymic masses, have been rarely observed. Also, intrapulmonary tumors and focal masses arising from congenital infections have been observed in utero.

Genitourinary Abnormalities

Embryology

The fetal kidneys begin to develop at approximately 7 menstrual weeks and between 7 and 11 menstrual weeks ascend into a permanent location in the flank of the fetus. After 16 weeks' gestation, virtually all amniotic fluid is produced by fetal urination. If normal amniotic fluid is present after 16 weeks, it implies at least one functioning kidney.

Sonographically the fetal kidneys can be identified adjacent to the spine in most second trimester fetuses. They appear as elliptical hypoechoic structures on either side of the lumbar ossification centers and are usually visible by 14–16 weeks. Later in pregnancy, fetal lobulations and fetal pyramids may be visualized.

Granum and colleagues indicate that the ratio of kidney circumference to abdominal circumference is usually 28–30% throughout pregnancy.[103] The bladder empties every 25 minutes and should be visible on sonography. Many anomalies in the kidneys can be identified in the early second trimester, and patients can appropriately be counseled. Some renal conditions, however, such as mild polycystic kidney disease, may not be visible until after 24 weeks.

Hydronephrosis

Hydronephrosis is the most common abnormality detected antenatally. Because an obstructed kidney may develop dysplastic changes, accurate assessment of degree of hydronephrosis is important. The different classification systems for hydronephrosis have been described, but it is generally

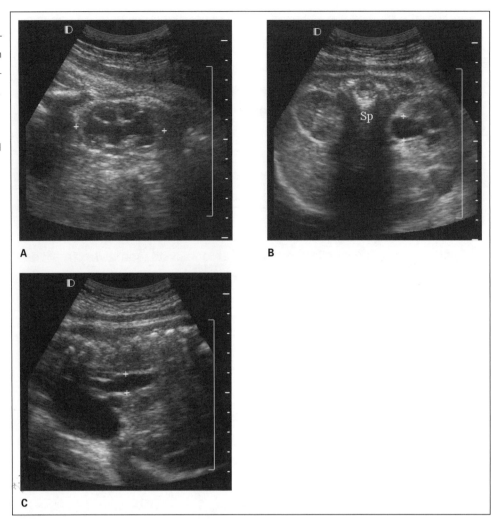

Figure 112.
Fetal renal hydronephrosis. **A** Sagittal sonogram of a fetal kidney demonstrating hydronephrosis. **B** Transverse sonogram of the fetal kidneys demonstrating unilateral hydronephrosis. **C** Longitudinal sonogram demonstrating a dilated ureter. Sp=spine.

agreed that a renal pelvis that measures greater than 8 mm in A-P diameter before 20 menstrual weeks and greater than 10 mm in A-P diameter after 20 weeks should be considered to represent hydronephrosis (figure 112). Further, there seems to be a general consensus that if the A-P diameter of the renal pelvis measures greater than 4 mm in diameter before 20 weeks and greater than 8 mm in diameter after 20 weeks, follow-up should be obtained to evaluate possible developing hydronephrosis. Other measurement techniques, including ratio of the A-P diameter of the fetal renal pelvis to the A-P diameter of the kidney, have also been used. By this criterion, the fetal renal pelvis exceeding 50% of the A-P diameter of the kidney is generally accepted to represent significant hydronephrosis.

Ureteropelvic Junction Obstruction

Obstruction at the ureteropelvic junction (UPJ) is the most common form of obstructive uropathy observed in the fetus and represents approximately two-thirds of cases. A ureteropelvic junction obstruction is twice as common in males as in females and may be bilateral in 30% of cases.

Reflux and Ureterovesical Junction Obstruction

If both the renal pelvis and the ureter are enlarged, the distal ureterovesical junction (UVJ) may be either obstructed or refluxing. Sonographically it is difficult to tell the difference. If there is primary functional obstruction of the distal ureter due to an aperistaltic segment, the condition is termed *primary megaureter,* but vesicoureteral reflux is much more common.

Pyelectasis and Aneuploidy

Mild hydronephrosis, also termed *pyelectasis,* is observed in 2% of normal fetuses, but the incidence increases to 17–25% in fetuses with trisomy 21. If hydronephrosis is the only finding in the fetus, the incidence of chromosomal anomalies is approximately 1%, but this increases dramatically if associated with other fetal abnormalities such as a cardiac defect or short femur.

Urethral Obstruction

Bladder outlet obstruction is another cause of hydronephrosis and hydroureter. In addition to hydronephrosis, bladder wall thickening is often observed, and the ureters may be tortuous. Also, perinephric urinoma, urine ascites, and sometimes urinothorax may be observed. If the obstruction is severe or complete, oligohydramnios may be observed. The most common cause of bladder outlet obstruction is posterior urethral valves. This occurs in males, and the dilated proximal urethra is usually observed. This finding is referred to as the "keyhole sign" (figure 113A). In females, urethral atresia or cloacal anomaly may cause bladder outlet obstruction. With severe bladder outlet obstruction, renal dysplasia with echogenic kidneys (figure 113B) or cystic changes in the renal parenchyma may be observed. Bladder outlet obstruction is probably the most common cause of obstructive renal dysplasia.

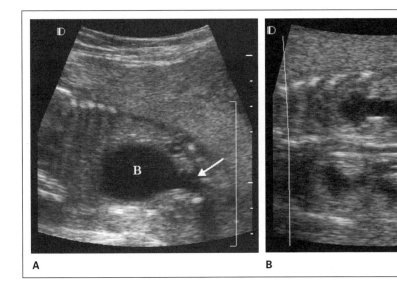

Figure 113A. "Keyhole sign." **A** Sonogram of fetal pelvis with enlarged, dilated bladder and urethra (arrow). **B** Renal dysplasia with hydronephrosis. Same fetus demonstrating bilateral hydronephrosis. Note that kidneys are diffusely echogenic because of dysplasia.

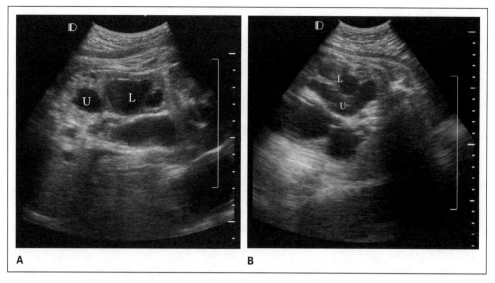

Figure 114.
Renal duplication. **A** Sagittal sonogram demonstrates duplicated collecting system. Note that the collecting system is divided into upper (U) and lower (L) pole parts. **B** Another sagittal sonogram of the same kidney demonstrates dilated segments of the upper (U) and lower (L) pole ureters.

Prune Belly Syndrome

Prune belly syndrome is a constellation of anomalies including large bladder, dilated ureters, undescended testes, and absent or atrophic abdominal wall musculature. There is some debate as to the cause of this abnormality, but many investigators believe that this condition may be caused at least in some cases by bladder outlet obstruction.

Renal Duplication

Another cause of hydronephrosis is renal duplication. In this condition the ureters are partially or completely duplicated, either unilaterally or bilaterally. The ureteral segment that arises from the upper pole is often obstructed with marked dilatation of the upper pole portion of the collecting system. In some cases this may appear to resemble a cyst in the upper pole (figure 114). The lower pole ureteral segment is usually not obstructed but may reflux. A common associated abnormality is an ectopic ureterocele, which appears as a cystlike extension of the distal ureter into the urinary bladder.

Renal Cystic Disease

The Potter classification of renal cystic disease is shown in table 4.

1 Autosomal Recessive Polycystic Kidney Disease (Potter's Type I)

Autosomal recessive polycystic kidney disease (ARPKD), previously referred to as *infantile polycystic kidney disease,* is an autosomal recessive condition that occurs in one in approximately 40,000 births. It is characterized by microscopic cysts. Sonographically it appears as diffusely enlarged

	Type I	Type II	Type III	Type IV
Nomenclature	Infantile polycystic kidney disease	Multicystic dysplastic kidney (MCDK) disease	Adult polycystic kidney disease	Renal cystic disease associated with hydronephrosis
Location	Bilateral	Unilateral 30%, with contralateral renal disease including hydronephrosis, renal agenesis, or MCDK	Bilateral	Dependent on etiology of hydronephrosis
Ultrasound appearance	Enlarged echogenic	Cysts of variable size; noncommunicating	Rare in utero, enlarged echogenic	Hydronephrosis with cortical cysts, may change in appearance during pregnancy
Amniotic fluid	Often oligohydramnios	Normal to oligohydramnios (if bilateral)	Usually normal	Normal to oligohydramnios depending on underlying cause
Prognosis	Poor	Good—dependent on contralateral kidney and associated malformations	Adult onset	Dependent on underlying cause
Risk in subsequent pregnancies	25%	Probably <5%	50%	Dependent on underlying cause

Table 4. Classification of major renal cystic diseases (Potter's syndromes).

Data from Porto M, McGahan JP: The fetal abdomen and pelvis. In McGahan JP, Porto M (eds): *Diagnostic Obstetrical Ultrasound.* Philadelphia, Lippincott, 1994, p 442.

echogenic kidneys (figure 115). In many cases, the medullary pyramids are more echogenic than the cortex and the periphery of the kidney is more hypoechoic. This peripheral halo of hypoechoic cortical tissue strongly suggests the diagnosis of autosomal recessive polycystic kidney disease, but is not observed in every patient.

All fetuses affected with autosomal recessive polycystic kidney disease have some component of liver disease, and biliary duplication cysts may be visible within the liver late in pregnancy. The degree of renal impairment is variable; in the most severe cases, findings may be observed as early as 16 menstrual

Figure 115.
Infantile polycystic kidney disease (IPKD).
A Transverse sonogram of a 34-week fetus with IPKD. Note the echogenic kidneys and mild pelviectasis.
B Sagittal sonogram of the same fetus.

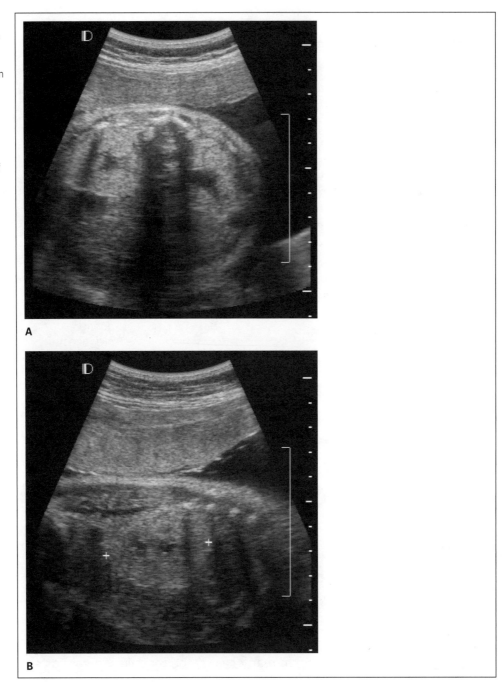

weeks and there may be oligohydramnios throughout most of the pregnancy. In milder cases, however, the findings may not be detectable until after 24 weeks or even after birth.

Another condition that may resemble autosomal recessive polycystic kidney disease is Meckel-Gruber syndrome. In this syndrome, the fetus may have encephalocele and polydactyly. The degree of abnormality of the kidneys is always quite severe, oligohydramnios exists, and the condition is fatal. In our experience, Meckel-Gruber syndrome occurs nearly as often as autosomal recessive polycystic kidney disease. Because of this, any fetus that has large echogenic kidneys should be examined for polydactyly and encephalocele.

Other conditions that may resemble autosomal recessive polycystic kidney disease in utero include glomerulocystic disease, trisomy 13, and congenital hypernephric nephromegaly.

2 Multicystic Dysplastic Kidney (Potter's Type II)

Multicystic dysplastic kidney (MCDK) arises as a result of ureteral obstruction early in the development of the kidney, probably before 8–10 menstrual weeks. The size of the dysplastic kidney may be large, normal, or small, and it may contain cysts of various sizes that do not communicate with one another (figure 116). In the usual situation, no significant parenchyma exists peripheral to the cysts in the kidney and the parenchyma that is observed lies between the cysts and is echogenic. There may or may not be a cystic area

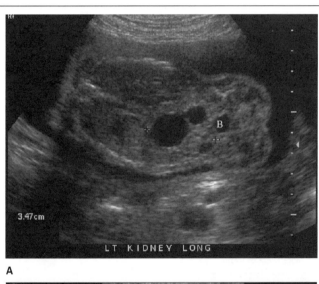

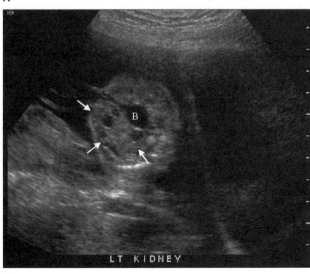

Figure 116.
Multicystic dysplastic kidney of the left kidney. **A** Sagittal sonogram of a fetus that has multicystic dysplastic kidney. Note kidney (cursors) and multiple cysts. B = bladder.
B Transverse of the same fetus. Note multiple cysts of the left kidney (arrows). B = bladder.

in the center of the kidney. In approximately 40% of cases, some abnormality is observed in the opposite kidney, most commonly ureteropelvic junction obstruction. Bilateral multicystic dysplastic kidney does occur rarely.

Sonographically, the cysts in multicystic dysplastic kidney may not be visible until early in the second trimester. Multicystic dysplastic kidney is differentiated sonographically from hydronephrosis in that the cysts do not communicate with one another.

3 Autosomal Dominant Polycystic Kidney Disease (Potter's Type III)

Autosomal dominant polycystic kidney disease (ADPKD) is typically a disease first noted after age 40. The severity of the disease is variable; however, in a few cases the condition may be noted in the fetus or neonate. The sonographic appearance of autosomal dominant polycystic kidney disease in the fetus and neonate is variable. In many cases multiple macroscopic cysts are identified in all or portions of the kidneys, and cysts may be observed in other organs, including the liver, spleen, and pancreas. There appear to be some cases of autosomal dominant polycystic kidney disease, however, in which there are extensive microscopic cysts with large echogenic kidneys resembling autosomal recessive polycystic kidney disease. In autosomal dominant polycystic kidney disease the risk of recurrence is 50% if one of the parents is affected.

4 Obstructive Renal Dysplasia (Potter's Type IV)

If a fetus has severe urinary or bladder outlet obstruction, cortical cysts may develop in the kidneys. These cysts are more commonly observed in fetuses that have posterior urethral valves or uretero pelvic junction obstruction. Usually, the renal parenchyma is echogenic, and renal pyramids are not visible. Macroscopic cysts may also be observed.

Meckel-Gruber Syndrome

Meckel-Gruber syndrome is a recessive condition. For the diagnosis of Meckel-Gruber syndrome to be made, the fetus must demonstrate two of the three predominant characteristics. The first characteristic is abnormal kidneys. The kidneys are large, echogenic (figure 117A, B) and resemble the kidneys observed in autosomal recessive polycystic kidney disease, but the malformation of the kidney is actually a form of multicystic dysplasia. In addition to the abnormal kidneys, the fetus must demonstrate either an encephalocele, polydactyly (figure 117C), or both. Numerous other malformations are observed in these fetuses, including holoprosencephaly and Dandy-Walker malformation. The renal disease is always severe, and oligohydramnios always exists. Therefore, this condition is always fatal at birth.

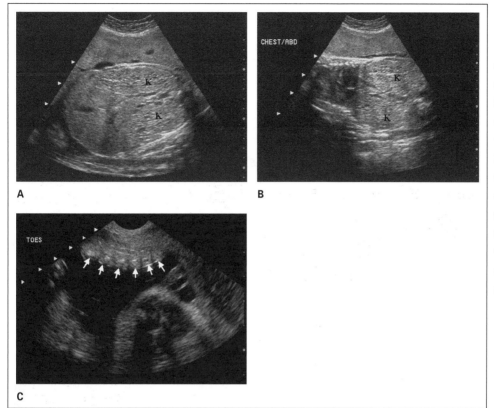

Figure 117.
Meckel-Gruber syndrome. **A** Transverse sonogram of fetal abdomen demonstrates bilateral enlarged echogenic kidneys (K) with visible cysts. **B** Sonogram of the same fetus demonstrates a small chest and large kidneys (K). **C** Sonogram of same fetus showing polydactyly of the toes (arrows).

Trisomy 13 is a common chromosomal abnormality, which will be discussed elsewhere, but the major malformations observed sonographically are typically omphalocele, polydactyly, and in many cases holoprosencephaly. Cystic disease in the kidneys is found in approximately 30% of patients at autopsy, but only a few show changes that are visible sonographically. In our experience, the changes are not as severe as typically observed in autosomal recessive polycystic kidney disease or in Meckel-Gruber syndrome.

Other Renal Abnormalities

1 Bilateral Renal Agenesis (Classic Potter's Syndrome)

Bilateral renal agenesis is a lethal anomaly, which occurs in approximately 1 in 4000 births[104] (figure 118). There is early failure of development of the ureteric buds. The kidneys do not develop significantly, and in the second trimester, there is oligohydramnios (figure 118A). The oligohydramnios results in the so-called Potter's sequence, which is a group of findings in the fetus resulting from longstanding oligohydramnios. These findings include flattening of the nose, low-set ears, prominent epicanthic folds, and limb contractures.

Pulmonary hypoplasia is the usual cause of death, which typically occurs within hours or days after delivery. Sonographically, the kidneys are not identified. Color flow Doppler may be helpful to establish that renal arteries are not

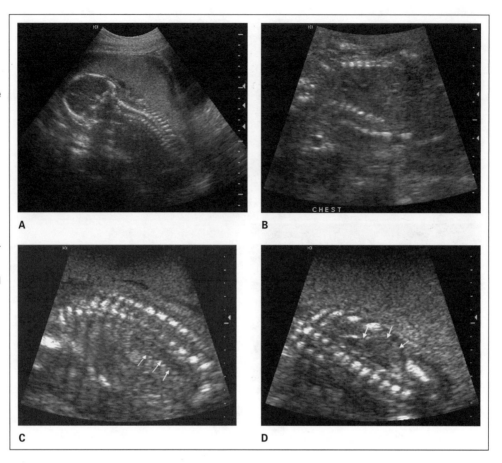

Figure 118.
Bilateral renal agenesis.
A Sagittal sonogram of a fetus with bilateral renal agenesis. Note the marked oligohydramnios. **B** Sagittal sonogram of the chest. Note that the chest diameter is smaller than the abdominal diameter. **C** Sagittal sonogram of the left adrenal (arrows). Note that the adrenal is long and flat and parallel to the spine. **D** Sagittal sonogram of the right adrenal (arrows).

present in these fetuses. The positive sonographic sign that suggests the presence of bilateral renal agenesis is the appearance of long, flattened adrenal glands in the renal fossae bilaterally (figure 118C and D). The adrenal gland is thin and long with an echogenic central core. Various terms have been used to describe this finding, including "lying down adrenals" and "oreo cookie sign." After noting the long flat adrenals in the renal fossae bilaterally, the sonographer should search to establish that no pelvic kidney exists and that the urinary bladder is not visible. The chest will be small (figure 118B), and a "bell-shaped" thorax is often observed. In some cases additional anomalies may be observed, including musculoskeletal, cardiovascular, genitourinary, and CNS anomalies. The most notable example of associated anomalies is *sirenomelia,* a condition in which the two lower extremities are fused.

2 Unilateral Renal Agenesis

Unilateral renal agenesis is three to four times more common than bilateral renal agenesis. The long flat adrenal gland will be observed in the empty renal fossa, and if the other kidney is normal, the bladder will appear normal and there will be normal amniotic fluid. In this condition, a careful search should be made of the lower abdomen for a single pelvic kidney.

3 Renal Ectopia

One or both kidneys may not ascend normally into the renal fossa. The incidence is 1 in 1200 births, and unilateral pelvic kidney[105] is more common than horseshoe kidney. In horseshoe kidney, both kidneys are ectopically located in the pelvis and fused together in the midline.

Associated anomalies that may be noted with ectopic kidney include skeletal, cardiovascular, gastrointestinal, and gynecological abnormalities. Horseshoe kidney is associated with Turner's syndrome and trisomy 18.

Neoplasms

1 Neuroblastomas

Neuroblastoma is actually a malignant tumor arising from the neural elements rather than the kidney but often presents as a mass in the region of the kidney and may invade the kidney. Neuroblastomas can occur anywhere along the spinal column, in the chest, abdomen, or pelvis.

2 Congenital Mesoblastic Nephroma

Congenital mesoblastic nephroma (CMN) is quite rare but is the most common primary renal tumor in the first months of life. Pathologic examination shows congenital mesoblastic nephroma to be distinct from Wilms' tumor. Arteriovenous shunting may occur within the tumor, causing heart failure in the fetus. Many cases demonstrate polyhydramnios.

Abnormalities of Genitalia

Numerous abnormalities of genitalia occur. In males the phallus may be short or bent, and occasionally the scrotum is bifid. In a condition called testicular feminization a male fetus will have genitalia that appear typically female. In females, ambiguous genitalia can also occur. In some cases, the clitoris may be quite prominent and the labia partially fused, suggesting atypical male genitalia. This often occurs in adrenal hyperplasia. In some cases of adrenal hyperplasia the genitalia may appear identical to normal male genitalia. There is also a condition called XX male in which the chromosomes are female but the genitalia are clearly and typically male in appearance.

1 Hydrocele

Hydrocele refers to fluid in the scrotum surrounding the testes. This may occur as an isolated finding with little or no clinical significance but also occurs in patients that have fetal hydrops.

2 Cryptorchidism

The testes do not typically enter the scrotum until after 30 weeks' gestation. If the testes do not descend at the normal time, the condition is called *cryptorchidism*. This may be seen as an isolated finding, or it may be associated with a variety of syndromes.

3 Hydrometrocolpos

There is a wide range of developmental anomalies of the uterus and vagina, including cloacal abnormalities in which the vagina, uterus, and urinary bladder all communicate. In milder conditions, obstruction of the hymen may occur with dilatation of the uterine cavity and vagina (*hydrometrocolpos*). Secondary hydronephrosis may also be observed.

4 Ovarian Cyst

A cyst in the pelvis of a female fetus is most likely an ovarian cyst. These cysts are caused by the high levels of circulating maternal estrogen and usually resolve postnatally.

Gastrointestinal Abnormalities

Embryology

Embryologically, the gastrointestinal (GI) tract is generally referred to in three parts (figure 119):

- The foregut, which includes the esophagus, stomach, liver, pancreas, and part of the duodenum.
- The midgut, consisting of the distal duodenum, jejunum, and proximal colon.
- The hindgut, consisting of the distal colon, rectum, and portions of the vagina and bladder.

During the 6th menstrual week, the stomach forms as a dilatation of a portion of the foregut. Between 8 and 12 weeks, there is herniation of the midgut into the base of the umbilical cord (see figure 103), where it normally undergoes a 270-degree rotation and then returns to the abdomen by 12–14 weeks.

Sonographically, the stomach should be visualized by 14 weeks but may be observed earlier endovaginally. Initially the bowel is somewhat echogenic, and no differentiation between the small bowel and colon is possible until after approximately 22 weeks, when the colon begins to fill with meconium. The large and small bowel gradually increase in diameter throughout pregnancy. At 20 weeks the colon measures approximately 3–5 mm in diameter and at term approximately 18 mm in diameter.

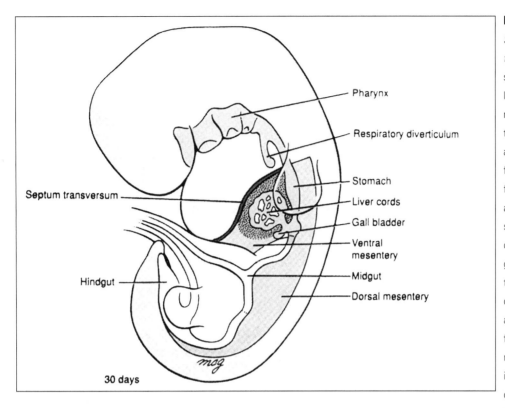

Figure 119.

Structure of the gut tube. The foregut consists of the pharynx, located superior to the respiratory diverticulum, the thoracic esophagus, and the abdominal foregut. The abdominal foregut forms the abdominal esophagus, stomach, and about half of the duodenum and gives rise to the liver, the gallbladder, the pancreas, and their associated ducts. The midgut forms half of the duodenum, the jejunum and ileum, the ascending colon, and about two-thirds of the transverse colon. The hindgut forms one-third of the transverse colon, the descending and sigmoid colons, and the upper two-thirds of the anorectal canal. Reprinted with permission from Larsen WJ: *Human Embryology,* 2nd edition. New York, Churchill Livingstone, 1997.

Position of the Stomach

As a part of routine obstetrical sonogram, the sonographer should determine the position of the stomach in the abdomen. Normally the stomach is in the left upper quadrant and on the same side of the fetus as the cardiac apex. If the stomach and heart are both on the right, the fetus has situs inversus and there is increased risk for Kartagener's syndrome. If the stomach and the heart are on opposite sides of the body, there is a high incidence of associated anomalies, especially cardiac. In these fetuses, polysplenia or asplenia may be present. The spleen may not be visible. An enlarged azygous vein may be observed in polysplenia.

Esophageal Atresia

Esophageal atresia refers to interruption of the esophageal lumen, typically in the chest. In most cases an abnormality of the trachea is also present with a tracheoesophageal fistula, which communicates either with the proximal or distal loop of esophagus. Ninety percent of esophageal atresias have a communicating tracheoesophageal fistula. Thirty to seventy percent of neonates with esophageal atresia have other congenital anomalies, typically of the VACTERL group (vertebral, anal, cardiac, tracheoesophageal, renal, limb). The primary sonographic finding associated with esophageal atresia is polyhydramnios in the second trimester.

Table 5.
Failure to visualize the stomach in the left upper quadrant: possible causes.

Normal stomach has just emptied.
The stomach has been displaced into the chest or into the umbilical cord.
Amniotic fluid is not being produced or fails to reach the amniotic cavity (renal agenesis, posterior urethral valves).
Esophageal atresia exists.
Microgastria is present.

Detection of the atresia is quite difficult sonographically, although it should be suspected in patients with severe polyhydramnios in mid-pregnancy. In such patients, a search for VACTERL-associated anomalies may help to strengthen the suspicion for esophageal atresia. Growth restriction is present in 40% of fetuses that have esophageal atresia.[106] If esophageal atresia is isolated, the survival rate is approximately 79%.[107] If other anomalies are also present, the survival rate is lower.

Nonvisualization of the Stomach

After 14 weeks the stomach is normally visualized sonographically, and if it is not visualized, re-examination should be considered. Persistent failure to visualize the fetal stomach may indicate fetal anomalies, including atresias or CNS abnormalities, with subsequent musculoskeletal defects, which impair swallowing (see table 5).

Occasionally echogenic material is identified within the stomach in the second trimester. This echogenic material may be due to swallowed bloody amniotic fluid. This is sometimes observed in women who have undergone amniocentesis.

Duodenal Atresia

Duodenal atresia is interruption of the GI tract in the second and third portion of the duodenum just beyond the duodenal cap. Sonographically a "double bubble" appearance with a dilated stomach and proximal duodenum can be visualized (figure 120), but this is typically not identified until after 24 weeks. Polyhydramnios will be noted. Approximately 30% of fetuses that have duodenal atresia will have Down syndrome, often accompanied by additional defects including cardiac anomalies.[108, 109] In general, associated anomalies, including skeletal, vertebral, cardiac, gastrointestinal, and renal anomalies, are observed in patients with duodenal atresia.

Small Bowel Obstruction

Small bowel obstruction may occur in the jejunum or ileum for a variety of reasons including atresias and volvulus. Because the bowel takes some time to dilate in utero, the diagnosis is not usually made early in pregnancy. If the

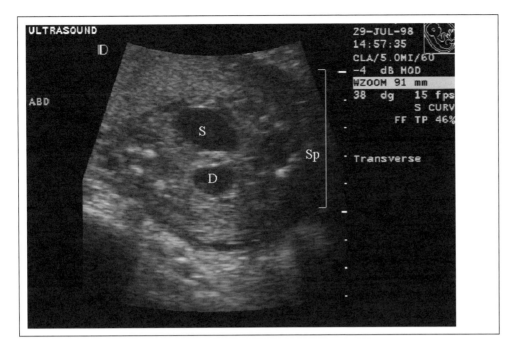

Figure 120.
Duodenal atresia. Transverse sonogram of a fetal abdomen. Note the "double bubble" sign. S = stomach, D = duodenum.

bowel is larger than 7 mm in the mid-abdomen in the second trimester, the possibility of bowel atresia should be considered (see tables 6 and 7). In some cases, bowel hyperperistalsis or intra-abdominal calcifications are identified. Ascites may be noted as well. The calcifications and ascites may be due to bowel perforation. The overall mortality for infants with jejunal or ileal atresia is usually 10% or less. Surgical resection is the typical treatment. Polyhydramnios may be observed if the small bowel atresia is proximal, that is, in the jejunum. If the bowel atresia is distally located in the ileum, polyhydramnios is less common because fluid is reabsorbed above the atresia.

Gestational Age (weeks)	Small Bowel Lumen (mm)		Colon Lumen (mm)		Average Length (mm)	
	Average	Largest	Average	Largest	Small Bowel	Colon
>40	4.4	6	18.7	28	11.3	63.0
35–40	3.7	8	16.8	26	11.0	70.0
30–35	2.9	6	11.4	16	9.8	55.0
25–30	1.8	3	8.0	13	7.9	37.0
20–25	1.4	2	4.4	6	4.5	19.0
15–20	1.2	2	3.6	5	4.5	9.8
10–15	1.0	1	1.5	2	2.4	10.0

Table 6.
Fetal bowel, lumen diameter, and length of contiguous bowel segment.

Reprinted with permission from Parulekar SG: Sonography of normal fetal bowel. *J Ultrasound Med* 10:211–220, 1991.

Table 7.
Risks associated with echogenicity of the fetal bowel.

Cystic fibrosis
Trisomy 13, 18, 21
Cytomegalovirus
Parvovirus
Intra-amniotic blood
Gastrointestinal obstruction
Severe intrauterine growth restriction
Unexplained intrauterine demise

Colon Atresia

Approximately 5–10% of bowel atresias occur in the colon and may be due to vascular insult. Colon atresias do not typically lead to polyhydramnios because fluid is absorbed from the proximal bowel.

One of the common types of colon atresia is anorectal atresia, which is associated with the VACTERL complex of malformations. Enlargement of the colon in the latter part of pregnancy to more than 18 mm in diameter is a sonographic sign that suggests anal atresia may be present (table 6). Another cause of dilated colon segments is Hirschsprung's disease, in which there are abnormal nerve connections in a section of bowel.

Meconium Ileus

In meconium ileus, abnormally thick viscous meconium collects in the small bowel and obstructs and dilates the ileum. The thick, sticky meconium is due to cystic fibrosis. Sonographically, dilated meconium-filled small bowel is noted and the colon is small or not visualized. If this finding is noted in utero, it is likely that the fetus has cystic fibrosis.

Meconium Peritonitis

If bowel atresia or perforation occurs in utero, bowel contents extend into the abdominal cavity, and calcifications may result from the peritoneal irritation. Meconium peritonitis may occur in patients with or without cystic fibrosis. In fetuses with cystic fibrosis, the degree of calcification is typically less. On occasion a meconium pseudocyst may occur with a calcified ring in the abdominal cavity. If the intra-abdominal calcifications are extensive, postnatal surgery may be necessary for bowel perforation and obstruction.

Echogenic Small Bowel

Echogenic small bowel is usually defined as bowel equal to or brighter in echogenicity than the adjacent bone in the ileum (figure 121). Echogenic

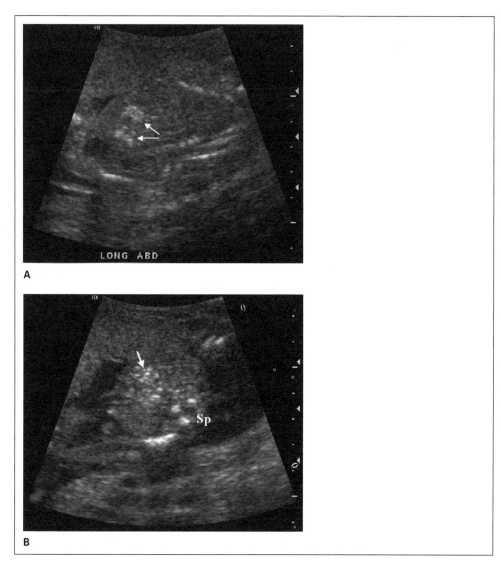

Figure 121.
Echogenic bowel.
A Sagittal sonogram of fetal abdomen demonstrates echogenic bowel (arrows). **B** Transverse sonogram of the same fetus. Note that the echogenic bowel (arrow) is as bright as the spine (Sp).

small bowel may occur as a result of a number of processes, including swallowing of bloody amniotic fluid from intra-amniotic bleeding or amniocentesis. Another cause of echogenic small bowel is cystic fibrosis. Hyperechoic bowel is present on antenatal sonography in 50–80% of fetuses that have cystic fibrosis.[110, 111] If hyperechoic bowel is identified and the gallbladder is not visualized in the second trimester, the fetus may require testing for cystic fibrosis.

Echogenic small bowel has been reported with trisomy 13, 18, and 21. If echogenic bowel is observed, a careful search is indicated for other anomalies, which may suggest chromosomal abnormalities. If other risk factors or other sonographic findings are noted, amniocentesis may be desired for chromosomal characterization (table 7).

Echogenic small bowel includes congenital infections, such as cytomegalovirus and toxoplasmosis. Growth restriction has been observed in approximately

18% of fetuses that have hyperechoic small bowel.[112] There is also an increased incidence of second and third trimester fetal demise with hyperechoic small bowel.

Bowel Duplication

Round, cystic, and long tubular fluid collections in the abdomen may be due to duplication of segments of the bowel. In some cases, peristalsis may be observed in these bowel duplications. Cysts adjacent to or within the biliary system (*choledochal cysts*) may also appear as rounded cystic masses in the abdomen, usually near the porta hepatis.

Fetal Liver

Enlargement of the fetal liver may occur in a number of conditions, including isoimmunization such as Rh disease, congenital infection, and such syndromes as Beckwith-Wiedemann and Zellweger. Normally the liver is quite homogenous; inhomogeneity is abnormal and may suggest hepatitis. Focal hypoechoic masses may be observed in the liver and may represent tumors of the liver, including mesenchymal hamartoma, hemangioendothelioma, or hemangioma. Although rare, hydrops may sometimes occur in these conditions. Calcifications in the liver may be observed in liver masses or may occur alone from intrauterine infection or vascular insult.

Fetal Gallbladder

Typically the fetal gallbladder is visualized by 14–15 menstrual weeks. Cholelithiasis occurs rarely in the fetus. Failure to visualize the fetal gallbladder may suggest cystic fibrosis. Agenesis of the gallbladder may occur occasionally with duodenal atresia or biliary atresia.

Fetal Spleen

The fetal spleen is a relatively small organ in the upper abdomen on the left and may occasionally be visualized in utero. Absent spleen has been reported on a few occasions in fetuses with asplenia or polysplenia. Enlargement of the spleen may be due to infection, such as cytomegalovirus.

Fetal Ascites

Ascites in the abdomen may be associated with many conditions, including immune and nonimmune hydrops, urinary tract obstruction, congenital infections, abdominal tumors, thoracic tumors, and bowel obstruction with perforation. In some individuals, the abdominal wall musculature may be confused with ascites, particularly in the upper abdomen. This finding is referred to as *pseudoascites*.

Skeletal Abnormalities

The normal fetal skeleton begins to form at 6–7 menstrual weeks, and the skeleton begins to ossify at 9 weeks in the clavicle and 10–11 weeks in the skull and vertebral bodies. By the end of the first trimester all the long bones, skull, spine, ribs, and pelvis have begun to ossify. The epiphyses and carpal bones do not show ossification until much later.

In general there is earlier ossification of bones in females than in males. When the bones are developing, the muscles are developing as well, and for normal joint development to occur, both the muscles and the bones must develop normally.

Abnormal Fetal Skeleton

A classification for general limb anomalies has been developed. According to this system, the limb defects are generally classified into seven categories, as follows.

   I.   Failure of formation of parts (arrest of development).

   II. Failure of differentiation (separation parts).

   III. Duplication.

   IV. Overgrowth (gigantism).

   V.   Undergrowth (hypoplasia).

   VI. Congenital constriction bands syndrome.

   VII. Generalized skeletal abnormalities.

If there is an abnormal environment during the normal differentiation process of embryogenesis, the portion of the limb that is changing most rapidly at that time will be affected. This may be a result of anoxia, drugs, hormones, infections, radiation, or hyperglycemia.

Short-Limb Skeletal Dysplasia

A particularly important group of abnormalities consists of fetuses that have noticeably short limbs in utero. Short-limb skeletal dysplasias can be separated into two general classes of conditions:

1. Dysplasias in which the fetal long bones are notably shortened by 20 weeks.

2. Fetal conditions in which the limbs are notably shortened only in later pregnancy.

For instance in *thanatophoric dwarfism,* the fetal long bone lengths may be normal until 12–13 weeks. In *achondroplasia,* the fetal limb lengths may be normal until 20–30 weeks.

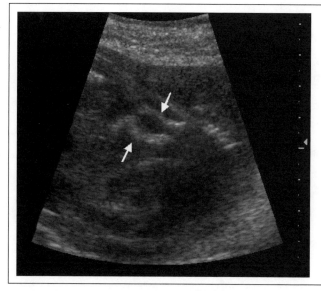

Figure 122.
Extremity bone shortening in dwarfism. Sagittal sonogram of the tibia and fibula in a fetus with thanatophoric dwarfism. Note that the bones are short and wide and slightly curved (arrows).

Skeletal dysplasias in which limbs are notably short before 20 weeks are usually lethal at birth (figure 122). Many of these conditions can be specifically diagnosed prenatally.

In a much larger group of skeletal dysplasias, fetal limb lengths are more mildly shortened; in this group, the limbs will not demonstrate significant shortening until the end of the second trimester. Only a few of these conditions can be specifically identified in utero.

Fetal Examination for Suspected Short-Limb Skeletal Dysplasia

In addition to the usual examination of the fetus, additional assessment is necessary if a short-limb skeletal dysplasia is suspected (table 8).

1. *All the long bones,* including both femoral, tibiae, fibulae, humeri, radiae, and ulnae, should be imaged and the lengths measured. Also, the morphology of the long bones and the sonographic reflectivity of the long bones should be evaluated.

2. *Fetal skull.* The shape and density of the skull should be evaluated. If the skull appears to be underossified, compressing the skull with the transducer may indicate whether the skull is abnormally flexible.

3. *Fetal ribs and chest.* If a fetal skeletal dysplasia is suspected, fetal chest circumference should be obtained at the level of the fetal heart, and the length and character of the ribs should be observed. Irregular or fractured ribs should be noted. The fetal scapula should be specifically imaged in transverse and longitudinal planes.

4. *Fetal spine.* The fetal spine should be imaged with particular attention to the ossified vertebral bodies.

Table 8. Sonographic assessment of bones.

Anatomic Site	Assess For
Long bones	Degree of limb shortening Pattern of limb shortening Degree of mineralization Presence of fractures, bowing, or angulation Abnormal shape or contour Limb reduction anomalies Hypoplastic or aplastic bones
Calvarium	Macrocranium Frontal bossing Craniosynostosis Compressibility/abnormal degree of mineralization
Thorax	Thoracic length and circumference Hypoplastic ribs "Bell-shaped" thorax of pulmonary hypoplasia Convex contour in cross section Scapula
Spine	Degree and pattern of mineralization Platyspondyly Anomalies of segmentation or curvature Caudal regression syndrome Myelodysplasia
Hands and feet	Postural deformities Abnormal number of digits Syndactyly
Facial features	Cleft lip and palate Hypertelorism and hypotelorism Flat nasal bridge/"saddle nose"

5. *Fetal hands and feet.* The fetal hands and feet should be carefully examined to evaluate the length of the fingers and toes, to check for polydactyly, and to check for positioning abnormalities such as clubfeet or rocker-bottom feet.

6. *Fetal face.* Later in pregnancy, there may be clues in the appearance of the fetal face that will help differentiate among skeletal dysplasias.

Lethal Skeletal Dysplasias

If a sonographer finds a fetus that has markedly shortened limbs before 20 weeks, this fetus is likely to represent one of two short-limb skeletal dysplasias.

1 Thanatophoric Dwarfism

Thanatophoric dwarfism (TD) is the most common short-limb skeletal dysplasia, with reported incidence of 1 in 6000 and 1 in 17,000 births.[113–115] It is caused by one of two single-point mutations in the FGFR3 gene (fibroblast growth factor receptor-3, located on chromosome 4). These two different types of thanatophoric dysplasias are similar but do not have exactly the same appearance. The most notable difference between the two is that one has curved long bones, especially femurs, and the other has straighter long bones and is more likely to have a cloverleaf skull.

Sonographic Findings

In thanatophoric dwarfism, all the long bones are markedly shortened and densely ossified. As noted above, there may be curving of the long bones (figure 123), particularly the femur, but this is not required. In addition, the thorax is small, with a chest circumference typically less than the 5th percentile for age (figure 124). The chest may be bell shaped in the coronal plane, and there may be a marked discrepancy in A-P chest diameter compared with A-P abdominal diameter. More specifically, the ribs tend to extend to the mid-axillary line (figure 125) rather than extending farther forward as is

Figure 123.
Thanatophoric dwarf femur. Longitudinal sonogram of fetal femur. Note bowing and cartilegenous epiphyses (arrows).

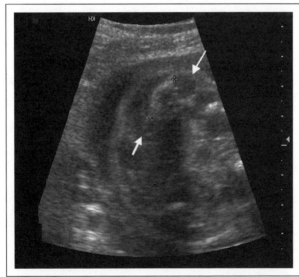

Figure 124A.
Small chest in a thanatophoric dwarf. Transverse sonogram of fetal chest.

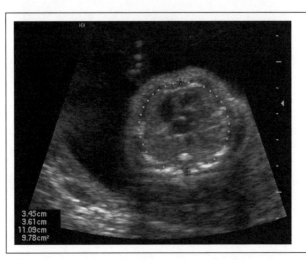

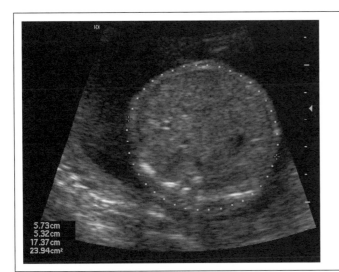

Figure 124B.

Small chest in a thanatophoric dwarf. Transverse abdomen. Note the chest is much smaller than the abdomen.

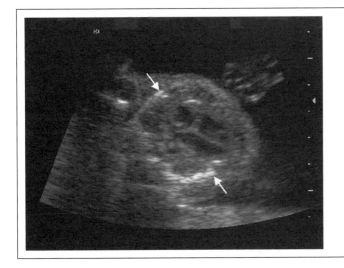

Figure 125.

Transverse sonogram of the fetal chest in a thanatophoric dwarf. Note the shortened ribs that end at the mid-axillary line (arrows).

normally observed. Evaluation of the fetal spine shows platyspondyly. The vertebral bodies are markedly flattened, with wide hypoechoic disc spaces between them (figure 126). Careful examination must be made to differentiate the vertebral bodies from the lateral masses of the spine because lateral masses will be larger than the vertebral bodies. The fetal skull may be brachycephalic or may show marked abnormality with a tri-lobed outline (cloverleaf or Kleeblattschadel) (figure 127). In this condition, there is marked bulging of the temporal bones and the frontal bone. Polydactyly is not observed in thanatophoric dwarfism.

2 Osteogenesis Imperfecta Type II

The second most common short-limb condition observed in utero is type II osteogenesis imperfecta. The incidence of osteogenesis imperfecta type II is approximately 1 in 54,000.[114] In this condition, there is abnormal formation of type I collagen, which may be caused by many different gene mutations

Figure 126.
Platyspondyly in a thanatophoric dwarf. Sagittal sonogram of the fetal spine reveals wide spaces between the ossified vertebrae.

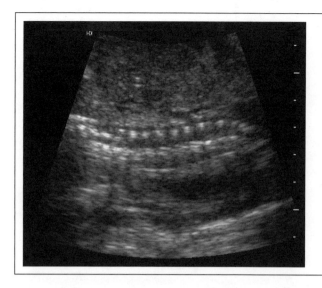

Figure 127.
Kleeblahtschadel cranium. Sonogram of a fetal head. Note the cloverleaf appearance of the cranium with lateral bulging of the temporal bones (arrows).

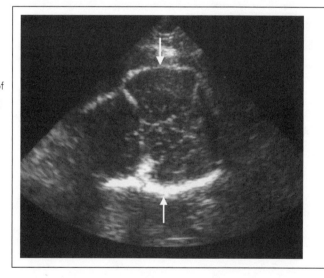

in one of two collagen genes. Type II osteogenesis imperfecta is usually caused by a new dominant mutation but rarely can be inherited in a recessive manner.

Sonographic Findings

The fetal long bones are shortened and irregular in outline, appearing crumpled because of multiple fractures (figure 128). If fractures are few, the long bones may appear translucent and the posterior surface of the bone may be visible (figure 129).

The fetal skull is often underossified and may be difficult to detect. The fetal head may be soft and pliable under the transducer (figure 130). The fetal spine is usually normally ossified, but rarely platyspondyly may be observed in osteogenesis imperfecta type II. The fetal chest usually demonstrates

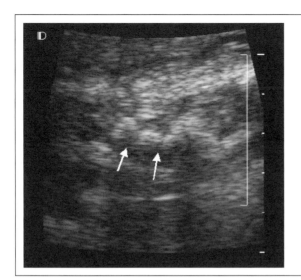

Figure 128.

Femur fracture in osteogenesis imperfecta type II. Longitudinal sonogram of a femur reveals bowing and fractures (arrows).

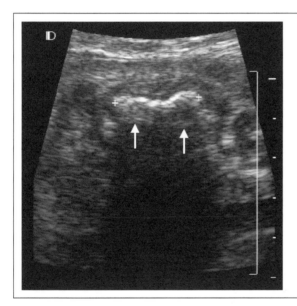

Figure 129.

Translucent bone in osteogenesis imperfecta type II. Longitudinal sonogram of fetal femur. Note the posterior surface of the bone is visible (arrows).

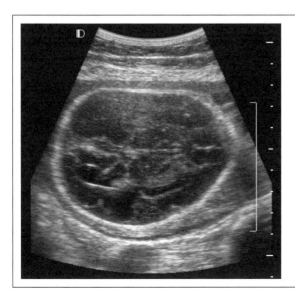

Figure 130.

Fetal skull in osteogenesis imperfecta type II. The skull is not well ossified and flattens with transducer pressure.

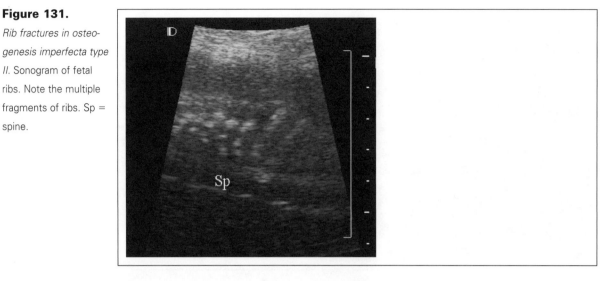

Figure 131.
Rib fractures in osteogenesis imperfecta type II. Sonogram of fetal ribs. Note the multiple fragments of ribs. Sp = spine.

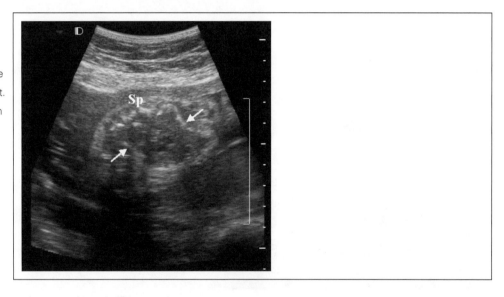

Figure 132.
"Caved-in" chest in osteogenesis imperfecta type II. Transverse sonogram of fetal chest. The ribs are longer than those in thanatophoric dwarfism, but there is concavity of ribs laterally (arrows). Sp = spine.

longer ribs than are observed in thanatophoric dwarfism. The ribs usually extend to the anterior axillary line. In many cases the ribs are irregular in outline with evidence of multiple fractures (figure 131). A characteristic appearance is seen in many cases of lethal osteogenesis imperfecta type II in which the ribs are "caved in" laterally (figure 132). This is due to motion of the fetal arms causing fractures of the ribs.

3 Other Lethal Skeletal Dysplasias

In addition to thanatophoric dwarfism and osteogenesis imperfecta type II, several other less common lethal skeletal dysplasias are relatively easy to diagnose sonographically. In all cases the bones are very short. In *achondrogenesis,* there is virtually no ossification of the vertebral bodies; however, the posterior elements of the spine may be visible. In *short-rib polydactyly syndrome,* the ribs are markedly shortened and the chest is very small in

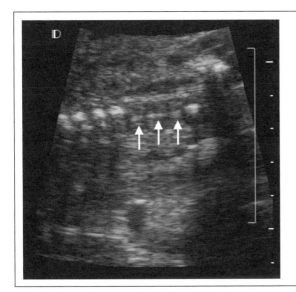

Figure 133.
Fetal spine hypophosphatasia. Longitudinal sonogram of lumbar vertebral bodies. Note that three bodies are unossified (arrows).

circumference. Typically the ribs reach only the posterior axillary line. Polydactyly of the fingers is also present, and the vertebral bodies are usually well ossified.

In *lethal hypophosphatasia,* the fetal long bones may be markedly shortened, with deep cupping of the metaphyses. In addition, the ribs may be short and fragmented. The skull may be markedly underossified. The spine may have groups of three ossified, then three unossified, then three ossified vertebral bodies, in an alternating pattern (figure 133).

Short-Limb Skeletal Dysplasias with Milder Limb Shortening

A few skeletal dysplasias with milder limb shortening may be diagnosed prenatally. The most common of these is *heterozygous achondroplasia,* which occurs 1 in 20,000–30,000 births.[113–115] In this condition there is mild platyspondyly and mild limb shortening. Other subtle findings, including narrowing of the interpedicular distance in the lumbar spine and frontal bossing of the skull, may be observed. This condition is somewhat difficult to diagnose prenatally unless one of the parents is an achondroplastic dwarf. If both parents are achondroplastic dwarfs, a recessive form of achondroplasia is sometimes observed, which is much more severe and is always lethal. The defective gene has been identified for achondroplasia and is the same FGFR3 gene that is affected in thanatophoric dysplasia, but a different single-point mutation is the cause of achondroplasia.

Camptomelic Dysplasia

Camptomelic dysplasia is a rarer dysplasia, reported to occur in 1 in 100,000–200,000 births.[116] The limb shortening is variable, but specific features may suggest the diagnosis, including a mid-femoral sharp bend in each

Figure 134.
Camptomelic dwarf.
A Longitudinal sonogram of a femur in a fetus with camptomelic dysplasia. Note the sharp angulation in the mid-femur. **B** Sagittal sonogram of the scapula in the same fetus. Note the very short length of the scapular blade (arrow).

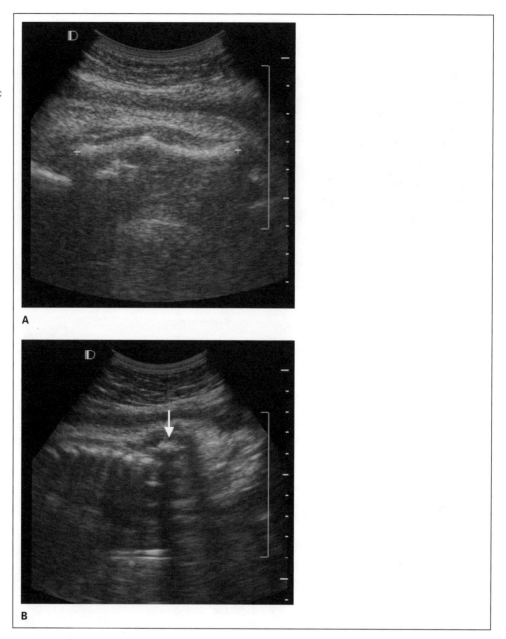

femur (figure 134A). Bends in the distal tibia may occur as well. Clubfeet are usually observed, and a short scapula is noted (figure 134B). The prognosis for this condition is variable, but many may die during early postnatal life. At least one survivor has been reported at age 17.[117] This condition is due to a mutation in the SOX9 gene on chromosome 17.

Mild Osteogenesis Imperfecta

Some cases of osteogenesis imperfecta are much milder and are not lethal at birth. These milder forms may not be detectable in utero, but some may be observed because of fractures or underossification of bones.

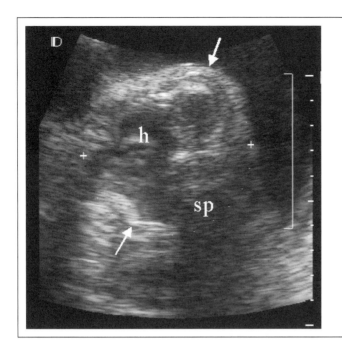

Figure 135.

Cloverleaf chest in ATD. Transverse sonogram of the chest of a fetus with asphyxiating thoracic dysplasia. Note the trilobed appearance of the chest. The ribs are short and bowed laterally (arrows). The heart (h) lies between the ossified ends of the ribs. Sp=spine.

Asphyxiating Thoracic Dystrophy (Jeune Syndrome)

A few cases of asphyxiating thoracic dystrophy have been detected prenatally. These fetuses typically have a relatively small chest and may have polydactyly. Renal disease is common in these individuals. The incidence is reported to be 1 in 72,000, and approximately 60% die from respiratory compromise.[114] In our experience, severely affected fetuses may show an unusual "cloverleaf chest" (figure 135).

Chondroectodermal Dysplasia (Ellis-Van Creveld Syndrome)

Another condition, which may be suspected in utero, is Ellis-Van Creveld syndrome. These fetuses have short limbs and have polydactyly of the feet in every case. There are changes in the hair, teeth, and nails, which are probably not observable sonographically. Congenital heart disease is present in 50% of cases. Mortality in infancy is approximately 50%, usually due to cardiorespiratory problems.[118]

Metatropic Dysplasia

Another rare condition that is diagnosable in utero is *metatrophic dysplasia*. In this condition there is markedly exaggerated enlargement of the metaphyses in the bones (figure 136A). The chest may be somewhat small, and there is platyspondyly (figure 136B).

Focal Limb Anomalies

In addition to generalized skeletal dysplasias, a number of anomalies of the extremities may occur alone or as a part of various syndromes.

Figure 136.
Metatropic dysplasia.
A Sagittal sonogram of femur in a fetus with metatrophic dysplasia. Note the marked widening of the metaphysis and large femoral condyles (C). **B** Sagittal spine, same fetus. Note platyspondyly.

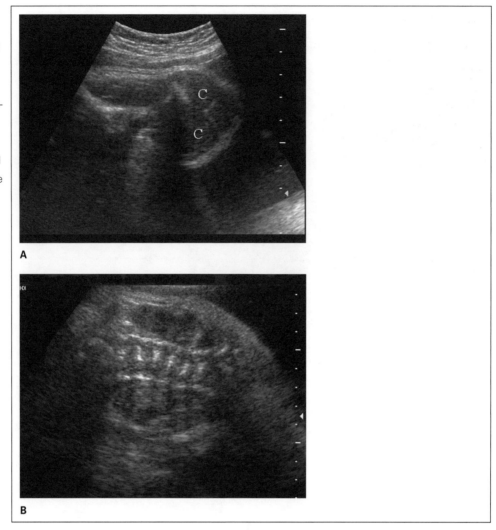

1 Radial Ray Abnormalities

Absence of the radius is a fairly common abnormality, which may be observed in a number of syndromes including trisomy 18 and many rarer syndromes. The radius may be absent without other anomalies or in association with vertebral anomalies and tracheoesophageal atresia. If the radius is absent, typically the thumb is also absent, and the fingers lie perpendicular to the ulna.

2 Clubfoot Deformity

Deformation of the foot can occur as a part of a syndrome or alone (figure 137). The incidence of clubfoot is 1–7 per 1000.[119] Clubfoot may be a finding associated with spina bifida. A similar deformity called *rocker-bottom foot,* in which there is hyperextension of the foot, is observed in trisomy 18.

3 Focal Femoral Hypoplasia

Occasionally isolated shortening of one or both femurs may be observed. This is sometimes observed in infants of diabetic mothers.

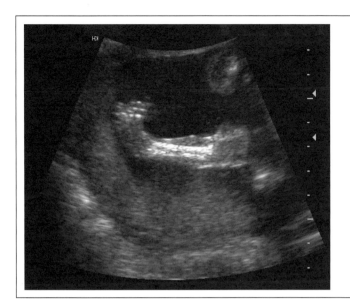

Figure 137.
Clubfoot. Longitudinal sonogram of the lower leg. Note that the toes are in the same plane as the tibia.

Cardiac Abnormalities

An extensive body of knowledge exists about fetal echocardiography. Echocardiography recognizes and documents a wide variety of fetal cardiac disease. Fetal echo helps determine if in utero treatment is necessary and is used to manage the delivery of fetuses with cardiac abnormalities.[120]

The incidence of congenital heart disease is approximately 1 in 100 live births.[121-123] Ventricular and atrial septal defects are the most common cardiac abnormalities to be imaged.[124] Other obvious cardiac abnormalities may be reliably visualized and documented using fetal ultrasound. Some of these include Ebstein's anomaly, tricuspid atresia, persistent truncus arteriosus, hypoplastic left heart syndrome, double-outlet right ventricle, single ventricle, atrioventricular canal, and transposition of the great arteries.

In this section we will discuss the initial assessment of the fetal heart and related anatomy on routine obstetrical examination. The discussion here will not be extensive enough to cover all the material on the fetal portion of an echocardiography examination. If a cardiac abnormality is detected on an initial obstetrical examination, or if there is strong suspicion on the basis of clinical data, a complete fetal echocardiogram is recommended and should be performed as a separate procedure from the obstetrical examination.

Indications

As a part of the routine obstetrical examination, particular attention should be given to assessment of the fetal heart when there are maternal and/or familial factors present for cardiac disease. Maternal risk factors include a history of diabetes mellitus, drugs, polyhydramnios, oligohydramnios, and collagen vascular disease. Phenylketonuria, and infections such as rubella, CMV, and coxsackie virus also preclude a careful examination of the fetal heart. Familial factors include left heart obstructive lesions and genetic syndromes (hypertrophic cardiomyopathy, DiGeorge, Holt-Oram, Noonan, marfans and tuberous sclerosis).[125]

Sonographic Findings

During an obstetrical sonogram, indications that a complete fetal echocardiogram would be helpful include[125-127]:

- Situs inversus.
- Asplenia.
- Dextrocardia.
- Enlarged heart.
- Obvious abnormal findings in the fetal heart.
- Sustained cardiac arrhythmia.
- Increased nuchal translucency found early in pregnancy.
- Small for gestational age.
- Extracardiac abnormalities.
- 2-vessel umbilical cord.

Fetal position may make the ultrasound exam difficult. An anterior location of the spine creates posterior shadowing, often obscuring images of the heart. However, once the sonographer has established fetal lie, the location of the liver, right and left kidneys, stomach, spleen, inferior vena cava, and aorta, in relationship to the spine in a transverse image, should be documented. This determines situs. A superior sweep of the beam in this plane into the thoracic cavity reveals a four-chamber view of the heart (figures 138A and B). It lies at an approximate angle of 45 degrees relative to midline, just above the diaphragm, in a more horizontal position at this stage of development. The right ventricle is the closest chamber to the fetal anterior chest wall. The stomach and heart are both normally located on the fetal left side, further proving cardiac sidedness. A sagittal view of the fetal body illustrates the abdominal and thoracic cavities and an optimal view of the heart and stomach with relationship to the diaphragm.

The heart should be examined during routine fetal sonography. Normally it occupies approximately one-third of the cross-sectional area of the fetal thorax. Traditional views of the heart may be attempted as fetal lie allows. The angle of the beam may not be traditional but it can project and document the

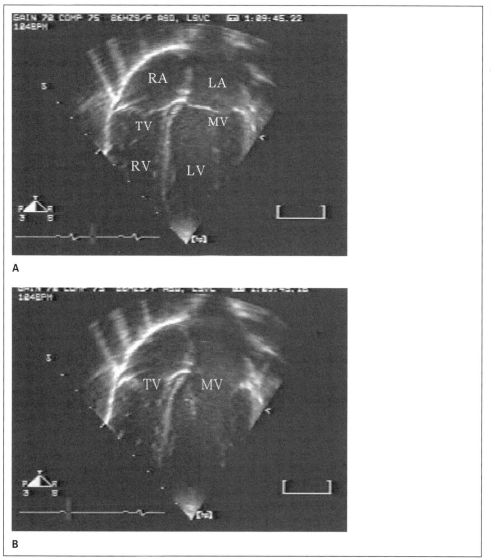

Figure 138.
Normal four-chamber view of the fetal heart.
A Systole. **B** Diastole.

same information. Standard views and beam orientation are shown in figure 139. In the four-chamber view, the two ventricles should be approximately equal in size, as should the two atria. The atrioventricular valves are often visualized, and the foramen ovale may be imaged in many cases. If observed, it should be bowing predominantly toward the left atrium. The right ventricle has a more irregular internal margin. The left ventricle is smooth-walled. Chordae tendinae may sometimes be imaged extending from the ventricular wall to the edges of the atrioventricular valves.

In the normal fetal heart, a short-axis view of the left ventricle will reveal two papillary muscles, neither of which is located on the interventricular septum.

The associated bicuspid mitral valve may be demonstrated just superiorly to the papillary muscles in this same plane. A sagittal plane through the normal fetal thorax is helpful to obtain a short-axis view of the heart. These images

Figure 139.
Sonographic views and approaches to the fetal heart and great vessels. The axis of the fetal heart is more horizontal compared with its postnatal lie in the chest (center). Note that all the views are shown as being obtained from the chest or the abdominal wall; however, it is also possible to achieve all these imaging planes from the back. **A** Four-chamber view showing both atria and the foramen ovale within the atrial septum, both ventricles, and the atrioventricular valves. **B** After slight clockwise rotation and tilt of the transducer toward the fetal left shoulder, the long axis comes into view. **C** Further clockwise rotation and tilt of the transducer results in sagitally oriented planes, which are valuable for depicting the aortic arch and the "ductus arch." **D** Perpendicular to the long axis, the short-axis views are obtained. At the base of the heart, the aorta lies centrally and is surrounded by the structures of the right ventricle and the pulmonary artery, as postnatally. **E** Further toward the apex, the left ventricular structure with two papillary muscles can be seen. Reprinted with permission from Silverman NH, Schmidt KG: Ultrasound evaluation of the fetal heart. In Callen PW (ed): *Ultrasonography in Obstetrics and Gynecology*, 4th edition. Philadelphia, Saunders, 2000, p 380.

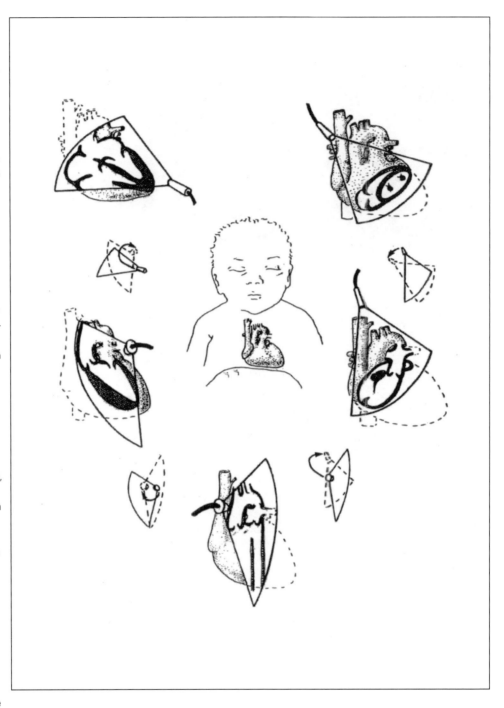

are desired to demonstrate atrioventricular canal and other cardiac anomalies. Although many other cardiac anomalies can occur, the following conditions are some of the more common and sonographically recognizable in the four-chamber view:

- Atrioventricular canal.
- Single ventricle.
- Ebstein's anomaly.

- Hypertrophied or dilated ventricles.
- Ventricular hypoplasia.
- Tricuspid or mitral valve atresia.

Assessment of the outflow tracts cannot be made from the four-chamber view. Specific evaluation of the outflow tracts may require off-axis images. Cardiac imaging of complex abnormalities such as D- and L-transposition, tetralogy of Fallot, persistent truncus arteriosus and double-outlet right ventricle needs to be performed in multiple views with segmental analysis and careful attention to proving great artery-ventricular association and orientation. This may be difficult and beyond the scope of the obstetrical exam. Additional images in the traditional and off-axis views, with color and pulsed-wave Doppler interrogation, would be necessary for a cardiologist to make a definitive diagnosis. This degree of imaging would normally occur during a fetal echo in the specialized setting of a pediatric cardiac echocardiography laboratory.[127]

If imaging is optimal in a short-axis view at the level of the aortic valve, the sonographer may demonstrate the crossing of the great arteries and the normal main pulmonary artery dividing into right and left branches. Rotating the notch of the transducer counterclockwise from the fetal orientation, moving slightly superiorly on the fetal chest, then directing the beam to the fetus' left may allow visualization of the ductus connecting the distal main pulmonary artery or proximal left pulmonary artery branch to the descending aortic arch. Sliding the transducer slightly superiorly may demonstrate the aortic arch and branches and a short-axis view of the right pulmonary artery. Structural abnormalities, which may be suspected on routine obstetrical sonography requiring additional images, include the following:

1 Atrial Ventricular Septal Defects

Atrial ventricular septal defects (figure 140) may not be visible if small. Isolated atrial septal defects may not be detectable in utero because blood flow in the fetus normally crosses the foramen ovale.[128]

2 Ebstein's Anomaly

In *Ebstein's anomaly,* the tricuspid valve is displaced deeper than normal into the right ventricle (color plate 11). Tricuspid regurgitation may be severe and the right ventricle overloaded. The right ventricular outflow tract may be compromised as well due to poor right ventricular function.[129–132] Pulmonary stenosis in varying degrees or atresia is an associated anomaly.[133–135] Atrial septal defects are also a common finding.[136]

Figure 140.
Atrial septal defect (ASD). Subcostal coronal view of the heart demonstrating an ASD (arrow). A large pericardial effusion is also present.

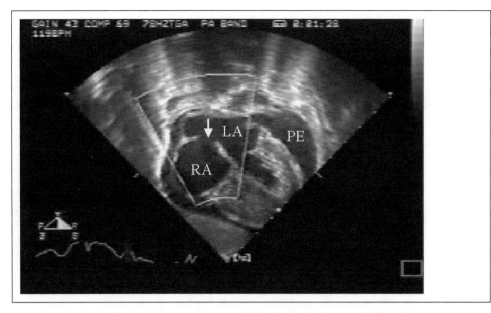

Figure 141.
Hypoplastic left heart syndrome. Apical four-chamber view in systole. Note the small left ventricle and mitral atresia (arrow).

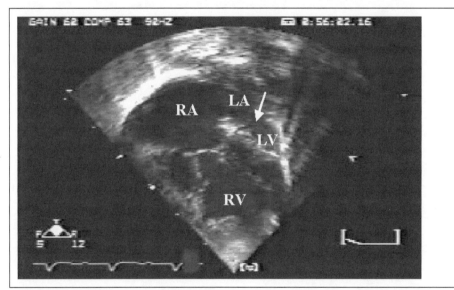

3 Hypoplastic Left Heart Syndrome

In *hypoplastic left heart syndrome* (HLHS), the left ventricle and atria are smaller than usual (figure 141), and typically there are abnormalities involving hypoplasia and stenosis or atresia of the mitral and aortic valves. Hypoplasia of the ascending aorta and aortic arch are common. Coarctation can result and is commonly found with a large patent ductus arteriosus (PDA).[137–139] The PDA may be seen in a high left parasternal window (figure 142).

4 Coarctation

Coarctation may be observed outside the constellation of left-sided obstructions (figure 143). It often presents with a bicuspid aortic valve.[140] A large

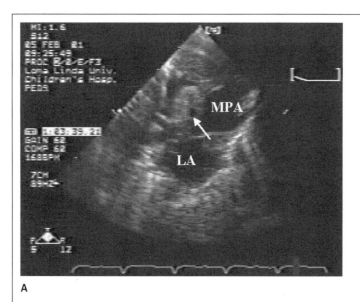

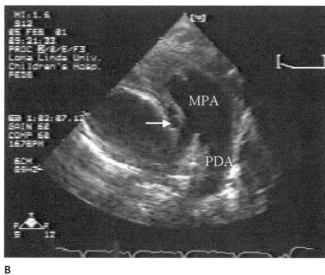

Figure 142.
Hypoplastic left heart syndrome. Dilated pulmonary artery, pinhole aorta. **A** Suprasternal notch (crab view). **B** High short-axis ductal view. Note the large main pulmonary artery, right pulmonary artery, and very small ascending aorta (arrow) in transverse.

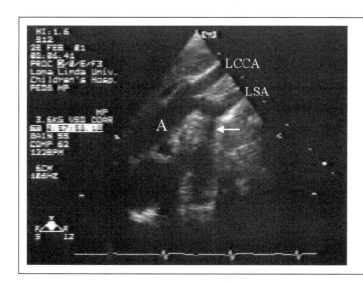

Figure 143A.
Coarctation of the aorta. Suprasternal notch long-axis view of the aorta. Note the coarctation (arrow) of the aorta just after the left subclavian artery (LSA) branches off from the aortic arch.

Figure 143B.
Coarctation of the aorta. Calipers measure the transverse arch and coarcted area (arrow).

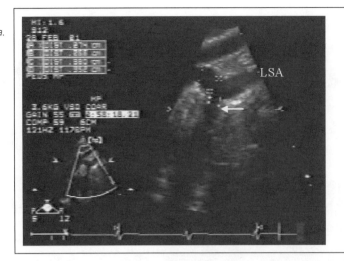

perimembranous ventriculoseptal defect requires interrogation of the aortic arch to rule out this pathology. Imaging a fetal coarctation may be extremely difficult.[141, 142]

5 Single Ventricle

In *single ventricle* the interventricular septum does not develop completely or at all. There may be either one or two atrial ventricular valves (figure 144). Physiologic or anatomic single ventricle is commonly found in double outlet right ventricle, double outlet left ventricle, univentricular atrioventricular connections and cardiac malpositions, and abnormalities of atrial and ventricular situs.

Figure 144.
Single ventricle. **A** Apical four-chamber view in systole. Note double inlet left ventricle (SV, single ventricle). **B** Slightly different view in systole also demonstrating double inlet left ventricle. **C** Apical four-chamber view in diastole demonstrates complete AVC with a single ventricle (SV). AVV (atrial ventricular valve).

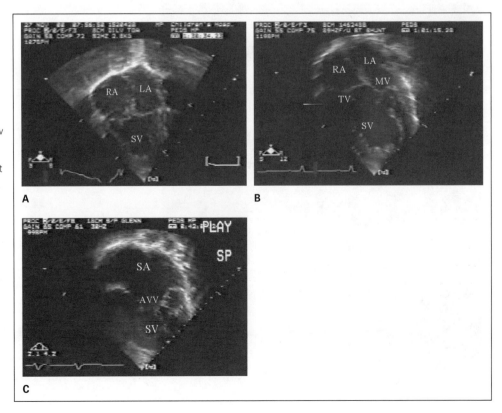

6 Persistent Truncus Arteriosus

In *persistent truncus arteriosus,* there is typically a single large vessel arising from the base of the heart anteriorly, which overrides the interventricular septum creating a large septal defect. The pulmonary arteries arise from this single vessel in different configurations (color plate 12). In some cases the left branch pulmonary artery may have anomalous origins or may be absent.[143–146]

7 Transposition of the Great Arteries

In *D-transposition,* the heart tube develops in a normal dextro-looping pattern. The ventriculoarterial orientation, however, is reversed from normal. The aorta rises from the right ventricle and the pulmonary artery from the left ventricle (figure 145). The morphologic and anatomic right ventricle is therefore pumping blood to the system while the morphologic and anatomic left ventricle is pumping blood to the pulmonary vasculature. Aside from a large patent ductus arteriosus and atrial septal defect, assuming a ventriculoseptal defect is not present, this pathology is not compatible with life. In *congenitally corrected*

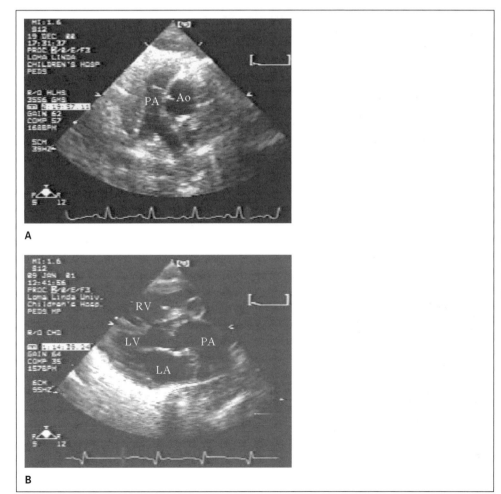

Figure 145.

Transposition of the great arteries. **A** Suprasternal notch approach (SSN) and short-axis view of the great vessels. Note the pulmonary artery (PA) and branch arteries are rightward of ascending aorta (AO) in diastole. **B** Left parasternal long axis view. Note the great vessels are parallel, with pulmonary artery (PA) off the LV.

or L-transposition of the great arteries there is atrioventricular discordance, as well as ventriculoarterial discordance. The right morphologic ventricle and tricuspid valve arise from the left anatomic atrium, and the left morphologic ventricle and mitral valve arises from the right anatomic atrium. The pulmonary artery is located on the right side of the heart but arises from the anatomic right, morphologic left ventricle. The aorta is situated on the left side of the heart, but arises from the left anatomic, right morphologic ventricle. The right morphologic ventricle again pumps blood systemically, however it is oxygenated blood from the left atrium.[147] The left morphologic ventricle pumps blood to the pulmonary vasculature. There are other cardiac anomalies that may present with this pathological condition that warrant imaging in a pediatric cardiac lab.

8 Tetralogy of Fallot

Tetralogy of Fallot presents with a large, anteriorly malaligned ventriculoseptal defect due to an overriding aorta, resulting in degrees of pulmonary valve hypoplasia to atresia. The right ventricular outflow tract may also be hypoplastic. It

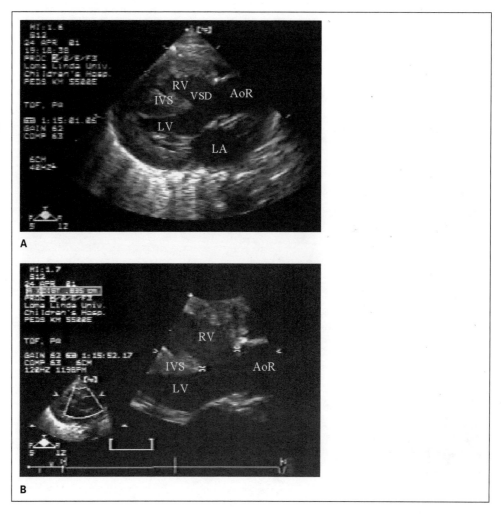

Figure 146.
Tetralogy of Fallot.
A Parasternal long-axis view in systole. Note the overriding aorta (AoR, VSD, and RV) hypertrophy. **B** Zoomed view.

can present with muscle bundles, creating a subvalvar stenosis and gradient. Right ventricular hypertrophy may not be present due to the various shunts found in the fetal circulation. The posterior aortic root retains continuity with the anterior leaflet mitral valve annulus orientation (figure 146).

9 Double-Outlet Right Ventricle

In *double-outlet right ventricle,* a ventriculoseptal defect is present. Both the aorta and pulmonary artery arise from the right ventricle (figure 147). Diagnosis is confirmed by documenting lack of continuity between the posterior aortic root and the anterior leaflet mitral valve (ALMV) annulus. In utero, it is proven more commonly with visualization of both great arteries committed primarily to more than 50% to the right ventricle.[148–150]

10 Cardiomyopathy

When *cardiomyopathy* (CMP) is present, the fetal heart may appear abnormally large, with either dilated chambers or thick ventricular septum and walls (figure 148). Atrioventricular valve regurgitation is common in dilated cardiomyopathy. When imaging what appears to be a hypertrophied left ventricle and septum, PW Doppler analysis should be made from the apex to the aortic valve in short increments to reveal a potential gradient. M-mode of the

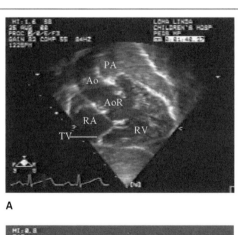
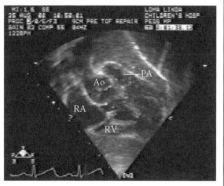

Figure 147.
Double-outlet right ventricle. **A** Subcostal coronal view of great vessels and RV. Note the aorta, proximal pulmonary artery, and tricuspid valve. **B** Subcostal coronal view. Note pulmonary and aortic valves. **C** Short-axis view zoomed on outlet view of both great arteries. Note both great arteries arising from RV.

Figure 148.
Dilated and hypertrophic cardiomyopathy. **A–B** Dilated cardiomyopathy. **C** Hypertrophic cardiomyopathy.

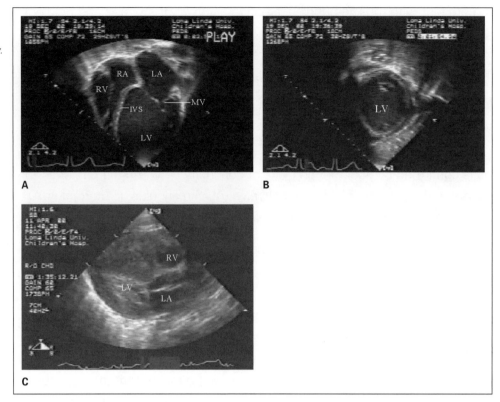

short or long axis left ventricle in either cardiomyopathy is helpful to determine chamber size, left ventricular wall and septum thickness, and to evaluate cardiac function.

11 Atrioventricular Canal

A primum atrial septal defect and inlet ventricular septal defect indicate *atrioventricular canal* (AVC). Complete AVC is a more obvious find. Color Doppler must be used to demonstrate the degree of atrioventricular valve regurgitation. Complete atrioventricular canal presents with a "gooseneck" deformity caused from narrowing of the left ventricular outflow tract. This occurs as the aorta is malaligned anteriorly and superiorly from its normal position in the fold between the annuluses of the two atrioventricular valves.[151] Atrioventricular canal may be balanced or unbalanced. It can present with two atrioventricular valves (color plate 13).

Many other cardiac anomalies can occur, but these are some of the more common and recognizable sonographic abnormalities in the fetal heart.

Situs Abnormalities

Situs inversus and *heterotaxia* may be an indication of a wide variety of fetal abnormalities. Cardiac anomalies are common. Careful and thoughtful attention must be given to segmental scanning of the fetal heart and related anatomy, as in any potential heart disease.

Cardiac Tumors

Rarely, echogenic masses may be observed within the fetal heart. Among cardiac tumors, rhabdomyoma is the most common. An association has been established between rhabdomyomas and tuberous sclerosis.[152, 153] Other tumors that may be imaged in the fetal heart include teratomas, fibromas, hemangiomas, and myxomas. None of these may be histologically diagnosed with ultrasound. However, the location, size, and echogenicity of each tumor need to be determined in multiple planes of imaging.

Abnormalities of Fetal Heart Rate and Rhythm

In the second and third trimester, the fetal heart rate may vary. An average heart rate in the fetus is 140 ± 20 beats per minute.[154] When fetal arrhythmias are observed, the sonographer should lift the transducer until the heart rate and rhythm return to normal and then proceed. The frequency and duration of these episodes should be noted if possible. Patients presenting with these types of fetal abnormalities should be referred to a pediatric cardiologist for further evaluation.

Syndromes

Thousands of syndromes have been described in humans. A *syndrome* is a collection of abnormalities that occur together, usually with a specific cause. Of all the syndromes that are known, there is a rather small group that are relatively common and that can be effectively evaluated with sonography.

Trisomy 21 (Down Syndrome)

Down syndrome is the most common syndrome observed in humans, with an overall incidence of approximately 1 in 600–800 newborns.[155] The incidence of Down syndrome increases with advancing maternal age; at the maternal age of 40, the incidence is approximately 1 in 75 pregnancies.[156] Using sonography to diagnose Down syndrome is relatively difficult, as most of the findings observed in Down syndrome are subtle and nonspecific. Because the sonographic findings in Down syndrome can be difficult to detect, other screening programs are used as the primary methods for detecting Down syndrome in younger women. When the mother is over the age of 35, the incidence of Down syndrome is approximately 1 in 275,[157] and in many states, all these woman are offered amniocentesis if they desire it. In younger woman, maternal serum alpha-fetoprotein (MS-AFP) or triple-screen tests on the mother's blood are performed as the primary screening method for Down syndrome.

Sonographic findings that suggest that Down syndrome may be present are:

1. Thickened nuchal fold.
2. Mildly shortened femur and/or humerus.
3. Mild fetal pyelectasis.
4. Echogenic bowel.
5. Hypoplasia of the middle phalanx of the 5th digit.
6. Mild brachycephaly.
7. Echogenic intracardiac foci.
8. Underossification of the nasal bone.
9. Duodenal atresia.
10. Heart defects.
11. Iliac angle.

1 Thickened Nuchal Fold

The nuchal fold is measured in a specific way on a specific image of the fetal head. The transverse view of the fetal head should be positioned so that in the anterior portion of the head the cavum septi pellucidi is visualized, and in the posterior portion of the head the cerebellum and occipital bone are visualized. On this view, the nuchal fold is measured from the outer edge of the occipital bone to the skin margin (figure 149). A measurement exceeding 6 mm is considered abnormal. The nuchal fold thickening tends to resolve in the late second trimester.

Figure 149.

Thickened nuchal fold. Sonogram of a fetal skull. Note thickened nuchal fold (arrows).

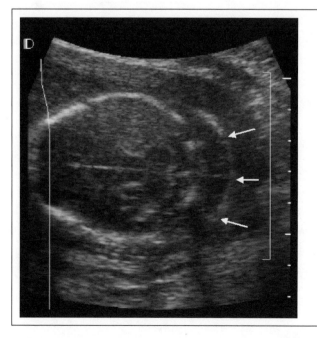

2 Short Femur and/or Humerus

It has been observed that some fetuses with Down syndrome have slightly shorter femurs than normal. Bromley and others produced regression equations comparing the biparietal diameter (BPD) to femur length.[158] The expected femur length is calculated from the equation 0.9028 × BPD − 9.3105 = expected femur length. Fetuses whose measured femur length was less than or equal to 0.91 times expected were shown to be at increased risk for Down syndrome. Similarly, slightly short humeri have been associated with increased risk for Down syndrome. The same authors calculated a regression equation for expected humeral length: 0.8492 × BPD − 7.9404 = expected humeral length. If the humeral length is less than 0.9 times (10% reduction) the expected, increased risk for Down syndrome exists. The positive predictive value for Down syndrome with the slightly shortened limb bones depends on the woman's underlying risk for Down syndrome on other bases.

3 Renal Pyelectasis

It has also been noted that some fetuses that have Down syndrome have slightly dilated renal pelves. Fetal pyelectasis in this context is defined as 4 mm or greater in A-P diameter of the renal pelvis (figure 150).

4 Echogenic Bowel

Hyperechoic bowel is rarely observed but is associated with an increase in chromosomal abnormalities, including Down syndrome, and is also associated with intrauterine growth restriction (IUGR).

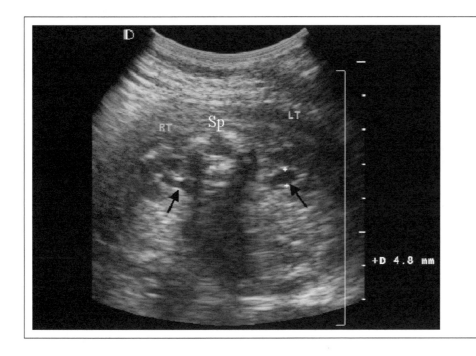

Figure 150.

Pyelectasis. Transverse sonogram of a fetal abdomen demonstrating left pyelectasis.

5 Hypoplasia of the Middle Phalanx of the 5th Digit

It has been observed that the middle phalanx of the 5th digit of the hand is smaller in Down syndrome individuals than in others. The 5th middle phalanx is 85% the size of the 4th middle phalanx in non–Down syndrome individuals and 59% the size of the 4th middle phalanx in Down syndrome fetuses.[159]

6 Brachycephaly.

Mild brachycephaly is also observed in many Down syndrome fetuses, but a cephalic index measurement has not been established for this purpose. Many of the Down syndrome screening programs take into account the frequently observed brachycephaly of the fetal head.

7 Echogenic Intracardiac Focus

A bright papillary muscle reflection is noted in some fetuses. This typically is visualized as a focal echogenic spot in the left ventricle at the level of the papillary muscle (figure 151). This finding has been associated with cardiac defects, which should be visible on the examination, but has also been associated with chromosomal anomalies such as trisomy 21. Right-sided or bilateral echogenic foci are more strongly associated with chromosome anomalies. About 18% of fetuses affected with trisomy 21 demonstrate one or more echogenic intracardiac foci, and if the finding is observed alone, there is a weak increase in risk of Down syndrome.[160] This finding by itself, however, is not a strong enough risk factor to trigger amniocentesis.

Figure 151.
Echogenic intracardiac focus. Sonogram of a fetal heart. Note the echogenic intracardiac focus (arrow).

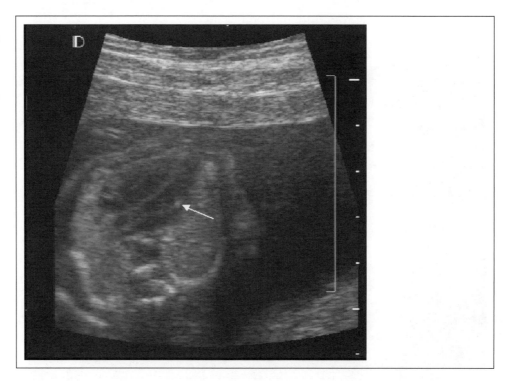

8 Underossified Nasal Bones

Recently, several groups of investigators have noted that the nasal bone is absent or hypoplastic in Down syndrome fetuses. In 60–70% of first and second trimester fetuses with Down syndrome, the nasal bone is unossified or underossified.[161, 163, 164, 165, 167] Bromley[166] has proposed using a ratio of biparietal diameter divided by nasal bone length. In that study, if the ratio was 11 or greater, the sensitivity for detection of Down syndrome was 69% with a false positive rate of 5%.

Other investigators have suggested that adding nasal bone assessment to nuchal translucency and biochemical markers increases sensitivity and decreases false positive rates for detection of Down syndrome.[162]

9 Duodenal Atresia

Duodenal atresia is seen in approximately 3% of Down syndrome fetuses. If the fetus observed has duodenal atresia, however, there is an approximately 30% risk that the fetus has Down syndrome (figure 152). This finding is not particularly helpful in detection of Down syndrome for termination, however, because the finding is typically not visible until 22–26 weeks. At this time elective termination is difficult to obtain in many states.

10 Heart Defects

Numerous cardiac defects have been observed in Down syndrome, most typically atrioventricular canal defects. If a fetus is observed to have a major cardiac defect, chromosomal analysis is indicated.

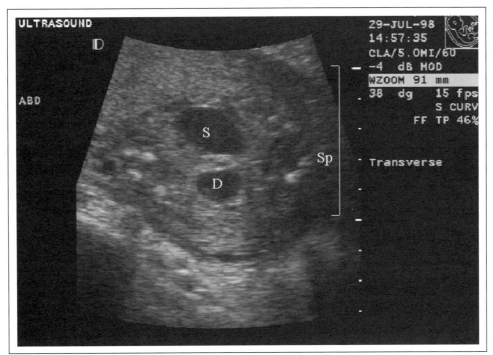

Figure 152. *Duodenal atresia.* Transverse sonogram of a fetal abdomen. Note the "double bubble" sign. S = stomach, D = duodenum.

11 Iliac Angle

In trisomy 21, it has been observed that the angle between the two iliac bones is slightly increased in fetuses that have trisomy 21. This measurement is difficult to interpret, however, because the angle of the ileum in the normal fetus changes as the scan plane moves from iliac crest down through the pelvis. The subjective observation of mildly increased angle in the iliac bones may be somewhat helpful.

Sonographic Scoring System for Fetal Anomalies Associated with Chromosomal Abnormality

Bernaceraf et al. in 1994 proposed a scoring system with risk of major chromosomal anomalies in the presence of specific abnormalities[168]:

Cardiac defect or duodenal atresia	2
Thickened nuchal fold	2
Short femur	1
Short humerus	1
Pyelectasis	1
Choroid plexus cyst	1
Echogenic bowel	1

According to this system, when a fetus has a score of 2 or more the mother is medically entitled to amniocentesis. The higher the score, the higher the risk for trisomy 21 specifically. This scoring system is particularly helpful for detecting fetuses with Down syndrome, as the other major chromosomal anomalies are more likely to be accompanied by multiple major structural abnormalities.

If only one sonographic marker is present, the decision to do amniocentesis can be made based on the risk of Down syndrome for a specific woman multiplied by the risk of Down syndrome associated with that finding (table 9).

Prognosis

The IQ of Down syndrome children is usually between 25 and 50, with a few individuals having IQ greater than 50.

Trisomy 18 (Edward's Syndrome)

The incidence of trisomy 18 is approximately 1 per 3,300 newborns.[169] The incidence of major structural anomalies is more common in trisomy 18 than in trisomy 13. Ninety to ninety-five percent of fetuses that have trisomy 18

Table 9.
Isolated sonographic markers and risk of Down syndrome.

Marker (Isolated)*	Likelihood Ratio for trisomy 21**
Nuchal thickening	11
Echogenic bowel	6.7
Short humerus	5.1
Short femur	1.5
Echogenic intracardiac focus	1.8
Pyelectasis	1.5
0 markers (normal scan)	0.4

*Choroid plexus cysts are not included in this list, as they have been associated with trisomy 18, and not trisomy 21.

**Factor by which risk of trisomy 21 is altered. For example, the presence of isolated nuchal thickening increases the odds of trisomy 21 by a factor of 11, while a normal scan (0 markers) reduces the risk of trisomy 21 by more than 50% (to only 40% of its pre-scan value).

Data from Nyberg DA, Souter VL, El-Bastawissi A, et al: Isolated sonographic markers for detection of fetal down syndrome in the second trimester of pregnancy. *JUIM* 20:1053–1063, 2001.

have cardiac anomalies, such as ventricular septal defect, atrial septal defect, or patent ductus arteriosus. Diaphragmatic hernia and omphalocele are also associated with trisomy 18, and agenesis corpus callosum is observed in less than 10% of infants. Cystic hygromas are sometimes observed in trisomy 18.

Another constellation of abnormalities observed in trisomy 18 includes positional abnormality of the hands and feet, including clenching of the hands with overlapping index finger, clubfeet, or rockerbottom feet. There is often limited motion of the arms and legs in utero.

Other abdominal abnormalities include omphalocele and renal abnormalities, including horseshoe kidney, pelvic kidney, ureteral duplication, and polycystic kidney. Skeletal anomalies, including radial agenesis, spina bifida, hemivertebrae, and scoliosis, may also be observed.

Choroid plexus cysts are present in a third of fetuses with trisomy 18 and are present in 1–2% of normal fetuses. Some observers suggest that larger or bilateral choroid plexus cysts are more highly associated with chromosomal abnormalities, but others contest this finding. Most observers suggest that isolated choroid plexus cysts are not sufficient findings to trigger amniocentesis. If choroid plexus cysts are observed in the fetus, however, the sonographer should carefully examine for other abnormalities.

Prognosis

Approximately 10% of trisomy 18 infants live past the age of one year.[170]

Figure 153.
Holoprosencephaly. Coronal sonogram of a fetal head demonstrating a single ventricle.

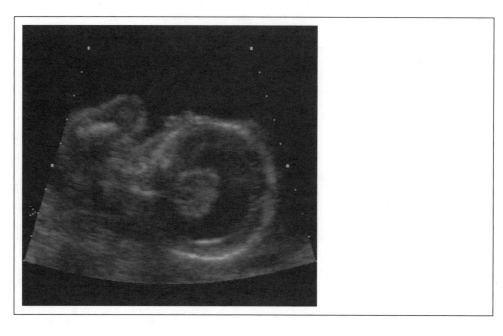

Trisomy 13

The incidence of trisomy 13 is approximately 1 in 5,000 pregnancies.[169] Trisomy 13 is also associated with extensive structural anomalies. One of the most notable is holoprosencephaly, with abnormality of the brain and face as described in the section on the brain and spinal cord (see "Fetal Brain and Cranium") (figure 153). Holoprosencephaly is found in more than 50% of patients that have trisomy 13. Polydactyly of the hands and feet is also commonly observed. Cardiac defects, including patent ductus, atrial septal defect, and dextroposition, are observed in 80% of patients with trisomy 13. Single umbilical artery (SUA) is also very common in trisomy 13. Omphalocele is observed in less than 50% of patients. Spina bifida is observed in less than 50% of fetuses that have trisomy 13. Thirty percent of patients are reported to have polycystic kidney disease at autopsy, but only rarely do trisomy 13 fetuses demonstrate sonographic findings suggesting polycystic kidney disease. Only 18% of individuals who have trisomy 13 survive past one year of age.

Turner Syndrome

Turner syndrome is a chromosomal syndrome in which one of the sex chromosomes is missing and the other sex chromosome is X, otherwise known as XO syndrome. Turner syndrome is not associated with advanced maternal age, and the missing sex chromosome is usually from the father. Most fetuses that have Turner syndrome are miscarried, and the incidence of Turner syndrome in newborns is 1 in 5,000.[171] Thus, more fetuses than newborns will be observed with Turner syndrome.

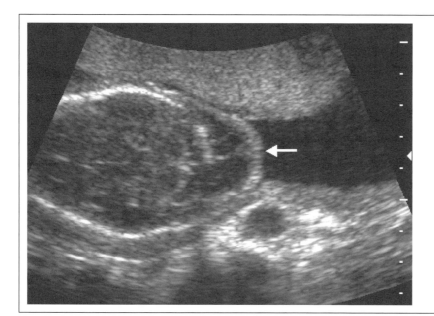

Figure 154.
Cystic hygroma. Axial sonogram of a fetal head and neck. Note the cystic changes at the neck (arrow).

Sonographically the most typical observation in Turner syndrome is cystic hygroma (figure 154). The degree of cystic hygroma is variable. The percent of Turner syndrome fetuses that have cystic hygroma is unclear. Other anomalies that may be observed in Turner syndrome include cardiac defects, usually aortic coarctation. Horseshoe kidneys may also be observed in some cases.

Hydrops, pleural effusions, and cystic hygroma are sometimes observed. The in utero prognosis for Turner syndrome seems to be closely related to the degree of fetal hydrops and pleural effusions. If the hydrops and pleural effusions are severe, these fetuses are more likely to miscarry.

In Turner syndrome, the fetuses are phenotypically female. After delivery, the ovaries degenerate. At adolescence there is little functioning ovarian tissue and these patients fail to develop reproductively. There is also a risk of mental retardation with Turner syndrome.

A similar syndrome with cystic hygroma and congenital heart disease with a male-appearing fetus is called *Noonan syndrome.*

Triploidy

Triploidy is a syndrome in which the fetus has three complete sets of chromosomes or 69 chromosomes. This apparently occurs in 1% of conceptuses, and most end in miscarriage.

From a sonographic point of view, there are two subsets of triploidy fetuses. One group has a fetus with a molar-appearing placenta; this group is usually called *partial hydatidiform mole.* The other group has a normal placenta and may have more fetal anomalies. Both groups apparently have significant growth restriction. The group with a more normal placenta may have more severe asymmetric growth restriction. The triploid fetuses that have a molar-appearing placenta typically have two paternal sets of chromosomes and one set from the mother, and the fetuses with a more normal-appearing placenta have two sets of chromosomes from the mother and one from the father.

The prognosis for these fetuses is dismal. Most die in utero, and the remainder die in the early neonatal period. The oldest recorded survivor is approximately 10.5 months.[172]

Sonographic findings in triploidy include molar-appearing placenta and major anomalies of most organ systems, including meningomyelocele, holoprosencephaly, absence of the corpus callosum, cleft lip and palate, hydrocephalus, congenital heart disease, renal anomalies, and abnormalities of the hands and feet.

Meckel-Gruber Syndrome

One of the most common syndromes that is not a major chromosomal abnormality is *Meckel-Gruber syndrome.* In this syndrome the fetus has large echogenic kidneys, which appear to be polycystic, although the pathologic malformation is multicystic dysplasia. The kidneys appear similar to severe cases of recessive polycystic kidney disease. In addition, the fetus may have an occipital encephalocele, polydactyly, or both. This syndrome is recessive. Other anomalies, including cleft lip and palate, micrognathia, hepatic cysts, and brain abnormalities including holoprosencephaly and Dandy-Walker malformation, have been observed. Omphalocele may be observed on occasion also. The prognosis is fatal because of marked oligohydramnios from renal dysfunction.

Table 10 summarizes the sonographic findings associated with common syndromes.

Table 10.
Common syndromes: incidence and sonographic findings.

Anatomic Site	Syndrome, Incidence, and Sonographic Finding					
	Trisomy 21 (Down Syndrome) 1 in 660 newborns (with advanced maternal age, 1 in 75 newborns)	**Trisomy 18 (Edward's Syndrome)** 1 in 3,300 newborns	**Trisomy 13** 1 in 5,000 pregnancies	**Turner Syndrome** 1 in 5,000	**Meckel-Gruber Syndrome**	**Triploidy** 1 in 10,000 newborns
Head	Thickened nuchal fold Mild brachycephaly	Agenesis corpus callosum Cystic hygromas Choroid plexus cysts	Holoprosencephaly	Cystic hygroma	Occipital encephalocele Cleft lip and palate Micrognathia Holoprosencephaly Dandy-Walker malformation	Holoprosencephaly Absent corpus callosum Cleft lip and palate Hydrocephalus
Chest	Echogenic intracardiac foci Heart defects	Cardiac anomalies (ASD, VSD, patent ductus) Diaphragmatic hernia	Cardiac defects (patent ductus arteriosus, ASD, dextroposition)	Cardiac defects (usually coarctation of aorta)		Congenital heart disease
Abdomen	Mild fetal pyelectasis Echogenic bowel Duodenal atresia	Omphalocele Renal abnormalities (horseshoe or pelvic kidney) Ureteral duplication Polycystic kidney	Single umbilical artery Omphalocele Polycystic kidneys	Horseshoe kidneys Hydrops and pleural effusions	Large echogenic kidneys that appear polycystic Hepatic cysts Omphalocele	Renal anomalies
Limbs/spine	Mildly shortened femur Mildly shortened humeri Hypoplasia of the middle phalanx of the 5th digit	Clenching of hand, overlapping index finger Clubfeet or rocker-bottom feet Skeletal anomalies (radial agenesis) Spina bifida Hemivertebrae Scoliosis	Polydactyly hands and feet		Polydactyly	Meningomyelocele Abnormalities of the hands and feet
Other						Partial hydatidiform mole IUGR Major anomalies of most organ systems

Coexisting Disorders

CHAPTER 9

Pelvic masses

Cystic masses

Complex masses

Solid masses

Maternal disorders presenting primarily with pain and swelling

Trophoblastic disease

. . . .

During pregnancy, a woman may experience a wide variety of coexisting diseases that are unrelated to the pregnancy. Conditions that are of interest in sonography can be divided into two general groups:

1. Conditions that result in a palpable pelvic mass that can be detected sonographically.
2. Conditions that result in pain in the abdomen, flank, leg, or pelvic area that are sonographically detectable.

Pelvic Masses

Pelvic masses may be detected either clinically or sonographically during pregnancy and may be unrelated to pregnancy. In a patient of large size, the mass may be difficult to detect either sonographically or clinically. In general, masses less than 5 cm in diameter are treated conservatively, whereas masses exceeding 5 cm in diameter may require surgical intervention. If there is suspicion of torsion, surgical intervention is usually required.

Cystic Masses

Corpus Luteum Cyst

As previously discussed, early in the pregnancy cycle a cyst develops in the ovary from which the egg ovulated. This cyst, the corpus luteum cyst, produces hormones until the placenta is established. The corpus luteum cyst is typically 2–3 cm in diameter but may be much larger, sometimes up to 10 cm. Usually it will regress by 16–18 menstrual weeks. Often there is increase in blood flow in the periphery of the cyst, and the cyst may contain internal echoes and septae as a result of hemorrhage. These cysts may be similar in appearance to paraovarian or peritoneal inclusion cysts. The latter cysts, however, should not arise from the ovary. Corpus luteum cysts are the most common ovarian masses observed in pregnancy.

Other Cystic or Partially Cystic Masses

1 Hydrosalpinx

Hydrosalpinx is an obstructed fluid-filled fallopian tube that typically occurs after a pelvic infection. Although it may be serpiginous (figure 155) in appearance, it sometimes appears as rounded, densely septated cysts and may be identical in appearance to a cystadenoma. Hydrosalpinx may occur unilaterally or bilaterally.

2 Paraovarian Cyst

A *paraovarian cyst* is a cyst that arises outside the ovary in the broad ligament area and may represent a Gartner's duct remnant. It may have septae and typically is asymptomatic.

Figure 155.
Hydrosalpinx. Transverse sonogram shows a fluid collection extending posterior to the uterus.

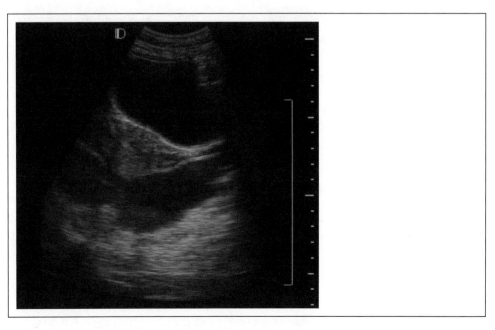

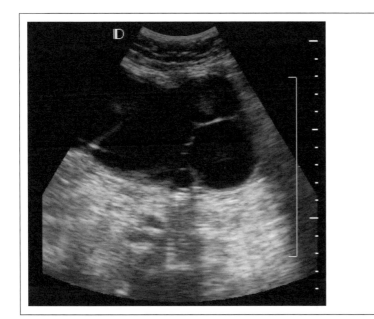

Figure 156.
Cystadenoma. Sagittal sonogram demonstrating a septated cystic mass.

In most cases a paraovarian cyst may be distinguished from an ovarian cyst by the fact that a paraovarian cyst occurs outside the ovary.

3 Cystadenoma

The most common cystic tumor of the ovary is a *cystadenoma*. Although cystadenoma may present as a simple cyst without evidence of septation or nodularity, typically a cystadenoma will be large and have thick or thin septae (figure 156) and may have nodules within the cystic component. The presence of nodules in the mass increases the likelihood of malignancy.

4 Torsion

Any adnexal mass or cyst may experience torsion with twisting of the vascular pedical and subsequent ischemia. Torsion typically causes severe pelvic pain. It can be difficult to diagnose torsion of an ovary or ovarian mass or adnexal mass. Doppler examination of normal ovaries may sometimes demonstrate normal blood flow, but some normal ovaries may not show significant blood flow; therefore, the absence of blood flow cannot be considered a reliable predictor of ovarian torsion. Conversely, the presence of blood flow in a suspected torsed mass or ovary does not exclude the possibility of partial torsion.

If torsion occurs in an ovary that does not have a significant mass, it is easier to diagnose. In this case, the venous obstruction typically occurs first and there is enlargement and edema of the ovary, and multiple ovarian cysts may be observed.

Table 11 lists the cystic pelvic masses associated with pregnancy.

Table 11.
Cystic pelvic masses associated with pregnancy.

Corpus luteum cyst
Hydrosalpinx
Paraovarian cyst
Cystadenoma
Ovarian torsion

Table 12.
Complex pelvic masses associated with pregnancy.

Cystadenoma
Dermoid
Teratoma
Pelvic kidney

Complex Masses

Complex masses contain both cystic and solid components. Some cystadenomas may present as complex masses. Pelvic inflammatory disease or ectopic pregnancy may also present as a complex adnexal mass. See table 12.

Dermoid Cyst

One of the most common complex masses in the adnexa is a *dermoid cyst*. A dermoid cyst is a tumor containing germ cells for teeth, hair, skin, and fat. Cystic areas may occur within them. A complex mass with bright echogenic foci and gray posterior shadowing usually represents a dermoid tumor (figure 157). Most dermoid tumors are benign, but occasionally they may be malignant. If more types of tissue are present, the tumor is called a *teratoma*.

Pelvic Kidney

A *pelvic kidney* may present as a solid or complex mass in the pelvis. If hydronephrosis is present, central cystic areas may be observed. The renoform appearance, presence of pyramids, and a hilar vascularity help establish the diagnosis of pelvic kidney. In addition, if there is a pelvic kidney, there usually is not a kidney in a normal position on that side of the patient. The renal fossa can be checked if there is a question.

Solid Masses

The most common solid masses encountered in pregnancy are enlarging *leiomyomas* of the uterine myometrium. These may vary in appearance and may be either hyperechoic or cystic centrally. They can be painful, particularly

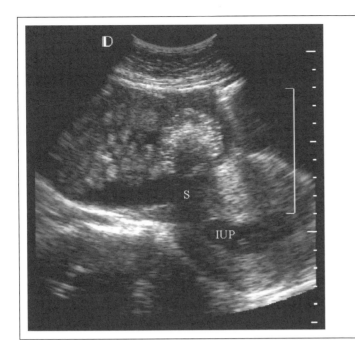

Figure 157.

Dermoid. Sagittal sonogram of dermoid tumor. Note shadowing (S). Note the intrauterine pregnancy posteriorly (IUP).

if they are undergoing central necrosis. A *focal myometrial contraction* (FMC) may mimic leiomyoma but will resolve within a few minutes and is usually not as well circumscribed as a uterine leiomyoma. If large fibroids are present in the uterus, their positions may be significant. If the placenta has implanted on a submucosal fibroid, it may lead to placental insufficiency. If the fibroid is in the lower uterine segment, it may obstruct the delivery and a c-section may be required. In general, uterine fibroids should be noted and measured during pregnancy. On follow-up examinations, the fibroids should be re-examined.

Rarely, *solid ovarian masses* may be observed in pregnant women. In many cases, there is clinical concern as to whether the solid mass is a fibroid arising from the uterus or truly an ovarian mass. If the solid mass distorts the uterus around it (claw sign), this suggests that the mass arises from the uterus and is not separate from the uterus. If no distortion of the adjacent uterus can be observed surrounding a solid mass, a solid ovarian tumor is more likely. The solid masses associated with pregnancy are listed in table 13.

Focal myometrial contraction
Leiomyoma
Solid ovarian masses

Table 13.

Solid pelvic masses associated with pregnancy.

Coexisting Maternal Disorders Presenting Primarily with Pain

A number of diseases may occur in pregnant woman that are not related specifically to pregnancy. In pregnant patients with pain, sonography is a particularly valuable imaging tool, as CT and x-ray studies are contraindicated. The patient may have pain in the upper abdomen, flank, leg, or pelvic area. Maternal diseases that can be successfully evaluated sonographically include the following:

1 Cholecystitis

Pregnant women may have gallstones and may develop cholecystitis. Pregnancy may be a possible cause of gallstones.

2 Pyelonephritis

Pregnant women typically have some degree of urinary obstruction due to the enlarging uterus and relaxing smooth muscle. It is normal to observe a mild degree of pelvicaliectasis in the right kidney, and sometimes dilatation of the collecting system in the left kidney is also noted. If a patient develops focal pain over the kidneys during pregnancy, pyelonephritis should be suspected. Urinalysis and urinary culture are helpful to establish the diagnosis.

3 Appendicitis

Appendicitis may occur in any patient of any age or gender. Appendicitis occasionally occurs during pregnancy, and under careful examination, the inflamed appendix can often be observed, even later in pregnancy. It should be remembered that the uterus enlarges and displaces the bowel, including the cecum, laterally and superiorly; therefore, the appendix may be higher in the abdomen in pregnant women.

4 Lower Extremity Deep Venous Thrombosis

The changes of pregnancy increase the likelihood of venous thrombosis in a number of ways, both by affecting clotting parameters and by increasing stasis in the pelvis and legs from direct pressure. Therefore, pregnant women are particularly likely to develop lower extremity deep venous thrombosis. In our experience, isolated pelvic thrombosis may occur early in pregnancy before the onset of venous obstruction. Sonography is helpful in establishing a diagnosis of lower extremity thrombosis and may be somewhat helpful in establishing a diagnosis of pelvic thrombosis.

5 Ureteral Calculus

If a pregnant patient experiences typical renal colic with spasmotic severe pain in the flank and pelvis, the possibility of ureteral calculus should be considered. In mid to late pregnancy, the uterus itself may act as a window for observation of the lower abdominal and pelvic course of the ureter. Ureteral calculus may be observed in the mid- or lower ureter and often can be observed at the ureterovesical junction. Thus, sonography may be helpful in the establishment of a diagnosis of ureteral calculus in pregnant women. In mid- to late pregnancy, a single view intravenous urogram has sometimes been used to evaluate for possible ureteral obstruction or ureteral stone; however, some degree of obstruction of the urinary tract is nearly always present in these patients, and the distal ureter may not be adequately evaluated.

Trophoblastic Disease

Another group of diseases related to pregnancy are abnormalities of the placenta. *Gestational trophoblastic disorder* (GTD) is a term applied to a spectrum of inter-related diseases originating from the placental trophoblast, which includes complete, partial, and invasive moles. All these diseases are characterized by marked edema and enlargement of the chorionic villi, with cystic structures developing within the villi. Molar pregnancy may account for as many as 1 in 40 miscarriages. These diseases are thought to be due to fertilization of an abnormal or normal egg with either an abnormal sperm or multiple sperm.

Classic Hydatidiform Mole

The *classic hydatidiform mole* (CHM) is caused by fertilization of an abnormal egg, which lacks any maternal DNA, with either two normal sperm or a single sperm with a double set of chromosomes from the father. Sonographically, a classic hydatidiform mole presents as a large echogenic placenta with many small but visible cystic areas within it. Terms such as "snowstorm" appearance or "bunch of grapes" have been applied to the sonographic appearance of this condition (figure 158). In classic hydatidiform mole, no fetus will be present, and enlarged theca-lutein cysts in both ovaries may be observed in some cases.

Theca-lutein cysts are due to very high beta hCG levels. Typically they are of uniform size, 2–3 cm in diameter (figure 159), arising in both ovaries. They are present in 25–45% of hydatidiform molar pregnancies. The overall appearance of the ovary is that of a large septated cystic mass. After evacuation of the molar pregnancy, the theca-lutein cyst may persist for 2–4 months.

Associated maternal findings include hypertension, hypothyroidism, hyperemesis, and bleeding. The beta hCG may exceed 1 million units. Rarely, other tumors such as a uterine dysgerminoma, sarcoma, or lymphoma may resemble the appearance of a classic hydatidiform mole.

Figure 158.
Classic hydatidiform mole. Sagittal (**A**) and transverse (**B**) images of an enlarged uterus demonstrating typical sonographic appearance of classic hydatidiform mole.

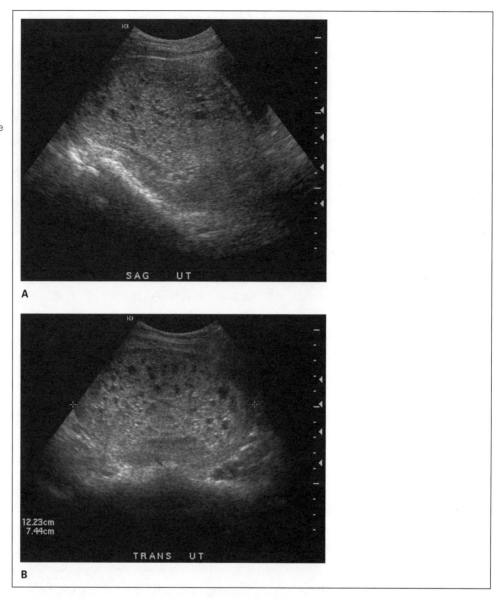

Figure 159A.
Theca-lutein cysts. Sagittal sonogram of an ovary with theca-lutein cysts.

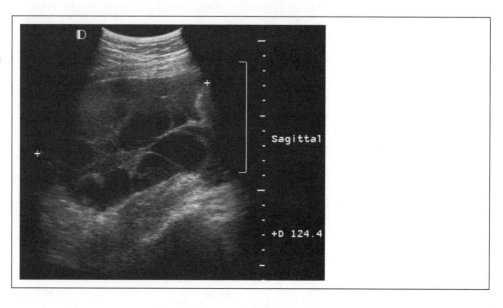

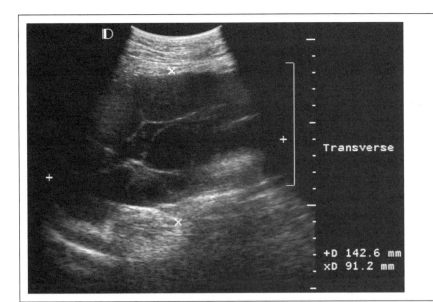

Figure 159B.
Theca-lutein cysts. Transverse sonogram of an ovary with theca-lutein cysts.

Partial Hydatidiform Mole

The traditional definition of a *partial hydatidiform mole* (PHM) is a molar-appearing placenta with an associated fetus. Most cases of partial hydatidiform mole are due to a triploid pregnancy; that is, a fetus that has three complete sets of chromosomes (69). In partial hydatidiform mole cases, two of these three sets are from the father and one from the mother. These two paternal sets of chromosomes may come either from two separate normal sperm or from one abnormal diploid sperm. The molar changes observed in the placenta (figure 160) are usually not as severe as in classic hydatidiform mole and become visible later in pregnancy. First-trimester and early second-trimester sonograms may appear essentially normal in a partial hydatidiform mole.

The prognosis for the fetus in a partial hydatidiform mole is poor, mortality rate is high, and most of the fetuses will be growth retarded. Fetal anomalies may also be observed.

There are cases of triploidy that do not present as partial hydatidiform moles in which the placenta is more normal in appearance. These fetuses seem to have more fetal anomalies and perhaps more severe growth restriction. In this group, the extra set of chromosomes is maternal in origin rather than paternal.

Rarely, partial hydatidiform mole may be observed with the normal number of chromosomes. Usually, these pregnancies show two paternal sets of chromosomes and no chromosomes from the mother. In other words, the genetics is very similar to a classic hydatidiform mole except that a fetus may develop as well.

Figure 160.

Partial mole. **A** Sonogram of a partial mole. Note the fetal abdomen (A), adjacent to the molar tissue (HM). **B** Sonogram of the same pregnancy also reveals molar tissue (HM).

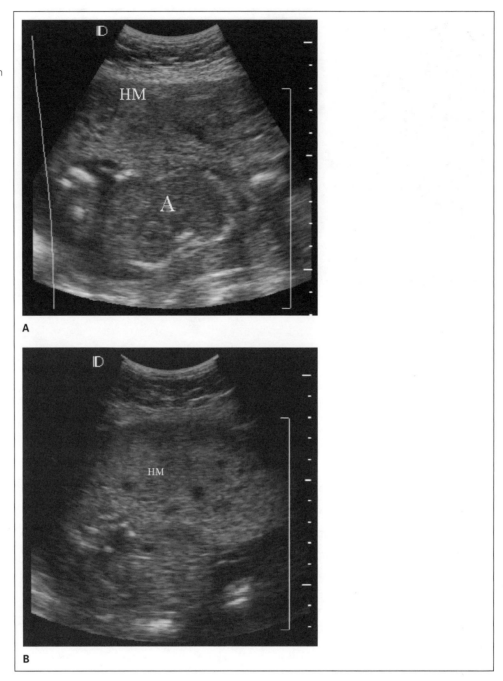

Classic Hydatidiform Mole with Normal Twin

In a few pregnancies, a fetus may be observed with molar-appearing placental material that does not represent a partial mole. In these cases there is a twin pregnancy consisting of a classic hydatidiform mole and a normal pregnancy (figure 161). On careful examination, normal placenta and molar placenta will both be observed. If the umbilical cord is followed to the placenta, one should note that the umbilical vessels from the fetus implant only on normal-appearing placenta and not on the molar portion (color plate 14).

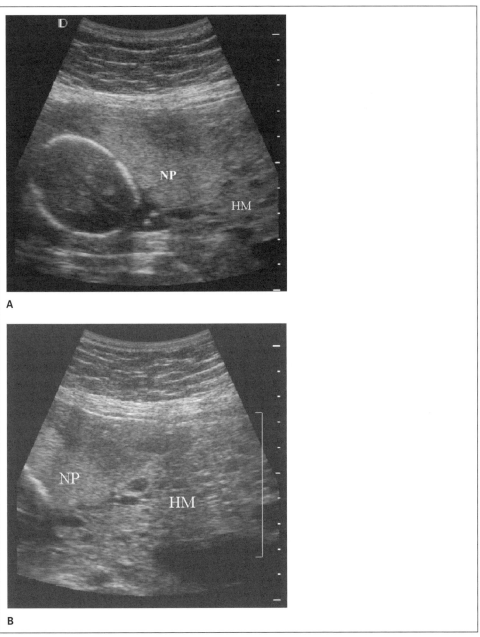

Figure 161.
Twin pregnancy with mole. **A, B** Fetal head and normal placenta (NP) with adjacent complete mole (HM).

Pseudo-Partial Hydatidiform Mole

Two conditions may resemble a partial hydatidiform mole in addition to the above described twin mole pregnancy.

1 Fetal Demise

After a fetus dies in mid-pregnancy, the placenta begins to degenerate, and the degenerating placenta may resemble a molar pregnancy. In this case, however, the fetus will have no heartbeat. Because fetal demise is common in partial mole, chromosomal assessment may be helpful to distinguish placental degeneration changes from changes in a partial mole pregnancy.

2 Beckwith-Wiedemann Syndrome

In some cases cystic changes may occur in the placenta of fetuses that have Beckwith-Wiedemann syndrome that may resemble a partial hydatidiform mole. In these cases, however, growth restriction of the fetus will not be observed, and other anomalies suggesting Beckwith-Wiedemann syndrome, such as omphalocele, may occasionally be observed.

Invasive Hydatidiform Mole (Chorioadenoma Destruens)

Invasive hydatidiform mole is described as penetration of molar tissue into the myometrium of the uterine wall. More commonly occurring in classic hydatidiform mole than partial mole, it may occur in either. At the time of delivery or D & C, the tissue attached to the uterine wall may be difficult to remove entirely. In some patients, the invasive nature of the mole may not be apparent until later. The patient may have heavy vaginal bleeding after delivery, or there may be subsequent rise in beta hCG after delivery. After uterine evacuation a persistent tumor may develop in 20–30% of patients who have the classic hydatidiform mole and 1–11% of patients who have partial hydatidiform mole. Invasive moles may spread to other organs by direct extension or by metastasis. Serial beta hCG levels should be obtained after termination of one of these pregnancies to evaluate for this eventuality. If persistent or recurrent elevation of beta hCG is noted, endovaginal sonography may help in evaluating the position and location of the myometrial invasion.

Choriocarcinoma

Choriocarcinoma is a highly malignant tumor of trophoblastic epithelium that metastasizes readily to the lungs, liver, and brain. Choriocarcinoma may occur after a molar pregnancy, after a miscarriage, or after a normal pregnancy. Approximately 50% of choriocarcinomas occur after a molar pregnancy. The primary tumor may be as small as 2–8 mm in size and still give rise to extensive metastasis. Choriocarcinoma and classic hydatidiform mole may have the same sonographic appearance.

PART II: Gynecology

PELVIC ANATOMY

PHYSIOLOGY

PEDIATRIC ABNORMALITIES

INFERTILITY

POSTMENOPAUSAL PELVIS

PELVIC PATHOLOGY

CHAPTER 10 Pelvic Anatomy

Embryology

Development of female pelvic organs during childhood

Normal adult pelvic anatomy

Sonographic technique

Sonographic appearance of normal pelvic organs

Indications for pelvic sonography

Contraindications to endovaginal sonography

. . . .

Sonography of the female pelvis is a valuable method for evaluating various medical conditions. The ability to image in longitudinal and transverse sections, the biologic safety of ultrasound, and the availability of both color and spectral Doppler have made sonography the primary initial imaging tool for evaluating female pelvic organs.

AIUM Guidelines

The American Institute of Ultrasound in Medicine (AIUM) has established minimum guidelines for performing routine gynecological sonograms. These guidelines have become an informal minimum legal standard for gynecological sonography.[2] (See Appendix B for a copy of the guidelines.)

Embryology

The embryologic development of the genital system begins in the 7th menstrual week, when the gonadal ridge develops on either side of the mesentery of hindgut. These gonadal ridges differentiate into an external cortex and an internal medulla. In a fetus that has XX chromosomes, the cortex of the gonadal ridge differentiates into the ovary and the medulla regresses. In an XY embryo, the cortex regresses and the medulla differentiates into the

Figure 162.
Embryologic development of paramesonephric duct. **A** Sketch of a ventral view of the posterior abdominal wall of a 9-week embryo showing the two pairs of genital ducts present during the indifferent stage of sexual development. **B** Lateral view of an 11-week fetus showing the sinus tubercle (mullerian tubercle) on the posterior wall of the urogenital sinus. It becomes the hymen in females and the seminal colliculus in males. Reprinted with permission from Moore KL, Persaud TVN: *Before We Are Born: Essentials of Embryology and Birth Defects,* 6th edition. Philadelphia, Saunders, 2003, p 251.

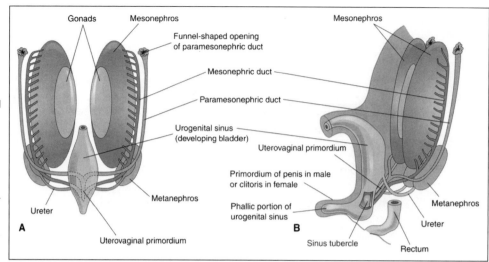

testis. In females, the cortex of the genital ridge produces primordial germ cells, which subsequently differentiate and become primary oocytes. All the egg cells develop within the ovary before birth, and no new oocytes develop after birth.

Lateral to the gonadal ridge on either side, the mesonephric (Wolffian) and paramesonephric (Mullerian) ducts develop as part of the mesonephric kidney. In males, the mesonephric duct develops into the seminal vesicles, vas deferens, and portions of the epididymis, and the paramesonephric duct resorbs. In females, the paramesonephric ducts (figure 162) develop into the fallopian tube, uterus, and portions of the vagina. If the development does not progress normally, the uterus and vagina may be partially or completely duplicated. In either gender, cystic remnants of the duct system that are not used to form the genital organs may persist.

Development of Female Pelvic Organs during Childhood

At birth, the uterus is quite prominent, measuring approximately 3.2 cm in length. The uterus is larger at birth than it will be later in infancy because of the maternal hormones of pregnancy. After birth the uterus regresses somewhat in size, but after age 2 the uterus remains at approximately 3.2 cm in total length (figure 163). The uterine corpus is usually smaller in A-P dimension and shorter in cephalo-caudad length than the cervix. At about 9–10 years of age, the uterus enlarges to approximately 4 cm in length, and by age 13, the uterus is approximately 5.4 cm in length. In early childhood, the ovarian size is approximately 0.7 to 0.8 cubic centimeters. By age 6, the ovarian volume increases to 1–1.2 cubic centimeters and at 8–11 years, the ovary increases in size from 2 to 2.5 cubic centimeters. After age 13 the ovarian size is approximately 4 cubic centimeters.

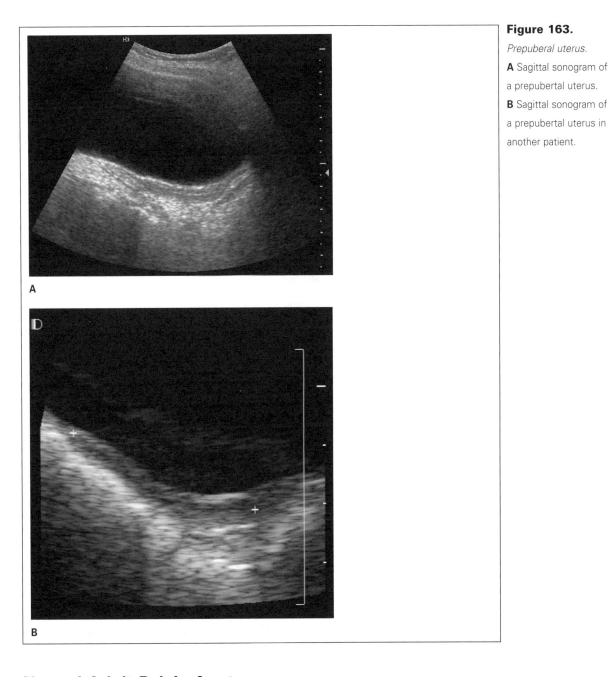

Figure 163.

Prepuberal uterus.
A Sagittal sonogram of a prepubertal uterus.
B Sagittal sonogram of a prepubertal uterus in another patient.

Normal Adult Pelvic Anatomy

The Uterus

1 The uterus lies in the mid-pelvis between the urinary bladder and the rectum (figure 164). There is normally a peritoneal reflexion, which extends down to the base of the bladder anterior to the uterus and down to the mid-cervix posteriorly. The posterior cul de sac is also referred to as the *pouch of Douglas*.

2 Lateral to the uterus there is a thick membranous ligament (the *broad ligament*) that extends from the lateral uterine margin to the pelvic sidewall. The superior margin of the broad ligament contains the round ligament.

Figure 164.
The uterus and surrounding anatomy. Reprinted with permission from the Netter Collection of Medical Illustrations, Volume 2, Section VI, Reproductive System.

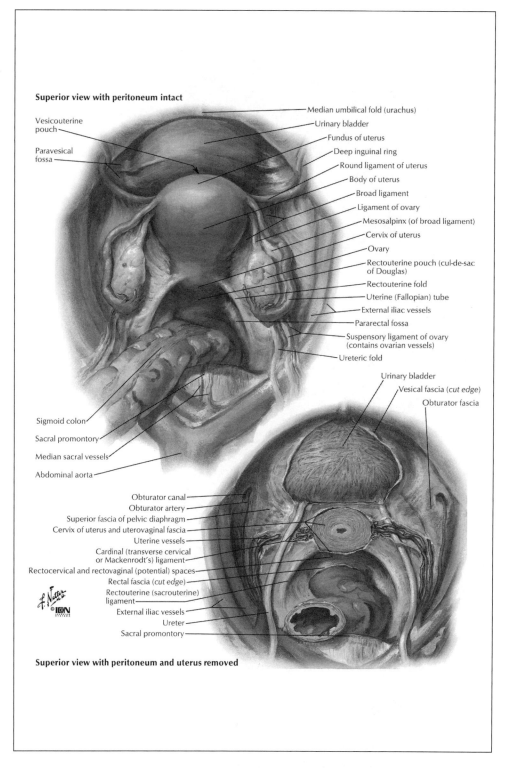

The broad ligament contains vessels, including uterine arteries and veins, which are the primary vascular supply of the uterus. The *round ligament* extends from the uterine fundus to the lateral pelvic sidewall and through the inguinal canal into the labia majora bilaterally. Another set of ligaments arise from the cervix laterally and extend posteriorly around the rectum to the sacrum. These ligaments are called the *sacro-uterine ligaments*.

3 The vagina extends antero-inferiorly posterior to the bladder and urethra and opens in the vulva. There is a 90-degree angle between the vagina and the uterine canal at the cervix.

4 The fallopian tubes extend from the lateral uterine fundus and curve laterally and inferiorly around the ovary, which normally lies posterior to the broad ligament. An ovarian ligament attaches the ovary to the uterine fundus, and the infundibulo-pelvic ligament attaches the ovary to the supralateral pelvic sidewall and contains the ovarian artery and vein. There is also a ligament between the ovary and the fallopian tube called the *mesosalpinx*. The fallopian tube is narrower at the uterine end. This portion is called the *isthmus,* and as the fallopian tube extends laterally toward the pelvic sidewall it widens out to form the ampulla. The end of the ampulla extends into fingerlike fimbria, which lie next to the ovary. The ovarian artery and vein extend medially beyond the ovary along the ovarian ligament and supply a collateral blood flow channel to the uterus through the cornual area. The cornual portion of the fallopian tube is the part that extends through the muscular wall of the uterus and into the endometrial cavity.

5 The ovarian artery arises from the aorta laterally just inferior to the renal artery bilaterally, and the ovarian veins return along the same route, entering the vena cava on the right below the right renal vein and entering the left renal vein near the kidney.

The uterine artery arises from the internal iliac artery and extends toward the uterus. The artery inserts on the cervix, and an extensive network of arteries and veins extends along the lateral anterior and posterior aspects of the uterus at that point. Anterior and posterior arteries extend in the uterine myometrium and are called the *anterior* and *posterior arcuate arteries*. Perpendicular to the arcuate arteries, radial arteries extend through the muscle and into the mucosa of the uterus.

6 The mucosal lining of the uterus is called the *endometrium.* Covering the entire internal surface of the endometrial cavity, the endometrium is continuous with the mucosa in the vagina and is continuous with the fallopian tube mucosa laterally. The endometrial thickness varies during the normal menstrual cycle and measures 4 mm in thickness on day 4, 8 mm on day 8, and 7–12 mm in thickness after ovulation (figure 165). The sonographic echogenicity of the endometrium also varies during the menstrual cycle. In the early proliferative phase, the endometrium is very thin and echogenic (figure 166). During the proliferative phase the endometrium thickens and becomes hypoechoic. The central endometrial line is echogenic and the peripheral margin of the endometrium is echogenic,

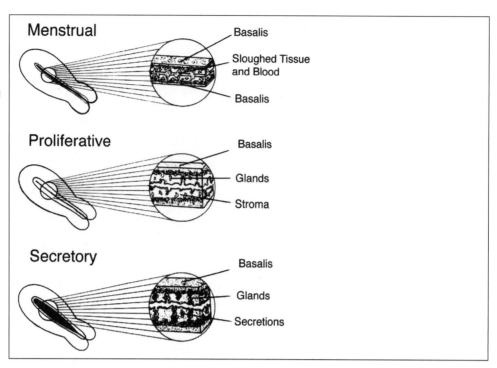

Figure 165.
Development of endometrium. Diagram demonstrating the phases of the menstrual cycle and changes that occur within the endometrium. Reprinted with permission from Fleischer AC, Kalemeris GC, Entman SS: Sonographic depiction of the endometrium during normal cycles. *Ultrasound Med Biol* 12:271, 1986. Copyright 1986 by World Federation of Ultrasound in Medicine and Biology.

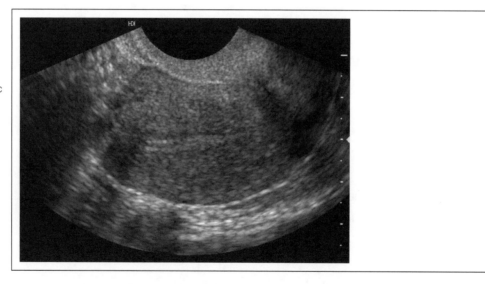

Figure 166.
Early proliferative phase. Sagittal sonogram of the uterus. Note the thin echogenic endometrial stripe.

but the endometrium itself is hypoechoic until after ovulation (figure 167). After ovulation, the endometrium becomes echogenic throughout its thickness and maintains echogenicity until menses (figure 168).

Cul de Sac Fluid

A small amount of cul de sac fluid is normally visualized during the menstrual cycle. The largest amount of free fluid is observed at mid-cycle at the time of ovulation. Normally, the fluid should be anechoic (figure 169). Debris or septations in the fluid are abnormal, suggesting hemorrhage, infection, or neoplasm.

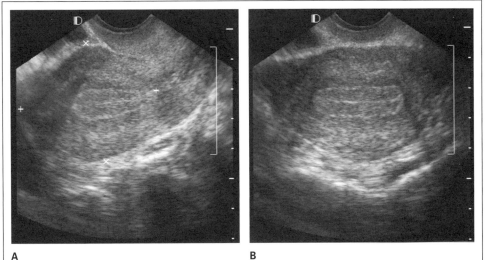

Figure 167.
Proliferative phase. Sagittal (**A**) and transverse (**B**) view of the uterus. Note the echogenic central line and hypoechoic endometrium.

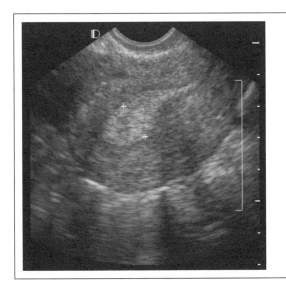

Figure 168.
Secretory phase. Sagittal sonogram of the uterus. Note the echogenicity throughout the endometrium.

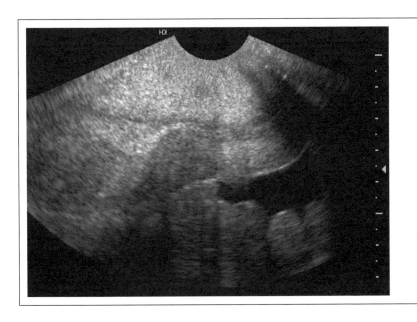

Figure 169.
Pouch of Douglas. Sagittal sonogram of the uterus and cervix. Note the fluid within the cul de sac.

Sonographic Technique

Three sonographic techniques are used to visualize structures in the female pelvis:

1. Transabdominal sonography
2. Endovaginal sonography
3. Sonohysterography

Transabdominal Sonography

In the early years, only transabdominal sonography was used to image pelvic organs. The examination is performed through a filled bladder, to use urine in the bladder as an acoustical window to visualize the uterus, ovaries, and pelvic sidewalls. Overdistention of the urinary bladder may distort the appearance of pelvic organs and may compress the cul de sac, obliterating small amounts of free fluid. The advantage of the transabdominal approach for imaging the pelvis is that the anterior portions of the pelvis, including the area anterior to the psoas muscle bilaterally and the upper pelvis along the lumbosacral portion of the spine, are visible from this approach.

With the development of endovaginal sonography, the importance of transabdominal sonography is declining, and in some ultrasound laboratories, transabdominal sonography is not performed routinely. In our view, however, transabdominal sonography is still required in at least some patients. Endovaginal sonography cannot adequately evaluate the upper part of the pelvis. Ovaries, pelvic masses, and ectopic pregnancies located in the upper pelvis may be missed on endovaginal sonography.

Endovaginal Sonography

Approximately 10 years ago, high-frequency probes were developed specifically for imaging in the vagina. These probes are typically sheathed with a plastic cover, and gel is used inside and outside the cover for acoustic contact. The transducers currently are usually 7–10 MHz in frequency and present a sector view from the tip of the transducer. With the patient in the supine position, the pelvis elevated from the bed on a pad, and the knees slightly flexed, the transducer is inserted into the vagina. The sonographer rotates the transducer to image the pelvic organs.

In general, endovaginal sonographic images are of higher quality than transabdominal images because high-frequency transducers can be used, and the detail of the images is better. The ovaries may not always be imaged on transvaginal sonography, however, particularly if they lie anteriorly in the pelvis. If the uterus is large, the fundus of the uterus may not be visible sonographically from this approach.

Sonohysterography

Sonohysterography is a variation of endovaginal sonography in which a catheter is inserted into the endometrial cavity and sterile saline is instilled into the cavity to better visualize the endometrium. This method is used primarily to resolve questions of possible endometrial abnormality. Endometrial polyps, irregular endometrium, and subendometrial fibroids may be visible on sonohysterography when the appearance on endovaginal sonography is indefinite.

Sonographic Appearance of Normal Pelvic Organs

1. The uterus is a pear-shaped, homogeneous, hypoechoic muscular organ. Some shadowing may be observed from the periphery of the uterus because of critical angle reflections from muscle bundles paralleling the surface of the uterus. The endometrium is typically an echogenic stripe of variable appearance as described. Blood vessels are typically visible adjacent to the uterus, especially near the cervix in the broad ligament. On some occasions, arcuate arteries may be visible as well, particularly with color flow imaging.

2. The ovaries are elliptical and of medium echogenicity, with peripheral small hypoechoic cysts that represent follicles. These follicles normally should be less than 25 mm in diameter. The ovaries are typically located laterally and posterior to the broad ligament.

3. The fallopian tubes are not normally visualized sonographically. These small muscular tubular structures are difficult to image and are usually visible only if they are abnormally distended.

4. The urinary bladder is visualized anterior to the uterus on transabdominal imaging, and portions of the urinary bladder may be visible on endovaginal sonography anterior to the cervix. Normally the bladder mucosa is barely visible as a hyperechoic structure on the internal surface of the bladder. The ureters may be visualized either transabdominally or endovaginally, and dilatation of the ureters, distal ureteral stones, or ectopic ureteroceles within the urinary bladder may be visible sonographically.

5. The sigmoid colon begins at the level of the lumbosacral junction of the spine and extends posteriorly through the pelvis. It extends posterior to the uterus, cervix, and vagina and is often visualized as an echogenic structure with posterior gray shadowing and possibly peristalsis. Abnormal conditions in the colon and distal ureter may also be identified in some patients.

Indications for Pelvic Sonography

Sonography is a valuable method for evaluating patients who have pelvic bleeding, pelvic pain, enlarged uterus, or pelvic mass. Uterine masses, endometrial abnormality, and ovarian masses can be detected and evaluated. Also, findings may be visible that suggest pelvic inflammatory disease, endometriosis, or possibly ectopic pregnancy. In addition, follicular maturity may be evaluated if needed.

Contraindications to Endovaginal Sonography

Endovaginal sonography is contraindicated in the following patients:

1. Premenarchal or virginal patients.

2. Patients who have undergone endovaginal radiation for cervical carcinoma. In these patients, the vagina is scarred and the endovaginal probe cannot be easily inserted to an adequate depth for imaging the pelvic structures.

3. Any patient who will not willingly undergo the endovaginal examination.

CHAPTER 11 — Physiology

Menstrual cycle

Human chorionic gonadotropin

Fertilization

. . . .

Menstrual Cycle

During the reproductive years of a woman's life, the typical cycle of interplay of hormones from the pituitary gland and ovary produces the cyclical changes of the menstrual cycle. The length of the cycle is variable but is usually approximately 28 days.

At the beginning of the menstrual cycle, the pituitary gland produces follicle-stimulating hormone (FSH). This hormone acts on the ovary to begin the development of ovarian follicles. The part of the menstrual cycle in which the follicles develop is called the *follicular phase* and lasts for the first 10–14 days of the menstrual cycle. During this time period, five to seven follicles usually develop in each ovary. By days 8–12, a single follicle becomes dominant and continues to enlarge. The other developing follicles in the same ovary begin to decrease in size at that time, and the developing follicles in the opposite ovary do not enlarge further. In 5–10% of women, two dominant follicles develop simultaneously, one in each ovary. The dominant follicle or follicles grow by 2–3 mm a day and by the time of ovulation reach a size of 18–25 mm in diameter. As the follicles develop, cells within the follicles begin to produce estrogen. The estrogen in turn acts on the endometrium of the uterus, which becomes thicker and more vascular.

As the dominant ovarian follicle becomes mature, the pituitary gland begins to produce luteinizing hormone (LH) as well. This hormone acts on the developing follicle, which begins to produce progesterone at about the time of ovulation.

The portion of the menstrual cycle that follows ovulation is called the *luteal* or *secretory phase* of the menstrual cycle. Under the influence of luteinizing hormones from the pituitary gland, the dominant follicle from which the egg recently ovulated begins to produce progesterone in larger amounts, along with the estrogen. The estrogen and progesterone act on the uterine endometrium, which becomes even thicker and more vascular. Also, secretory glands develop in the endometrium. If pregnancy does not occur, the endometrium then sloughs during menstruation.

There is a typical sonographic appearance of the endometrium during the menstrual cycle:

1. Initially, in the early follicular or proliferative phase, the endometrial stripe in the uterus is thin and echogenic.

2. As the endometrium develops before ovulation, it thickens, and the sonographic appearance changes, with the endometrium becoming hypoechoic.

3. In the late follicular or proliferative phase, the endometrium has a three-layer appearance, with the endometrial surface appearing echogenic, the mid-endometrium hypoechoic, and the deep endometrium echogenic.

4. After ovulation, the endometrium increases in thickness and becomes diffusely echogenic, probably as a result of proliferation of secretory glands.

See table 14 for endometrial thickness throughout the menstrual cycle. See also figures 164–167 for the sonographic appearance of the endometrium during the aforementioned phases.

Table 14. Normal variation in endometrial thickness throughout the menstrual cycle.

Phase of Cycle	Days of Cycle	Endometrial Thickness
Menstrual phase	Days 1–4	1–4 mm
Early proliferative phase	Days 5–9	5–9 mm
Late proliferative (periovulatory) phase	Days 10–14	10–14 mm
Secretory phase	Days 15–28	15–28 mm

Pregnancy Tests

Modern pregnancy tests are based on detection of human chorionic gonadotropin (hCG) in the urine or serum. A blood test for a beta subunit of human chorionic gonadotropin is more accurate than a typical home pregnancy test but is not necessarily more sensitive. The blood test is usually performed as a radioimmunoassay.

Home pregnancy tests are urine tests using color reaction to detect human chorionic gonadotropin in the urine. The sensitivity of the home pregnancy test depends on the concentration of the urine. In general, the sensitivity of home pregnancy tests ranges from 25 mIU to 100 mIU. Most laboratories will report a positive pregnancy test from a beta human chorionic gonadotropin blood test with a result greater than 15 or 20 mIU. Pregnancy tests are usually positive 1–2 weeks after conception.

Human Chorionic Gonadotropin

Human chorionic gonadotropin (hCG) is a hormone produced by the placenta to maintain the corpus luteum until the placenta is well established. Normally, an hCG level of less than 5 mIU per ml indicates the absence of pregnancy. In many laboratories, 20 mIU is considered a level to indicate pregnancy. This level should be reached by approximately the third menstrual week, or approximately one week before the first period is missed. In the early part of pregnancy, the hCG level should double every 2–3 days. A maximum is reached at between 9 and 12 weeks, and then the hCG gradually falls through the rest of pregnancy. At term the human chorionic gonadotropin level is still between 30,000 and 170,000 mIU/ml.

Fertilization

After ovulation, fertilization usually occurs within 24 hours. Sperm usually live 48–72 hours.

Once the egg is fertilized (zygote), it begins to divide into more and more cells. In the second and third days after ovulation, the cell multiplication progresses from 2 to approximately 16 cells. When there are 12–15 cells, the developing structure is called a *morula*. The morula enters the uterus about 4 days after fertilization. Very soon thereafter, a fluid space develops within the developing zygote. This fluid space is called the *blastocyst cavity.* By approximately 5–6 days, the blastocyst attaches to the uterine endometrium. At the periphery of the blastocyst an inner cell mass develops, and at implantation the inner cell mass produces a synciotrophoblast, which penetrates into the uterine wall as the very early precursor to the placenta. By about 8 days after ovulation, the bilaminar embryonic disc is developing, with the primary yolk sac forming on one side of the disc and the amnion on the other. By 14 days, the secondary yolk sac has formed and separated from the primary yolk sac. At the same time, the synciotrophoblast is burrowing into the wall of the uterus, forming the chorion frondosum. As the gestational sac enlarges, the synciotrophoblast that is adjacent to the amnionic cavity thins and forms the smooth chorion, which lies directly under the decidua capsularis. In the next few weeks the fluid between the amnion and chorion in the amniotic cavity resorbs, and the chorion and amnion are usually fused by approximately 15–16 menstrual weeks.

Pediatric Abnormalities

CHAPTER 12

Sexual ambiguity

Precocious puberty

Hematometra/hematocolpos

Other Abnormalities

. . . .

Sexual Ambiguity

A number of genetic defects may lead to ambiguous or incorrect development of the genitals. These conditions are important to sonographers because parents of the developing fetus are interested in gender assignment. Ambiguous genitalia may be variable in appearance. In males, the scrotum may be bifid and the penis may be small or malformed. In females, the clitoris may be large and the labia may be fused. In females with a 46 XX karyotype, this condition is usually called *female pseudohermaphroditism,* and if the individual is 46 XY, the condition is labeled *male pseudohermaphroditism*.

The most common cause of female pseudohermaphroditism is *congenital adrenal hyperplasia*. This condition is associated with genetic defects in the enzymes that produce the sex hormones. A variety of enzymatic defects in steroidogenesis may occur, but the most common is steroid 21 hydroxylase deficiency. This occurs in approximately 1 in 5 to 15,000 births.[173] In females it results in male-appearing genitalia. The genitalia may be ambiguous or may closely resemble normal male genitalia. In males, this condition may lead to precocious puberty findings. A number of other steroid enzyme defects may also lead to ambiguous genitalia in both males and females.

In fetuses in which the bladder and peritoneum do not form normally, such as in bladder extrophy, the genitalia may be absent or markedly abnormal.

A very rare cause of ambiguous genitalia is true hermaphroditism. In these individuals, there is a mosaicism, with some cells containing XX sex chromosomes and others containing XY chromosomes. These individuals will often have ambiguous genitalia, and on microscopic examination of the gonads, both sperm and ova production are present.

Precocious Puberty

If a girl develops secondary sexual characteristics such as breast development or pubic hair or begins to menstruate before the age of eight, she should be evaluated for possible precocious puberty.

True Precocious Puberty

In true precocious puberty, the girl will develop secondary sexual characteristics, as well as enlargement of the ovaries and uterus. In true precocious puberty, the ovary will be enlarged, with its volume exceeding 1 cubic centimeter, and functional cysts are often present. Also, the uterus will be enlarged, measuring 4–5 cm in length, and there is a change in the proportion of the uterus, with the fundus enlarging relative to cervical size. The fundus-to-cervix ratio should be between 2:1 and 3:1 in precocious puberty. In this condition, the cause is usually unknown, but intracranial tumors, particularly hypothalamic tumors, are the cause in some cases.

Pseudo Precocious Puberty

In *pseudo precocious puberty,* the hormones do not arise as a result of stimulation from the hypothalamus and pituitary gland. The usual cause is an ovarian tumor, including granulosa theca cell tumor and sometimes other causes such as functional ovarian cyst, dysgerminoma, teratoma, or choriocarcinoma. Sonographically, a mature uterus and ovarian mass will be identified. In a few cases, adrenal tumors may be the cause and rarely, hepatoblastoma of the liver.

Premature breast or pubic hair development may occur without enlargement of the ovaries or uterus. These cases are referred to as isolated premature thelarche "breast development" or isolated premature adrenarchy "pubic or axillary hair development."

Hematometra/Hematocolpos

In other parts of this book the embryology of the female genital organs is discussed and the anomalies that may be observed such as didelphys uterus, bicornis uterus, and subseptus.[174]

Hematometracolpos is an abnormality in which the caudal opening of the vagina is obstructed by a complete hymen. If this occurs in the later part of pregnancy or postnatally, the uterus and vagina will be distended with blood. Often low-level echoes may be seen within it. Other cystic lower abdominal pelvic masses may appear similar on occasion, particularly in severe pelvic anomalies such as abnormalities of cloacal development.

Other Abnormalities

"Wrong Gender"

In another group of conditions, the genitalia may appear relatively normal but contradict the genetic assignment of gender. A condition called *testicular feminization* or *androgen insensitivity syndrome* occurs in genetic males that develop normal female-appearing genitalia and subsequent body habitus. Conversely, in a condition called XX male syndrome, a genetic female may develop normal external male genitalia.

Testicular Feminization Syndrome

Testicular feminization occurs in 1–20,000 to 1–50,000 live births.[175] These individuals appear to be normal females externally but have 46 XY chromosomes. Internally, the vagina ends blindly, the uterus and fallopian tubes are absent or rudimentary, and gonads are intra-abdominal. The biochemical cause of this condition is not well understood but results in insensitivity of cells to testosterone.

XX Male

A single gene on the Y chromosome produces the *testes-determining factor* (TDF). This single gene when present on the Y chromosome results in the production of male genitalia. In XX male syndrome, this testes-determining factor gene is translocated to an X chromosome; thus, the individual is chromosomally female with 46 XX karyotype but is phenotypically male. These individuals are typically infertile and may develop medical problems in later life. They resemble XXY males, otherwise known as *Klinfelter syndrome*. The incidence of XX male syndrome is 1 in 20,000–30,000 newborn boys.[176] If the testes-determining factor gene is defective, a reverse condition may occur in which a genetically XY individual may appear female.

Infertility

CHAPTER 13

Indications for sonography in infertility

The infertility work-up

Causes of infertility

Medications and treatment

Assisted reproductive technology

. . . .

Infertility is defined as the inability to conceive a child after 12 months of unprotected intercourse. About 14% of couples in the United States have an infertility disorder.[177] Infertility may be due to problems of female reproduction, problems with male reproduction, or both. Approximately two-thirds of the cases of infertility are due to a female disorder and approximately one-third due to a male disorder. The most common causes of female infertility are tubal disease, endometriosis, cervical factors, and luteal phase abnormalities. Causes of male infertility include low sperm density and motility, abnormal sperm, and the presence of antisperm antibodies.

Another contributing factor to reduced fertility in many couples is postponement of childbearing. The conception rate for older couples decreases for a number of reasons. For instance, eggs from older women and sperm from older men do not remain viable as long, so the likelihood of fertilization decreases. Additionally, older women are more likely to experience endometrial abnormalities and such intraperitoneal diseases as endometriosis.

Indications for Sonography in Infertility

Ultrasound can aid in the diagnosis and treatment of infertility in a number of ways. For instance, sonography can be used to monitor the ovulatory cycle to identify abnormalities of the ovulatory process. Although radiographic contrast hysterosalpingography is the traditional method used to evaluate tubal disease, sonography can also be used to establish tubal patency. Fluid or a contrast agent is injected into the intrauterine cavity and tubes to evaluate tubal patency. Abnormalities of endometrial maturation, uterine anomalies and uterine fibroids can also be evaluated sonographically.

As a part of treatment for infertility, sonography can be used to follow the development of the ovarian follicles before harvesting of eggs, and it can be used as a part of the procedure for inserting fertilized or unfertilized eggs into the fallopian tube or uterine cavity.

The indications for sonography in infertility are:

1. Serial monitoring of follicular development
2. Guided follicular aspiration
3. Assessment of endometrial development
4. Assessment of tubal patency

The Infertility Work-Up

The infertility investigation begins with a detailed history and physical examination of both members of the couple. Although male factors are the cause of infertility in a minority of the cases, male causes of infertility are usually investigated first because the tests are less invasive and less expensive. Semen is analyzed and the sperm are studied for motility, density, morphology, signs of infection, and antisperm antibodies. If the semen analysis is normal, attention turns to the female factors.

Causes of Infertility

1 Disorders of Ovulation

Ovulation disorders account for approximately 18% of all infertility problems.[178] Taking a careful history will help suggest whether or not an ovulatory problem is likely. If a woman has normal menstrual cycles, ovulatory problems are less likely. If ovulation disorders are suspected, a full endocrinological work-up is usually performed. Even in couples where the woman is apparently ovulatory, basal body charts and luteal phase progesterone testing may be helpful. In these patients, ultrasound for follicular development may be helpful for confirmation.

Anovulation

Three general classes of conditions lead to anovulation:

1. Failure of the hypothalamus and pituitary to produce hormones stimulating ovulation
2. Failure of the follicle to rupture, as is seen in unruptured follicle syndrome or dysfunctional dominant follicle
3. Polycystic ovary syndrome

Hypothalamic and Pituitary Causes of Anovulation

If the hypothalamus and pituitary gland cannot produce luteinizing hormone and follicular-stimulating hormone (Kallmann syndrome), gonadotropin-releasing agonist (GnRHa) can be administered with an intravenous infusion pump. Another approach is to use human menopausal gonadotropin (hMG) to induce ovulation. When the dominant follicle reaches 20 mm in diameter, human chorionic gonadotropin (hCG) is administered to trigger ovulation. Sonography may assist in the evaluation of follicular development in these cases, particularly if human menopausal gonadotropin is used. Patients receiving human menopausal gonadotropin are more likely to develop hyperstimulation than patients on an infusion pump.

Failure of Ovulation

One cause of failure of ovulation that has been proposed is *luteinized unruptured follicle syndrome* (LUF). In this condition, the follicle enlarges to a normal diameter but fails to rupture and release the oocyte. The margins of the follicle are hazy with indistinct borders; the wall of the follicle thickens and resembles a corpus luteum cyst. The luteinized unruptured follicle gradually regresses at the time that the normal corpus luteum would regress.

Dysfunctional Dominant Follicle

In some women, the follicle enlarges much more than a normal follicle enlarges, stays enlarged for a few days, and then gradually regresses without follicular rupture. In this condition, the thickening of the follicle wall normally seen in luteinization does not occur. The wall appears thin with a sharp echo from the margin. The follicle then regresses in size. The menstrual cycle is not necessarily prolonged, and the degree of menses at the end of the cycle is variable.

▋2▐ Polycystic Ovary Syndrome (Stein Leventhal Syndrome)

Polycystic ovary syndrome (PCOS) is a common cause of infertility. Women who have polycystic ovary syndrome tend to be obese and have endocrine abnormalities. Traditionally the diagnosis of polycystic ovary syndrome is a

Figure 170.
Polycystic ovary syndrome. Sagittal sonogram of the left ovary in a patient with polycystic ovary syndrome. Note the large ovarian size with abundant central stroma and numerous small peripheral follicles.

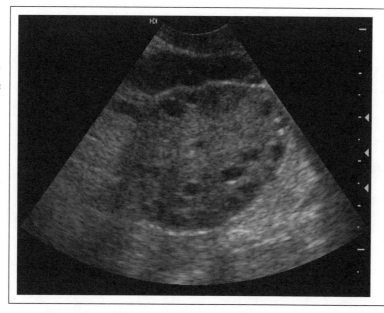

clinical one with endocrine assessment. Sonographic abnormalities have been reported in the ovaries. The ovaries are often rounded and enlarged and may be hyperechoic. In polycystic ovary syndrome, many more follicles are observed than are observed in normal ovulating women. Ten or more follicles in a single image may be observed (figure 170). Also, the follicles are usually peripheral and are all small and nearly the same size, measuring approximately 3–6 mm in diameter. An irregular outline of the ovary has sometimes been described as well.

In polycystic ovary syndrome, a single dominant follicle does not usually form. If hormonal stimulation is used, all the follicles enlarge. These women are particularly likely to develop ovarian hyperstimulation syndrome. Monitoring the ovaries with ultrasound is particularly important if hormonal stimulation is used in patients who have polycystic ovary syndrome. In polycystic ovary syndrome, the luteinizing hormone/follicle-stimulating hormone (LH/FSH) ratio is increased, and levels of circulating androgens are increased.

3 Tubal Factor

The fallopian tubes may be obstructed and prevent passage of the ovum into the uterus. Obstruction may be due to pelvic inflammatory disease, previous abortion, use of an intrauterine device (IUD), previous tubal surgery, endometriosis, or appendicitis. The conventional method of evaluating tubal patency and intrauterine anatomy is radiographic contrast hysterosalpingography. Recently, sonography has been used with the instillation of water or contrast into the endometrial cavity and fallopian tubes. Sonography can demonstrate patency of the fallopian tubes by demonstrating flow of fluid or contrast through the tube while it is being injected. In some cases, laparoscopy may be needed for further assessment.

If the tube is obstructed distally, surgical lysis of adhesions, fimbrioplasty, and tuboplasty may be performed. Proximal tubal obstruction is typically treated by cannulization of the tube by using a catheter through the uterus and cornu. This procedure is similar to angioplasty.

4 Cervical Factor

If the mucus in the cervix is of poor quality, it may act as a barrier to the sperm because of high viscosity or because of the presence of antisperm antibodies.

5 Abnormalities of the Uterus

Congenital abnormalities of the uterus, including uterus subseptus, bicornuate, and uterus didelphys can be evaluated by using either radiographic hystersalpingography or sonography. See "Pelvic Pathology" above.

Leiomyomas

Uterine fibroids or leiomyomas are benign growths of smooth muscle tissue that arise in the myometrium of the uterine wall. If fibroids are large, and particularly if they lie in the subendometrial position, they may impair fertility. Leiomyoma in the lower uterine segment may obstruct delivery. In some cases, myomectomy is performed in an attempt to improve fertility.

Endometrial Evaluation and Infertility

Normal endometrial development is critical for successful pregnancy. If the endometrium is too thin at the time of ovulation or if the endometrium does not develop in synchrony with ovulation, implantation may not occur. Observation of the thickness and echogenicity of the endometrium during the ovulatory cycle can assist in the infertility evaluation. The average normal endometrial thickness at ovulation is 8–10 mm. In polycystic ovary syndrome, the endometrium may be very prominent and thick, apparently because of high levels of luteinizing hormone. In luteal phase deficiency, the endometrial lining does not grow properly in the luteal phase because of inadequate progesterone production.

Medications and Treatment

Ultrasound Use in Infertility Procedures

A number of treatments may be used to assist infertile couples in the development of pregnancy. In general, these methods are referred to as *assisted reproductive technology* (ART). If ovulation is the problem, the ovaries may be stimulated with clomiphene citrate, human menopausal gonadotropin (hMG), or gonadotropin-releasing hormone agonists (GnRHa).

Clomiphene citrate is an estrogen analogue, which binds to the estrogen receptors in the hypothalamus. With clomiphene binding to the receptors, the feedback of estriol from the ovary is blocked, leading to the production of follicle-stimulating hormone by the hypothalamus, and ovulation occurs.

Human Menopausal Gonadotropin

Human menopausal gonadotropin (hMG) contains high levels of follicle-stimulating hormone and luteinizing hormone and may be injected to induce ovulation if a hypothalamic problem exists.

Gonadotropin-Releasing Hormone Agonists

Gonadotropin-releasing hormone agonists (GnRHa) are synthetic analogues of gonadotropin-releasing hormone, which stimulate the ovary to produce follicles. Gonadotropin-releasing hormone agonists produce a more normal follicular development of a dominant follicle compared with clomiphene citrate or human menopausal gonadotropin. Several different synthetic analogues have been developed.

Sonographic Follicular Monitoring

Sonography plays a major role in careful assessment of the ovaries bilaterally to determine the number and size of follicles present. Several sonograms are performed around the expected time of ovulation to determine which ovary will produce the dominant follicle. The dominant follicle produces the ovum for that cycle and generally measures 1.8–2.5 cm just before rupture.

Sonography may also be used to monitor follicle development when clomiphene citrate, human menopausal gonadotropin, or gonadotropin-releasing hormone agonists are being used. One of the objectives of the monitoring is to determine whether too many follicles are being stimulated and whether *ovarian hyperstimulation syndrome* (OHS) is developing. In ovarian hyperstimulation syndrome, there is weight gain, enlargement of ovarian cysts, ascites, and pleural effusions. In severe cases, the patient may develop hypotension, oliguria, electrolyte abnormalities, hemoconcentration, ovarian torsion, and thromboembolic complications (see the boxed insert). When multiple follicles develop, multiple pregnancy or ectopic pregnancy may be the result, even if ovarian hyperstimulation does not occur.

Ovarian hyperstimulation syndrome is characterized by:

1. Weight gain.

2. Cystic ovarian enlargement.

3. Ascites.

4. Pleural effusions.

In more severe forms:

1. Hypotension.

2. Oliguria.

3. Electrolyte abnormalities.

4. Hemoconcentration.

5. Thromboembolic complications.

6. Ovarian torsion.

Assisted Reproductive Technology

In Vitro Fertilization

The first child conceived by in vitro fertilization was due to the efforts of Dr. P. Steptoe and delivered on July 25, 1978. In vitro fertilization is indicated if there is irreversible tube occlusion, unexplained infertility, endometriosis, fertilization defects, or male factor infertility (see the boxed insert).

Indications for In Vitro Fertilization

1. Irreversible tubal occlusion.

2. Unexplained infertility.

3. Endometriosis.

4. Fertilization defects.

5. Male factor infertility.

If one of these factors is discovered on infertility work-up, stimulation of the ovary can be performed with the use of Clomid or Pergonal. When the three largest follicles reach 1.6–1.8 cm in diameter and estradiol levels are satisfactory, human chorionic gonadotropin is given to mature the follicles. Under direct ultrasound visualization, the oocytes can be aspirated from the follicles and incubated with sperm. Two to four of the developing embryos are inserted into the uterus near the fundus. If necessary, the embryos may be inserted into the uterus under direct ultrasound visualization. With IVF, the delivery of a normal infant occurs in approximately 21% of attempts.[179]

Gamete Intrafallopian Transfer

In gamete intrafallopian transfer (GIFT), oocytes are aspirated from stimulated follicles and immediately placed under laparoscopic visualization into the fallopian tube along with viable sperm. These elements are inserted into the fallopian tube from the abdominal approach through the fimbriated end of the tube. This procedure is used in couples who have at least one functional fallopian tube and evidence of cervical disorders or unexplained infertility. In some cases, the gamete intrafallopian transfer procedure may be performed under ultrasound visualization instead of by laparoscopy. The GIFT technique results in delivery of a normal-term infant in 28% of attempts.[179]

Zygote Intrafallopian Transfer

The zygote intrafallopian transfer (ZIFT) procedure is a variant of in vitro fertilization in which the oocytes are retrieved transvaginally, fertilized in vitro, and then inserted into the fallopian tube either laparoscopically or through a transcervical tube at one day of age instead of at day 2 or 3. It has been speculated that ZIFT might be more successful than GIFT because the embryo develops normally in the fallopian tube, but the validity of this assertion is still being evaluated.

Postmenopausal Pelvis

CHAPTER 14

Anatomy and physiology

Indications for sonography

Pathology

Therapy

. . . .

Anatomy and Physiology

Menopause occurs when no follicles remain in the ovaries that can respond to the follicular-stimulating hormone (FSH) produced by the pituitary gland. The ovary is no longer able to produce follicles and ovulate, and therefore estrogen and progesterone are no longer produced in adequate quantities.

Because no estrogen or progesterone is present, menstruation ceases and the uterus decreases in size. Specifically, the muscular body of the uterus diminishes in size and approaches the size of the cervix in A-P dimension. Normally, the postmenopausal endometrium is thin. The ovaries also decrease in size, apparently primarily because of lack of developing follicles.

The Uterus

As noted previously, after menopause the uterus rapidly decreases in size, particularly during the first 5 years following menopause. As the muscular body of the uterus continues to shrink, its size approaches the same A-P diameter as the cervix. The endometrial thickness is normally less than 8 mm. In women who have vaginal bleeding, an endometrial thickness of 5 mm or greater should be considered suspicious. The endometrium is measured excluding the hypoechoic inner layer of the uterine muscle surrounding it. If a woman is on hormone therapy after menopause, the appearance of the uterus and endometrium will not differ from that of a menstruating woman.

The Ovaries

As noted previously, the ovaries decrease in size after menopause owing to a lack of functioning follicles. The ovaries should not exceed 8 cubic centimeters of volume or 2 cm in greatest dimension, and neither ovary should be twice the size of the other one. Because few cysts and no follicles are visible in postmenopausal ovaries, the ovary may be difficult to identify and differentiate from other pelvic structures such as bowel.

Indications for Sonography

Three main reasons exist to perform sonography in postmenopausal women:

1. To evaluate the endometrium in a patient who has vaginal bleeding
2. To evaluate the uterus and ovaries in a woman who has a palpable pelvic mass
3. To screen for endometrial or ovarian cancer in high-risk women

Pathology

Ovarian Cancer

The incidence of ovarian cancer increases with age. Small cystic structures are identified within the ovaries, especially during the first 5–10 years after menopause, but should not exceed 5–10 mm. If a simple cyst exceeds 10 mm in size, follow-up is probably indicated, and if septations or nodules within the cyst are noted, surgery may be appropriate.

In the premenopausal woman, CA125, a serum marker for ovarian cancer, is difficult to interpret because many other conditions may also cause elevation of CA125. In postmenopausal women, however, the use of CA125 is more valuable in the detection of ovarian cancer because there are fewer other conditions that cause elevation.

The Sonographic Examination

When scanning the postmenopausal pelvis, views of the uterus, adnexa, and cul de sac should be obtained. In many laboratories, transabdominal views are obtained routinely. Endovaginal sonography should also be performed with the consent of the woman. Endovaginal sonography is particularly helpful in evaluating the thickness and homogeneity of the endometrium. Also, much clearer pictures of the ovaries can usually be obtained endovaginally. Sonohysterography may be performed if there is suspicion of abnormality of the endometrium. In this procedure, a small catheter is introduced into the uterine cavity, and fluid is instilled through the catheter to demonstrate the surface of the endometrium.

If an adnexal mass is visualized, the size and internal characteristics of the mass should be evaluated. Most but not all ovarian tumors are cystic. Doppler evaluation of adnexal masses may be somewhat helpful. If the resistance is lower, there should be a higher suspicion for malignancy. For instance, if a benign-appearing cyst is identified in the adnexa with a low resistive index in the postmenopausal patient, the finding is suspicious for malignancy.

Therapy

Hormonal Replacement

About 30% of postmenopausal women under the age of 65 use hormones after menopause.[180] The hormones can protect from fractures due to osteoporosis and may improve a woman's general well being. The use of hormones, however, especially estrogen, increases the proliferation of the endometrium. For this reason, most postmenopausal women who still have a uterus take combined estrogen and progesterone hormone treatment, either with a combined daily dose or with a sequential dose of first estrogen and then progesterone over a month-long cycle. In these women, the endometrial thickness varies with the cycle.

Hormone use in postmenopausal women will increase the uterine size but should not affect ovarian size.

Tamoxifen

Tamoxifen is an estrogen analogue that displaces estrogen in breast cancer cells. If the breast cancer is estrogen sensitive, tamoxifen can therefore inhibit the effect of estrogen on breast cancer. However, tamoxifen has an estrogenlike effect on the receptors in the uterus and endometrium, causing endometrial thickening, polyps, hyperplasia, and possibly malignancy. The typical sonographic appearance of tamoxifen is its effect on the endometrium, resulting in numerous cystic changes at the base of the endometrium.

Megestrol Acetate

Megestrol acetate is a synthetic progesterone. It has antiestrogen effects and suppresses estrogen. This drug is sometimes used to treat endometrial carcinoma. Lazebnik and others reported the sonographic appearance of the endometrium in a woman treated with megestrol acetate.[181] The endometrium was thickened and homogenous. No cystic changes were noted. Although the endometrium is thickened with the use of megestrol acetate, endometrial malignancy is not a likely result. In fact, megestrol is sometimes used to treat endometrial carcinoma. Uterine fibroids may incease in size with megestrol acetate treatment.

Pelvic Pathology

CHAPTER 15

Uterine pathology

Vaginal pathology

The ovary

Endometriosis

Polycystic ovary disease

Inflammatory pelvic conditions

Other pelvic masses

Urinary masses

Sonographic imaging of contraceptive devices

Upper abdominal findings associated with pelvic disease

. . . .

Uterine Pathology

Congenital Malformations

During embryologic development, the uterus and fallopian tubes develop from the paramesonephric ducts. The vagina forms from the urogenital sinus. In the course of the development of the uterus from the paired paramesonephric ducts, various malformations may result. For instance, there may be complete duplication of the uterus and vagina, called *uterus didelphys.* The malformation may be slightly less severe, with two separate uterine horns and two cervices but one vagina and a fused midline portion of the uterus. This condition is called *uterus bicornis bicollis.* If a bicornuate uterus exists but only one cervix, the malformation is called *uterus bicornis unicollis.*

Figure 171.

The more commonly diagnosed uterine abnormalities. Reprinted with permission from Richenberg J, Cooperberg P: Ultrasound of the uterus. In Callen PW (ed): *Ultrasonography in Obstetrics and Gynecology,* 4th edition. Philadelphia, Saunders, 2000, p 824.

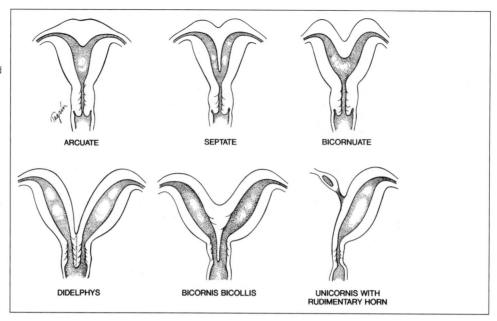

If the top of the uterus is smooth and not significantly notched in the midline and there is a septum that extends throughout the uterus, the malformation is called *uterus septus*. If there is a midline septum, which does not extend into the cervix, the malformation is called *uterus subseptus*. If only one uterine horn develops and there is one cervix, the malformation is called *uterus unicornis unicollis* (figure 171).

Conditions associated with duplication include increased incidence of spontaneous abortion, complications with pregnancy, renal anomalies (especially unilateral renal agenesis), and an obstructed duplicated horn that may present as a pelvic mass or hematometra. Clinically, patients may present with infertility and recurrent first trimester miscarriages or with hematometrocolpos.

Sonography, including three-dimensional sonography and sonohysterography, can delineate the internal anatomy of these malformations. Magnetic resonance is also a helpful imaging technique in evaluating these conditions.

Genital Anomalies Associated with In Utero Exposure to Diethylstilbesterol (DES)

Females with in utero exposure to diethylstilbesterol may develop uterine anomalies, including cervical stenosis and narrowing of the endometrial canal in the mid-uterus. Typically the upper part of the uterus is less affected. On hysterosalpingography the endometrial cavity may appear "T-shaped." In utero DES exposure is also associated with later development of adenocarcinoma of the vagina.

Uterine Masses

1 Leiomyomas

Leiomyomas, often informally called *fibroids,* are the most common pelvic masses in women. The incidence of uterine leiomyomas increases with age until menopause, and leiomyomas are more common in black women. It is estimated that 20–30% of all women will develop leiomyomas.[182] Thirty percent of hysterectomies are performed because of the presence of leiomyomas, although now myomectomy and angiographic embolization are becoming more popular.

Sonographically these tumors resemble the myometrium of the uterus. In many cases the tumors are well circumscribed (figure 172) and appear as rounded masses of approximately the same echogenicity as the surrounding myometrium. The echogenicity can be variable, however, and some fibroids

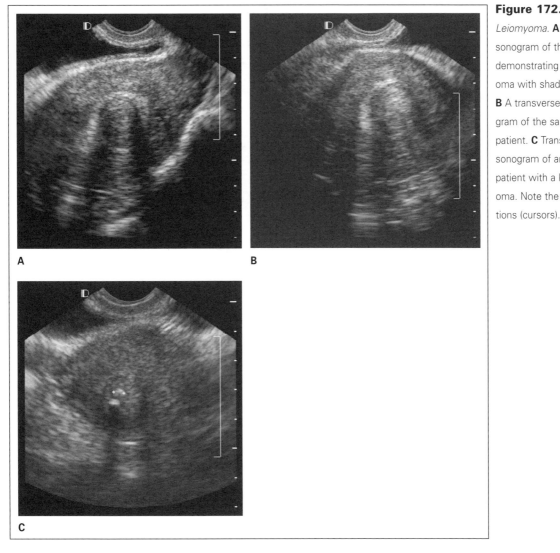

Figure 172.

Leiomyoma. **A** Sagittal sonogram of the uterus demonstrating a leiomyoma with shadowing. **B** A transverse sonogram of the same patient. **C** Transverse sonogram of another patient with a leiomyoma. Note the calcifications (cursors).

Figure 173.

Leiomyoma. **A** sagittal sonogram of the uterus demonstrates a well-circumscribed leiomyoma. **B** Transverse sonogram of the same patient, again demonstrating leiomyoma.

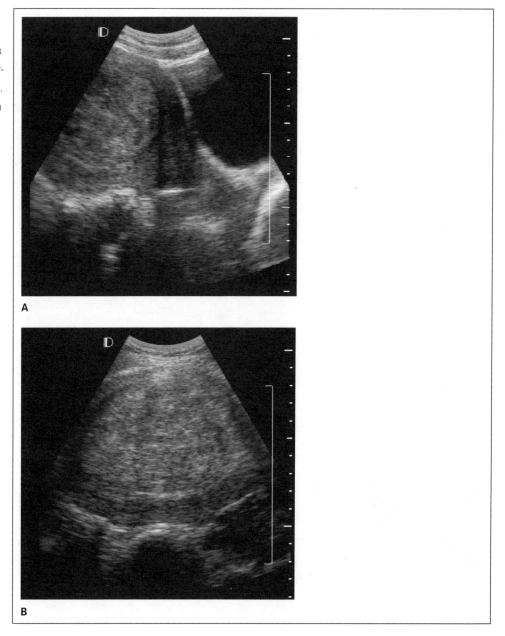

are significantly more echogenic (figure 173) than surrounding uterine muscle while others are somewhat more hypoechoic. Linear areas of posterior shadowing are often observed arising at the edge or within a uterine leiomyoma (figure 174). These shadows are likely due to critical angle reflections at the edges of rolls of muscle fibers. In some cases, calcifications may occur within the tumor in normal women. The uterus may be diffusely involved, and the tumors may not be separable or clearly defined on sonography. Usually the tumors arise from the fundus and mid-body of the uterus.

Fibroids arising in the cervix are rare but occur in perhaps 5–8% of cases.[183] Most leiomyomas are intramural or subserosal. Only about 5–10% lie in a

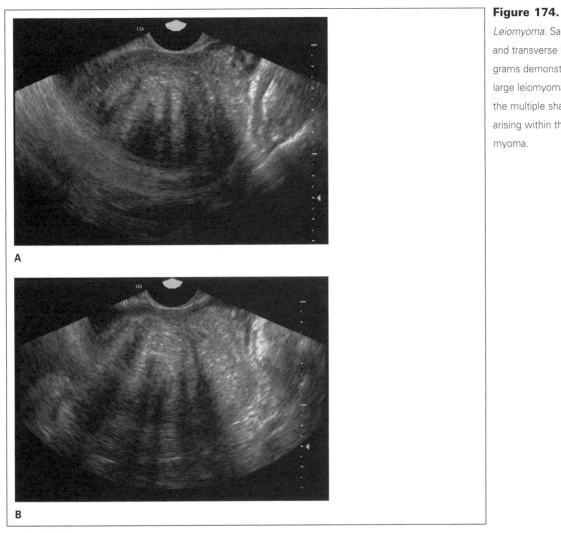

Figure 174.
Leiomyoma. Sagittal (**A**) and transverse (**B**) sonograms demonstrating a large leiomyoma. Note the multiple shadows arising within the myoma.

submucosal position adjacent to the endometrium.[183] These submucosal fibroids may aggravate bleeding at the time of menses.

The cause of fibroids is not entirely understood, but there is definitely estrogen dependence. Patients who are undergoing hormone replacement therapy or taking tamoxifen have been seen to correlate with growth of the leiomyomas.

Sonographically, a leiomyoma or fibroid is considered to be submucosal if the visible margin of the tumor lies close to the mucosa with some deviation of the endometrial echo. In many instances, a few slightly enlarged blood vessels will be found at the periphery of myomas.

With increased hormone levels such as occurs in pregnancy, the leiomyomas may enlarge and, if they grow fast enough, may become more symptomatic and necrotic in the center.

2 Leiomyosarcoma

Leiomyosarcoma is the very rare malignant form of leiomyoma. It constitutes approximately 1% of uterine malignancies.[184] Sonographically, leiomyosarcomas will appear quite similar to leiomyomas. One clue that a tumor may be malignant is rapid increase in size of a myoma without a hormonal explanation.

3 Adenomyosis

Adenomyosis is a condition in which glands of the endometrium form within the muscle of the uterine wall. Although this represents ectopic glandular tissue within the uterine muscle, the appearance resembles ill-defined fibroids within the uterus. Sonographically, the signs that may be observed include asymmetric wall thickness of the uterus, cystic changes within the myometrial area, coarse mottling of the myometrium, and multiple areas of faint posterior shadowing arising in the thickened portion of the uterine wall (figure 175). The diagnosis of adenomyosis by sonography is difficult and somewhat controversial, but a growing consensus exists that sonography can sometimes at least suggest the diagnosis. Magnetic resonance imaging is helpful for further evaluation. The clinical symptoms are typically pain and bleeding abnormalities associated with menses.

Endometrial Pathology

1 Endometrial Hyperplasia

Endometrial hyperplasia is the most common cause of bleeding in perimenopausal women. As a woman approaches menopause, hormonal changes occur, and endometrial thickening may result because of unopposed estrogen

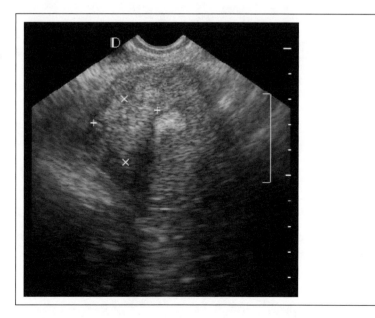

Figure 175.
Adenomyosis. Transverse sonogram of the uterus. Note the thickened and inhomogeneous portion of the uterine wall (cursors).

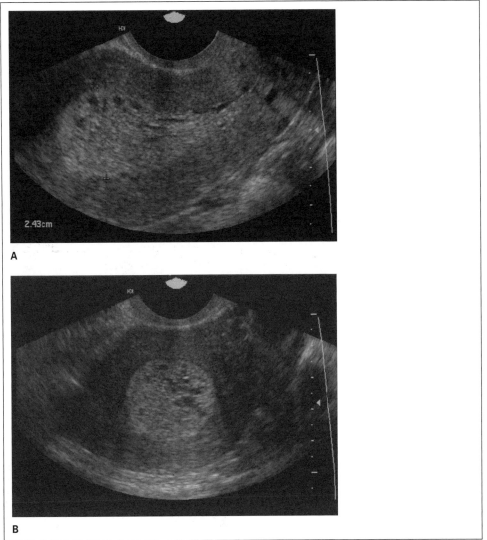

Figure 176.
Endometrial hyperplasia.
A Sagittal sonogram of the uterus. Note the thickened endometrium (cursors). **B** Transverse sonogram of the same patient. Again note the bright echogenic thickened endometrium.

stimulation. Sonographically, there is marked thickening of the endometrium in these patients (figure 176), and the thickening may be indistinguishable in some cases from endometrial polyp or carcinoma. For this reason, if the endometrium is thickened in a perimenopausal woman who is bleeding, endometrial aspiration biopsy is usually performed.

The use of tamoxifen for the treatment or prevention of breast cancer results in a thickened irregular endometrium within the uterus, sometimes with polyp formation and sometimes with subendometrial cystic changes.

Endometrial polyps represent overgrowth of endometrial glands and stroma covered by endometrial epithelium. Polyps may be pedunculated or sessile and are usually multiple and located in the fundus. Patients may be asymptomatic or present with vaginal bleeding or mucous discharge.

Sonohysterography is often helpful to evaluate suspected endometrial polyps or focal endometrial irregularity. Endometrial polyps are present in 38% of

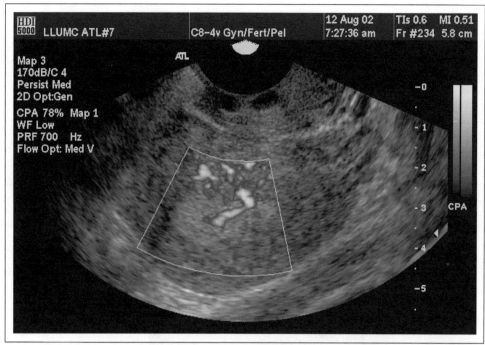

Figure 177.
Endometrial polyp. This endovaginal sonogram shows thickening of the endometrium. Note the single vessel entering the endometrium. At surgery, an endometrial polyp was identified and removed.

patients who have postmenopausal bleeding and differentials include hyperplasia, polyp, fibroid, or carcinoma.[185] If sonohysterography is not available, color or power Doppler imaging may be helpful. If a single vessel is identified entering the area of endometrial thickening, the diagnosis of endometrial polyp should be considered (figure 177).

2 Endometritis

Infection of the endometrium may occur after a dilation and curettage (D & C) procedure, pelvic inflammatory disease, or postpartum. When endometritis is present, the endometrium may appear thick and shaggy. There may be debris in the endometrial cavity, and on occasion air bubbles may be observed within the uterus.

3 Endometrial Carcinoma

Endometrial carcinoma is now the most common gynecological malignancy, with 33,000 new cases occurring each year in the United States.[186] There appears to be an association between endometrial carcinoma and a history of estrogen replacement. Patients usually present with postmenopausal bleeding. Sonographically, the endometrium may be thickened, measuring 5–8 mm in thickness, and there may be irregularity of the endometrium or myometrial distortion (figure 178). The tumors are typically diffusely or partially echogenic, with only 10–15% appearing isoechoic. Some patients who have endometrial carcinoma may not have a thickened endometrium, however.

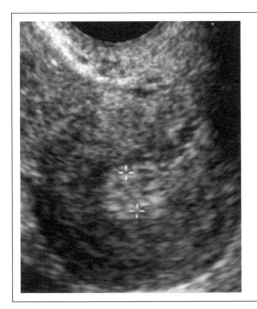

Figure 178.

Endometrial carcinoma. Sagittal view of the uterus demonstrating a prominent endometrium with irregular borders and complex internal echoes. Courtesy of Beryl Benacerraf, MD.

Sonohysterography or hysterosalpingography evaluation of the uterus is probably indicated in these cases.

An increased incidence of endometrial carcinoma exists in patients who are receiving tamoxifen for cancer. If the sonographic images suggest an irregular endometrial margin, which appears to extend into the muscle, this suggests endometrial invasion. Biopsy is often performed with suction and curettage.

4 Endometrial Adhesions

In women who have a history of infection or surgery, *endometrial adhesions* (Asherman syndrome) may sometimes be observed. Endometrial adhesions may be a cause of infertility or recurrent pregnancy loss. These adhesions are difficult to identify sonographically without inserting fluid into the uterine cavity. The sonographic evaluation is best performed using sonohysterography during the secretory phase of the cycle.

The Cervix

Common cervical masses include nabothian cysts, which are filled with fluid and show through transmission (figure 179). Solid masses in the cervix are usually fibroids. The primary method for detecting cervical carcinoma is a pap smear. Cervical carcinomas are typically squamous cell type, although rarely endometrial tumors are observed in the cervix. Sonography is not particularly helpful in the diagnosis of cervical carcinoma. The pap smear is a better screening test, for the disease can be detected when the lesions are still microscopic. If the cervical carcinoma is advanced, an ill-defined hyperechoic mass in the cervix may be observed, but magnetic resonance imaging is a better and more effective test for focal and distant extension of cervical carcinoma.

Figure 179.

Nabothian cyst. Sonogram of the cervix. Note the through transmission posterior to the nabothian cysts.

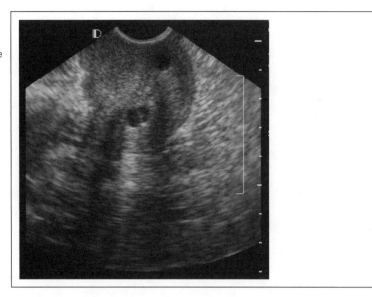

Figure 180.

Hematometracolpos. Sagittal sonogram of the uterus. Note the fluid within the uterus (U) and vagina (V).

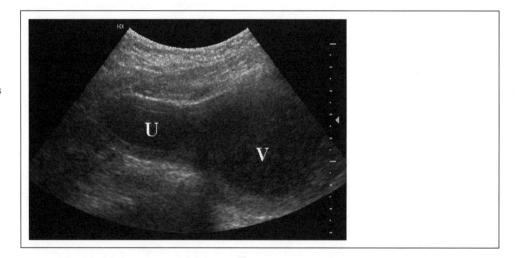

Vaginal Pathology

The most common abnormality of the vagina is imperforate hymen, resulting in hematometracolpos (figure 180). Another abnormality is Gartner's duct cyst that occurs in the wall of the vagina. These are mesonephric duct remnants from the structures that normally form into male genital organs. Epithelial tumors of the vagina and labia occur rarely.

The Ovary

Normal Sonographic Anatomy

The ovaries are usually but not always visible on either transabdominal or transvaginal sonography in menstruating women. The position of the ovaries is variable. The ovary may lie above the uterus posterior to the broad ligament or inferior and adjacent to the cervix. During the normal menstrual cycle, several small follicles usually develop in each ovary. One follicle becomes dominant and usually enlarges to 2.0–2.5 cm in diameter before ovulation. The follicles may be as small as 14 mm or as large as 29 mm in diameter at ovulation. The usual size of the ovary is approximately $1 \times 2 \times 3$ cm, with volume of 6–12 cubic centimeters. Occasional calcifications may be observed in the normal ovary.

After menopause, the ovaries decrease in size, and the average volume varies from 1 to 6 cubic centimeters. An ovarian volume exceeding 8 cubic centimeters in a postmenopausal woman is considered abnormal. Small anechoic cysts less than 3 cm in size may be observed in 15% of postmenopausal women. These cysts may change or disappear over time. Even in postmenopausal women, unilocular cysts less than 5 cm in size are usually not malignant. If a cyst is greater than 5 cm in size, or if it contains septations or nodules, surgery is indicated. Postmenopausal ovaries normally contain multiple peripheral echogenic foci; these foci aid in the identification of the ovaries.

Nonneoplastic Lesions

1 Functional Cysts

Functional cysts of the ovary include follicular cysts, corpus luteum cysts, and theca-lutein cysts. A *follicular cyst* is a mature follicle that fails to involute at ovulation. Because 2.5 cm is the upper limit of a normal developing follicle, only cysts larger than 2.5 cm are considered to be follicular cysts. Follicular cysts are usually unilateral, thin-walled, asymptomatic, and regress spontaneously. Ovarian cysts that are less than 3 cm in size generally resolve spontaneously. Ovarian cysts that are 3–5 cm usually require follow-up in 6–8 weeks, and many times these patients will be placed on birth control pills. When an ovarian cyst is greater than 10 cm, typically they do not resolve and have a higher malignancy potential requiring surgery.

A *corpus luteum cyst* is formed when hemorrhage occurs within the corpus luteum after ovulation. It can be larger and symptomatic. During pregnancy, the corpus luteum cyst usually reaches maximum size at approximately 10 weeks and resolves by 16 weeks. Increased blood flow and thickening of the wall (color plate 15) is often noted in corpus luteum cysts. Low resistance blood flow is noted.

A functional cyst or a corpus luteum cyst may contain internal hemorrhage. *Hemorrhagic cysts* are often symptomatic and may cause acute onset of pelvic pain. The sonographic appearance of hemorrhagic cyst depends on how long after the hemorrhage the sonogram is obtained. The hemorrhage may be bright and echogenic with through transmission, of medium echogenicity (color plate 16) or nearly anechoic with very thin septae.

Figure 181.

Theca-lutein cyst. Sagittal (**A**) and transverse (**B**) sonograms of a theca-lutein cyst. Note the septations.

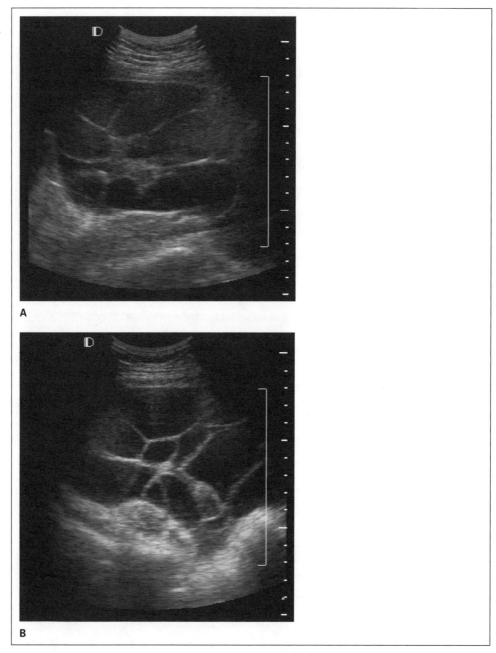

Transvaginal sonography improves the visualization of hemorrhagic cysts. A fluid-fluid level within the cyst is suggestive for hemorrhage. If follow-up sonograms are obtained, the internal appearance of the cyst should change over days to weeks.

Large bilateral multilocular ovarian cysts (figure 181) may occur if there are high levels of human chorionic gonadotropin circulating in the mother's blood. Typically, *theca-lutein cysts* are associated with a hydatidiform mole. The cysts may hemorrhage, rupture, or torse and may persist for days to weeks.

(Following evaluation of mole tissue, the theca-lutein cysts may take 2–4 months to regress.) Similar cystic changes are observed in multiple gestations and in patients treated for infertility.

2 Paraovarian Cysts

Paraovarian cysts occur in the broad ligament, not in the ovary. They account for 10% of all adnexal masses and are most common in the third and fourth decades of life.[187] Sonographically they have an appearance typical of cysts but do not lie within the ovary. They frequently are located superior to the uterine fundus and may contain internal echoes as a result of hemorrhage.

3 Peritoneal Inclusion Cysts

Peritoneal inclusion cysts are a form of pelvic adhesion in which fluid is trapped between fibrotic adhesions. Usually there is a history of trauma, abdominal surgery, pelvic inflammatory disease, endometriosis, or some combination of the above. Peritoneal inclusion cysts may reach 20 cm in size and are lined with mesothelial cells. They are sometimes referred to as *benign cystic mesothelioma or benign encysted fluid.* Sonographically, the typical appearance is that of an intact ovary surrounded by septations and fluid.

4 Ovarian Torsion

Ovarian torsion usually occurs in the first three decades of life and is associated with mobile adnexa. In 50–80% of cases, an ovarian tumor is the site of torsion.[188] Paraovarian cyst is another common mass that leads to torsion. Most ovarian tumors that lead to torsion are benign, such as dermoids. Ovarian torsion occurs more commonly on the right side because the sigmoid colon on the left impedes the development of torsion.

Clinically, patients present with acute or recurrent episodes of abdominal pain and occasionally a palpable mass. The symptoms may resemble appendicitis.

The sonographic appearance of ovarian torsion depends on whether or not an ovarian mass is present and on the duration and degree of torsion. If no ovarian mass is present, the ovary often enlarges, becomes edematous, and usually demonstrates multiple small follicles (color plate 17). If a mass is present within the ovary, edema may not be as evident.

The presence of a Doppler signal within an ovarian mass or an ovary does not exclude partial torsion. Absence of Doppler signal within the ovary may be observed in severe torsion, but some normal ovaries may not show arterial waveforms within them. If partial torsion occurs, there may be absence of diastolic flow in the arterial signal (color plate 17C) and venous flow may not be visible.

Table 15.
Classification of ovarian tumors.

Tumor Type	Tumor
Surface epithelial-stromal tumors	Serous cystadenoma
	Serous cystadenocarcinoma
	Cystadenofibroma
	Mucinous cystadenoma
	Mucinous cystadenocarcinoma
	Pseudomyxoma peritonei
	Endometroid tumors
	Clear cell tumors
	Transitional cell (Brenner) tumor
Germ cell tumors	Cystic teratoma (dermoid cyst)
	Struma ovarii
	Mature solid teratomas
	Dysgerminoma
	Yolk sac tumor
Sex-cord stromal tumors	Granulosa cell tumor
	Fibroma and thecoma
	Sertoli-Leydig tumor (arrhenoblastoma, androblastoma)

Neoplastic Ovarian Masses

Ovarian tumors can be divided into three general classes, as indicated in table 15:

1. Surface epithelial-stromal tumors
2. Germ cell tumors
3. Sex-cord stromal tumors

A few other tumors do not fit neatly into this classification system.

Surface Epithelial-Stromal Tumors

Surface epithelial-stromal tumors, the first major category of ovarian tumors, account for approximately 60% of all ovarian neoplasms and about 80–90% of primary ovarian malignancies.[189] The following tumors belong to this class:

■ Serous Cystadenoma

Most *serous cystadenomas* are unilocular and may reach 30 cm in size. Peak incidence is in the fourth and fifth decades of life. In some cases of benign serous cystadenomas, septa are visible. Sonographically, benign serous cystadenomas are sharply marginated, anechoic masses with thin internal septations (figure 182). Rarely, papillary projections from the septa are visible.

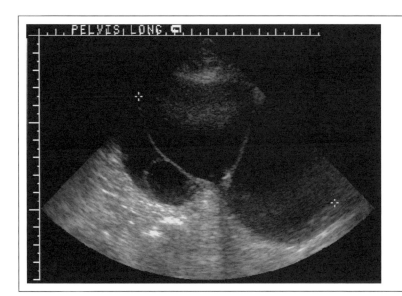

Figure 182.
Cystadenoma. Sagittal sonogram of a cystadenoma. Note multiple septations.

2 Serous Cystadenocarcinoma

Typically occurring between ages 45 and 65, *serous cystadenocarcinoma* accounts for approximately 40–50% of all malignant ovarian neoplasms.[190] Sonographic findings that suggest cystadenocarcinoma include numerous septae and large papillary masses arising from the internal surfaces of the tumor (color plate 18). Papillary masses on the periphery of the tumor may also be observed, and ascites is sometimes present, suggesting mesenteric metastasis.

3 Cystadenofibroma

A *cystadenofibroma* resembles a cystadenoma or cystadenocarcinoma but contains dense solid areas of tissue similar to fibroids or fibromas. These tumors are nearly always benign and usually occur after age 40.

4 Mucinous Cystadenoma

Mucinous cystadenoma comprises 20–25% of all benign ovarian neoplasms.[191] Mucinous cystadenomas usually occur in the third to fifth decades of life and are bilateral in only 2–3% of cases.

The sonographic appearance of mucinous cystadenoma is similar to that of serous cystadenoma, with the exception that the septa are more numerous. In some cases fine echoes may be observed in the dependent portions of the tumor because of the thicker contents (figure 183). This finding is inconsistent, however.

5 Mucinous Cystadenocarcinoma

The fluid in mucinous cystadenocarcinomas contains more proteinaceous material than serous tumors. As in the serous tumors, papillary excrescences,

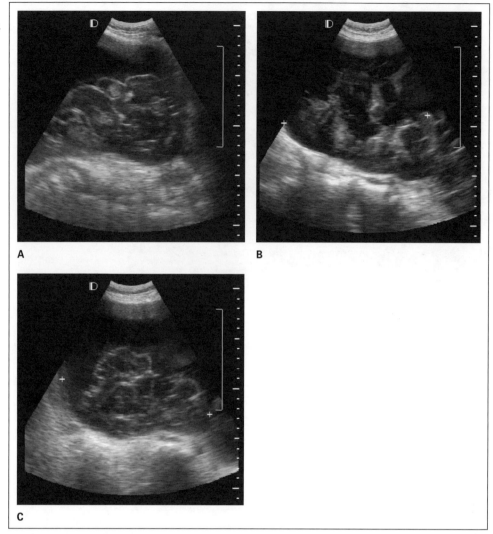

Figure 183.
Mucinous cystadenoma. Sagittal (**A** and **B**) and transverse (**C**) sonograms of a mucinous cystadenoma. Note the low-level echoes within the septated segments.

thick septa, solid areas, and hemorrhage are more common in malignant tumors. Sonographically, mucinous cystadenocarcinomas closely resemble serous malignant tumors. In some cases, debris in the fluid is more visible in mucinous tumors.

6 Pseudomyxoma Peritonei

Pseudomyxoma is a condition in which extensive mucinous material is present throughout the abdomen. This may be due to extension or spread of a malignant or mucinous tumor, or it may be due to rupture of a benign mucinous tumor or rupture of a mucocele of the appendix. Pseudomyxoma peritonei may also arise from mucinous tumors from other organs such as the bowel.

7 Endometroid Tumors

Endometroid ovarian tumors are lined with cells resembling the endometrium. Eighty percent of ovarian endometroid tumors are malignant.[192] The sonographic appearance of malignant endometroid tumors resembles the other

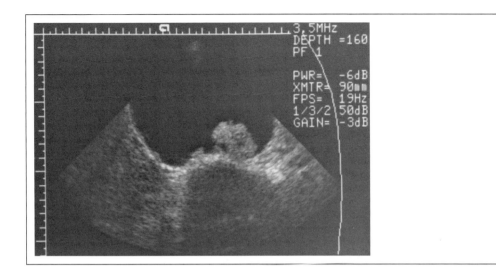

Figure 184.
Endometroid. Transverse sonogram of an endometroid tumor. Note the papillary mass.

cystic tumors. A cystic mass containing papillary projections is a typical appearance (figure 184), but occasionally an endometroid tumor may appear as a predominately solid mass. Twenty-five to thirty percent of endometroid tumors are bilateral.[193]

8 Clear Cell Tumors

Clear cell tumors are thought to arise from the mesonephros. They are as large as 15 cm in diameter and may occur at any age. In 15–20% of cases they are bilateral.[194] They are associated with endometriosis in the pelvis. Most clear cell tumors are frankly invasive and constitute 5–10% of all malignant ovarian epithelial stromal tumors.

9 Transitional Cell (Brenner) Tumor

Mostly benign, *transitional cell tumors* constitute 1–2% of all primary ovarian tumors.[195] The age of peak incidence is the fourth to the eighth decades, and 6–7% are bilateral. Typically these tumors are small, well circumscribed, and solid. Occasionally cystic components or calcifications may be observed. The appearance of transitional cell tumors resembles that of an ovarian fibroma.

Germ Cell Tumors

Germ cell tumors constitute the second general class of ovarian neoplasms. In children and adolescents, 60% of ovarian tumors are of germ cell origin and one-third are malignant. In adults, 95% of germ cell tumors are benign and consist of mature cystic teratomas (dermoid cysts).[196] The following are germ cell tumors:

1 Cystic Teratoma (Dermoid Cyst)

Dermoid cysts make up 5–25% of all ovarian neoplasms and occur most commonly during the reproductive years.[197] A dermoid cyst arises from the

Figure 185.
Dermoid with "tip of the iceberg" sign. Note echogenic mass with shadowing.

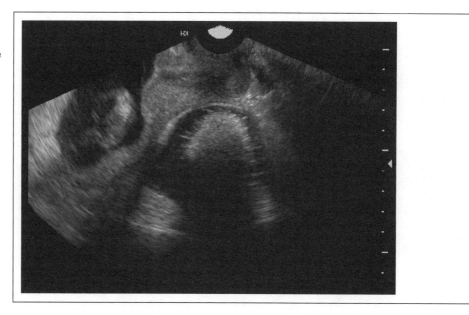

ectoderm; a teratoma usually contains elements arising from all three germ layers: *ectoderm, mesoderm,* and *endoderm.* Nearly all of them are benign. Eight to fifteen percent are bilateral, and the tumors vary in size, becoming as large as 40 cm in some cases. These tumors usually are cystic, with hair, fluid, and fat within them. Symptoms observed in cystic teratoma include abdominal pain, mass, swelling, and bleeding. Torsion can occur. Treatment is excision.

The sonographic appearance of dermoid cysts is variable. Some teratomas are primarily cystic in appearance, and many have a large echogenic area with posterior shadowing. This shadowing has been called "tip of the iceberg" sign (figure 185). This echogenic shadowing mass is due to hair and fat within the cystic mass. In some cases debris within the fluid or fine septations are noted. This may be related to hair within the cystic component. Calcifications are sometimes observed, typically due to bones or dental elements within the dermoid. In some cases, a rounded echogenic mass is noted at one end of the cystic tumor; this finding is called a *dermoid plug* (figure 186).

Other conditions may mimic dermoid cysts on sonography. Pitfalls include pedunculated fibroids, extraovarian lipomatosis masses, other cystic neoplasms with echogenic mural nodules, ectopic pregnancy, fluid-filled distended bowel, and inflammatory disease such as tubo-ovarian abscess (TOA) or perforated appendicitis with appendicolith.

2 Struma Ovarii

Struma ovarii are a special form of teratoma in which virtually all the tissue in the tumor resembles thyroid tissue. These tumors produce thyroid hormone.

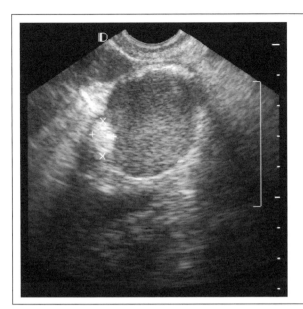

Figure 186.
Dermoid plug. Note echogenic mass (cursors).

3 Mature Solid Teratomas

Occasionally benign teratomas may present as a predominantly solid mass. Their appearance resembles immature teratomas, but they grow slowly in comparison.

4 Immature Teratomas

Immature teratomas are malignant lesions that comprise less than 1% of all ovarian teratomas.[198] Malignant teratomas occur primarily in the first two decades of life, and they are virtually unknown after menopause. The tumors are usually large, up to 28 cm, and are predominately solid but may contain cystic areas.

5 Dysgerminoma

Dysgerminoma is a malignant germ cell tumor that comprises approximately 1–2% of primary ovarian neoplasms and 3–5% of ovarian malignancies.[199] It occurs primarily in the second and third decades and may be observed in pregnancy. Ten to 17% are bilateral. Dysgerminomas are typically solid with a multilobular texture (figure 187). Approximately 5% of dysgerminomas produce human chorionic gonadotropin (hCG). The cells that occur in dysgerminomas are histologically identical to seminoma of the testis. The tumors typically grow rapidly, but metastatic spread is lymphatic and usually occurs late.

6 Yolk Sac Tumor

Yolk sac tumor (endodermal sinus tumor) is the second most common malignant germ cell neoplasm after dysgerminoma. It occurs most frequently in the second and third decades of life. It is nearly always unilateral and varies in

Figure 187.

Dysgerminoma. (Courtesy Beryl R. Benacerraf, MD, Harvard Medical School.)

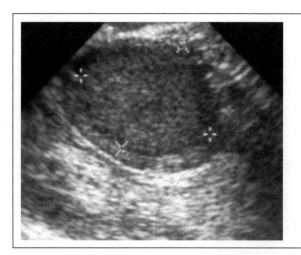

size from 3 to 30 cm. An elevated serum AFP level may be present. The mass is typically encapsulated, round, oval, or globular. It may appear similar sonographically to a dysgerminoma. Yolk sac tumors are highly malignant, metastasizing early via the lymphatics. They also invade surrounding structures.

Sex-Cord Stromal Tumors

The third general class of ovarian neoplasms are sex-cord stromal tumors. They account for 8% of all ovarian tumors.[200] Half of all sex-cord tumors are fibromas. The following tumors belong to this group:

1 Granulosa Cell Tumor

Granulosa cell tumors arise from cellular elements of the Graafian follicle and are hormonally active, producing estrogen. The high estrogen levels associated with this tumor lead to endometrial carcinoma in 10–15% of patients. Nearly all granulosa cell tumors are unilateral and most occur in postmenopausal women. These tumors have low malignant potential in the ovary.

2 Fibroma and Thecoma

Fibroma and thecoma tumors arise from ovarian stroma and may be difficult to distinguish from each other either sonographically or pathologically. Tumors that have more thecal cells are classified as thecomas, and those that have more fibrous tissue are classified as theco-fibromas or fibromas (figure 188). These tumors are benign.

Fibromas make up approximately 4% of ovarian neoplasms, are usually unilateral, and occur most commonly in menopausal and postmenopausal women. Rarely, they produce estrogen. More commonly they are asymptomatic and reach a large size. Ascites is reported in about half of the patients who have fibromas larger than 5 cm. Meig's syndrome (ascites and pleural effusion) occurs in 1–3% of patients who have fibromas.

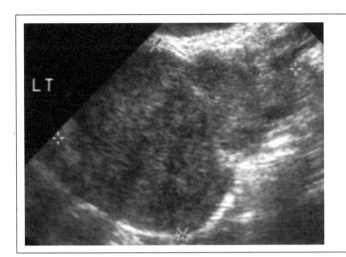

Figure 188.
Fibroma. Courtesy of Beryl R. Benacerraf, MD, Harvard Medical School.

Sonographically fibromas are hypoechoic masses with marked posterior shadowing and resemble leiomyomas except they arise from the ovary. Their appearance is similar to that of Brenner tumors and pedunculated uterine fibroids.

Thecomas are usually unilateral, always benign, and frequently show clinical signs of estrogen production. Sizes typically vary from 5 to 10 cm, and 70% occur in postmenopausal females.

3 Sertoli-Leydig Tumor (Arrhenoblastoma, Androblastoma)

Fewer than 0.05% of all ovarian tumors are Sertoli-Leydig tumors. These tumors usually occur in women under 30 and are typically unilateral and 5–15 cm in size. These tumors arise from cells similar to those of the embryonic testis and may produce male hormones. In about a third of the cases, symptoms of virilization are observed, including hair loss, breast atrophy, and enlargement of the clitoris. (In some cases these tumors may produce estrogen.) Ten to twenty percent of these tumors are malignant.

Metastatic Tumors

Approximately 5–10% of ovarian neoplasms are metastatic in origin. The most common primary sites are the breast and gastrointestinal tract. A *Krukenberg tumor* is a tumor that contains mucin-secreting "signet ring" cells and is usually gastric or colonic in origin. There are several routes of potential spread of tumor to the ovary.

1. The tumor may extend directly from the fallopian tube, colon, or retroperitoneum.

2. Malignant cells may travel through the endometrial cavity and fallopian tube to the ovary.

3. Tumors may spread from more distant sites by blood or lymphatic dissemination.

4. Surface implantation of tumors that spread through the peritoneal cavity is another route of metastasis to the ovary.

Endometrial carcinoma may metastasize to the ovary but would be very difficult to distinguish from primary endometroid carcinoma.

Metastasis to the ovary may present as bilateral solid masses that may become necrotic and show complex cystic change. If so, the tumors may resemble cystadenocarcinoma of the ovary.

Lymphoma may involve the ovary and is often bilateral. Sonographic appearance is similar to lymphoma elsewhere in the body as a solid hypoechoic mass.

Ovarian Carcinoma Screening

Ovarian carcinoma is the fourth leading cause of cancer death in women in the United States and makes up 25% of all gynecologic malignancies.[201] Ovarian carcinoma has the highest mortality rate of gynecologic malignancies because the diagnosis is usually made late. Ovarian carcinoma is much more common than endometrial or cervical carcinoma in premenopausal woman. Risk factors for the development of ovarian carcinoma include increasing age, nulliparity, infertility, family history of ovarian cancer, and history or previous breast, endometrial, or colon cancer. Ovarian cancer is also more common in Ashkenazi Jews.

CA125 is a high-molecular-weight glycoprotein recognized by the OC125 monoclonal antibody. CA125 is elevated in approximately 60–95% of women who have epithelial ovarian cancer but is less effective for detecting early disease and does not detect mucinous or germ cell tumors.[202] Furthermore, elevation of CA125 may be observed in benign conditions in menstruating women, including fibroids, pelvic inflammatory disease, and endometriosis. For these reasons, CA125 level measurement is not an effective method of screening for ovarian carcinoma in premenopausal women.

Numerous studies have been performed to evaluate the sonographic appearance of the ovaries and color Doppler to evaluate for ovarian malignancy, but these trials have not generally been shown to be cost-effective. However, postmenopausal screening for ovarian cancer using CA125 elevation as an indication for sonographic evaluation is more effective. The specificity obtained exceeded 99%.[203]

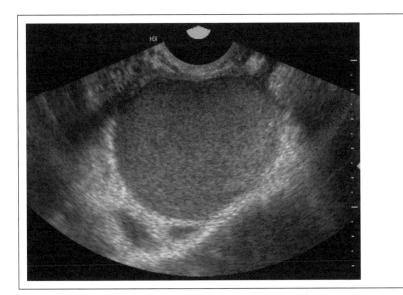

Figure 189.

Endometrioma. Sonogram of endometrioma. Note low-level echoes and through transmission.

Endometriosis

Endometriosis is defined as the presence of functioning endometrial tissue outside the endometrium and uterus. This condition typically affects women in the reproductive years and causes dysmenorrhea, dyspareunia, lower abdominal pelvic and back pain, and infertility. The endometrial implants may occur on the ovary, uterine ligaments, rectovaginal septum, cul-de-sac, and pelvic peritoneum. The only sonographically detectable forms of endometriosis consist of cystic masses containing endometrial tissue. These may occur within or outside the ovary. The cysts sonographically appear to contain fine low-level echoes in most cases. In some cases, the endometriomas (chocolate cysts) may be echogenic with posterior through transmission (figure 189) or may show fine stranding within the cyst, depending on the timing of the hemorrhage. Sonographically, endometrial implants on the surface of organs are not usually detectable.

Polycystic Ovary Disease

Polycystic ovary disease is an endocrinologic disorder. Typically the luteinizing hormone (LH) level is elevated and the follicle-stimulating hormone (FSH) level is depressed. Sonographically, the ovaries are sometimes enlarged. Numerous small cysts of approximately 3 mm in size are noted in the ovaries, and no large dominant cysts are identified. Usually the sonographic appearance consists of 10 or more cysts in a single image at the periphery of the ovary, with prominent central stroma in the ovary (see figure 170). Less commonly, multiple cysts 2–4 mm in diameter are noted distributed throughout the stroma. An irregular outline of the ovary is sometimes observed.

Stein-Leventhal syndrome, including oligomenorrhea, hirsutism, and obesity, is only one presentation of the spectrum of clinical disease called polycystic ovary disease.

Inflammatory Pelvic Conditions

Pelvic Inflammatory Disease

Bacteria are the usual agent of ovarian infections in Western countries. Ovarian involvement in pelvic inflammatory disease (PID) is nearly always secondary to infection first of the salpinx. Initially the ovary and tube may be still recognizable, but eventually the condition may progress to tubal-ovarian abscess (TOA). The symptoms are typically abdominal or pelvic pain and, less frequently, fever, vaginal discharge, bleeding, or urinary symptoms. Early in

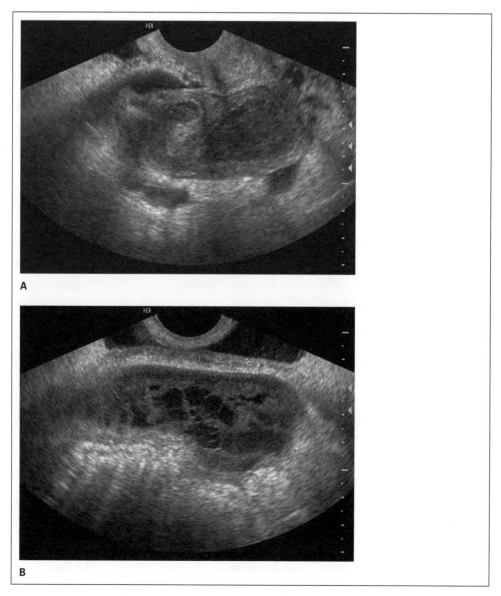

Figure 190.
Pelvic inflammatory disease. **A** Sagittal sonogram of the left fallopian tube. Note thickened wall and debris within the tube. **B** Transverse sonogram of a nearby abscess. Note debris and septations within the abscess.

the disease, sonographic findings may be minimal, but some findings (figure 190) have been described that suggest pelvic inflammatory disease:

1. Thickening of the fallopian tube to 5 mm or greater.

2. "Cogwheel" sign: a transverse view of the fallopian tube shows the fallopian lumen resembles a "cogwheel."

3. A fluid collection with incomplete septa correlating with folds or kinks in a dilated tube.

4. "Beads on a string" sign: multiple 2- to 3-mm nodules at the margins of the fluid-filled structure.

5. Diffuse cystic areas suggesting abscess with thickened walls and obstruction of architecture of both adnexa. Often there will be increased blood flow at the margins of these fluid spaces.

Laparoscopy with tubal culture may be performed for confirmation.

Other Pelvic Masses

The most frequent cause of pelvic mass on pelvic exam is probably an enlarged colon filled with fecal material. Typically, sonography can identify the presence of enlarged colon with fecal material. Peristalsis may be visible.

In some cases a true bowel mass such as a carcinoma of the rectosigmoid cecum or ileum will be present and mimic an adnexal mass. Again, careful sonographic examination should be able to delineate the origin of the mass.

Inflammatory bowel disease, sometimes with associated abscesses, may also be confused with adnexal mass or pelvic inflammatory disease.

Another common condition that can be confused with inflammatory disease of the adnexa is appendicitis. Visualization of an inflamed appendix and visualization of normal adnexal structures is helpful for differentiating these conditions.

Right or left colon diverticulitis may also simulate adnexal inflammatory disease. Sonography can often distinguish these conditions.

Urinary Masses

The pelvic kidney may present as a clinically palpable pelvic mass and is easily distinguished from other pelvic organs by sonography. An enlarged bladder or bladder diverticulum may be confused with a cystic pelvic mass. Careful sonographic examination should be able to distinguish these conditions. If necessary, post-void imaging may be helpful.

Dilated distal ureters may resemble adnexal cysts on transverse scans, but the ureters should become tubular in appearance on sagittal imaging.

Sonographic Imaging of Contraceptive Devices

An intrauterine device (IUD) is a physical structure placed in the endometrial cavity to impair fertility. Over the years, various shapes of IUDs have been produced. Currently, two intrauterine devices may deliver hormones directly to the endometrium.

Sonographically, an IUD appears as a highly echogenic usually linear structure within the endometrial cavity or body of the uterus. In some cases parallel echoes from the anterior and posterior surface of the IUD may be visible (figure 191). If the IUD is eccentric in position, the possibility of migration of the IUD into the myometrium should be considered. If blood clots or retained products of conception are present in the uterus, identification of an IUD may be more difficult.

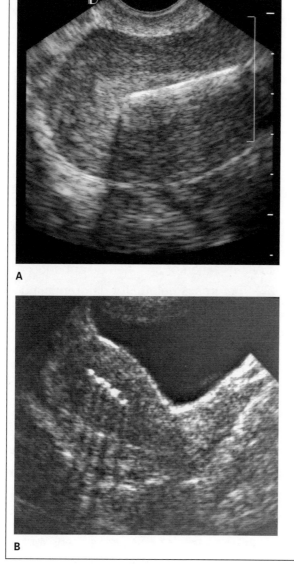

Figure 191.
Intrauterine device.
A Sagittal sonogram of intrauterine device. Note the linear echogenic structure within the endometrial cavity.
B Another type of IUD (Lippes Loop). Note the multiple reflectors within the uterine cavity.

Upper Abdominal Findings Associated with Pelvic Disease

In some patients who have pelvic disease, sonographic findings may be visible in the upper abdomen. These abdominal findings may sometimes be the first signal that there is a problem in the pelvis. Unilateral or bilateral hydronephrosis may be observed in a patient who has a pelvic mass that is compressing the ureters. Metastases in the liver from uterine or ovarian primaries are very uncommon. A pelvic colon tumor would be a more likely source. Generalized ascites and omental masses may be observed in ovarian malignancy.

Patient Care Preparation and Techniques

PART III

SONOGRAPHER'S INTERACTION WITH THE PATIENT

PERFORMING THE EXAMINATION

SUPINE HYPOTENSION

INFECTIOUS DISEASE CONTROL

PHYSICAL PRINCIPLES

ARTIFACTS

BIOEFFECTS

Patient Care Preparation and Techniques

CHAPTER 16

Sonographer's interaction with the patient

Performing the examination

Supine hypotension

Infectious disease control

Physical principles

Artifacts

Bioeffects

. . . .

Sonographer's Interaction with the Patient

Before beginning an ultrasound examination, it is important to review any medical information available regarding the patient's condition. The sonographer should carefully review the request for the examination, the reason for the request, and the medical chart, if available, for relevant laboratory data.

When the patient is in the examination room, the sonographer should introduce himself or herself and explain to the patient in simple language what examination is to be performed and how the procedure will be done. At this time, the sonographer may ask any medical questions about the reason for the examination, the symptoms the patient is experiencing, and any previous testing or procedures that have been done.

Performing the Examination

The examination should be performed according to clear and specific protocols. The sonographer should know which images are required and should label the images clearly. The exam protocol may vary depending on indication, patient history, and clinical presentation.

For pelvic examinations, the endovaginal technique should be explained to the patient. For instance, the patient may find it helpful if the sonographer explains that images taken by the endovaginal approach are often clearer and show pelvic detail more accurately. Explaining to the patient that the transducer is about the size of a tampon and that it will be covered with a sterile condom is helpful. If the patient has a latex allergy, a nonlatex condom should be used. The patient may insert the probe if that is her preference.

When an endovaginal examination is performed by a male sonographer, it is advisable to have a female chaperone in the room. The patient may refuse the examination if she does not wish to undergo endovaginal sonography. Endovaginal sonography is not generally performed on virginal patients and is not advisable in patients who have received pelvic radiation for cervical carcinoma. In the latter group of patients, the vagina will be scarred, and the endovaginal approach is likely to be painful and unsuccessful. If a patient is confused and unable to cooperate, endovaginal sonography is not advisable.

Supine Hypotension

During the second and third trimesters of pregnancy, a woman may experience light-headedness and shortness of breath during an obstetrical sonogram. These symptoms are often due to pressure of the enlarged uterus on the inferior vena cava, with reduction of venous return of blood. If the patient experiences these symptoms, turning the patient on the left side (away from the vena cava) will relieve pressure. Placing a cool damp cloth on the forehead or the neck may be helpful as well.

Infectious Disease Control

A number of housekeeping procedures help prevent transmission of bacteria and other infectious agents from staff to patient. Regularly wiping down the equipment with a bactericidal agent is helpful. Regular cleaning of exam tables is also beneficial. Transducers should be cleaned with a bactericidal agent between examinations, and endovaginal transducers should be soaked in such an agent between examinations. A condom must be placed over an endovaginal transducer before examination. If an open wound is present and sonography is required either within the wound or immediately adjacent to the wound, a sterile transducer cover and sterile gel should be used. In some clinical settings, thin plastic covers are routinely placed over transducers for all examinations.

Physical Principles

Sonography images the internal body structures by a method different from any of the other usual imaging methods, such as computerized tomography (CT), magnetic resonance imaging (MRI), or radiography. In sonography, a very high-frequency sound source emits focused sound beams that travel into the body and are reflected by interfaces within and between body organs. The sound reflections are then received electronically and processed to make an image of the internal structures of the body. In general, transducers producing higher frequencies of sound will give better detail of the internal structures of the body. However, higher-frequency signals are also more strongly attenuated within the body; therefore, lower-frequency transducers may be necessary to visualize deep structures.

Artifacts

Sonographic artifacts are details in a sonogram that do not accurately represent anatomic details in the patient. Many sonographic artifacts have been observed and reported, and a detailed discussion of these artifacts is beyond the scope of this book; however, a few of the more common sonographic artifacts will be reviewed briefly.

Reverberation Artifact

The reverberation artifact will be observed if there are multiple reflections within the body structures between the transducer and the body part being examined. For instance, hazy gray echoes in the anterior aspect of the urinary bladder are often due to sound bouncing back and forth between different layers of the abdominal wall before entering the bladder and when returning to the transducer. A similar finding is observed in the anterior half of the fetal skull, again as a result of reflections back and forth between the surface of the skull and more superficial soft tissues.

Refraction Artifact

If a sector transducer is used to image pelvic structures through the distended urinary bladder, two images of the structures posterior to the urinary bladder may sometimes be observed. For instance, a small gestational sac within the uterus may appear to be two gestational sacs. This artifact is due to a lens effect from abdominal wall structures. In this case, two different sound beams directed in slightly different directions are refracted and directed at the same point deeper in the pelvis. If this occurs, the sonogram may depict two images of the gestational sac. This artifact occurs only at the midline in the pelvis on transverse views, and moving the transducer to the right or to the left will eliminate the artifact.

Bioeffects

As noted previously, sonographic imaging is unlike any other imaging method in radiology. Ionizing radiation is not used, and the images produced use focused sound waves that reflect back to the transducer and are received to form an electronic image.

After extensive investigation for the past 40 years, significant biological effects have been observed using ultrasound on living tissue in mammals; they can be divided into two basic mechanisms:

1. Thermal heating
2. Cavitation

Thermal Heating

As ultrasound is transmitted into the body for imaging purposes, a gradual increase in temperature of the tissues being examined takes place. There seems to be general agreement that if the temperature increase within the tissue is less than 2°C, no significant biological effects will be observed. No significant biological effects have been observed for increases of 4°C for up to 16 minutes and 6°C for up to 1 minute. In general, it is recommended that unfocused ultrasound beam intensities not exceed 100 milliwatts per square centimeter for unfocused beams and 1 watt per square centimeter for focused beams. If these power limits are observed, no significant biological effects would be expected, even in the first trimester of pregnancy.

Higher power levels are sometimes used in diagnostic imaging for purposes other than fetal imaging. For instance, power levels used in Doppler studies of the vascular system and in echocardiography may exceed these limits.

Cavitation

The bioeffects observed in cavitation are more complex. The term *cavitation* or *acoustic cavitation* relates to interaction of small gas bubbles within water or tissue in the body and the ultrasound beam. The change in bubble size observed while interacting with the ultrasound beam is a complex process, and temperatures exceeding 5,000 degrees Kelvin may occur for an instant at the point of collapse of a bubble. A standardization of power measurement in the context of cavitation is characterized by the mechanical index (MI). In general, normal tissue, such as kidney tissue, does not show evidence of cavitation with mechanical indexes up to 4. However, air-containing tissues such as lung can show evidence of tissue damage with a mechanical index as low as 0.3.

Over the past 40 years, numerous clinical studies have been performed to evaluate for possible bioeffects of normal ultrasound imaging during pregnancy. These studies have shown no evidence of significant biologic effects on fetuses of pregnant women undergoing routine diagnostic sonography.

PART IV: Case Studies for Self-Assessment

OBSTETRICS

GYNECOLOGY

ANSWERS & EXPLANATIONS

Case Studies for Self-Assessment

CHAPTER 17

Obstetrics

Gynecology

Answers & Explanations

. . . .

Obstetrics

1 A 1 cm thick placenta would most likely be associated with:

   A. Gestational diabetes

   B. Erythroblastosis fetalis

   C. Intrauterine growth restriction (IUGR)

   D. Chorioangioma

2 The following Doppler images were obtained from the fetal cord and middle cerebral artery (MCA):

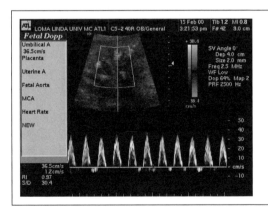

These images demonstrate:

   A. Normally low-resistance cord and high-resistance head Doppler

   B. Abnormally high-resistance cord and low-resistance head Doppler

   C. Normally low-resistance cord and head Doppler

   D. Abnormally high-resistance cord and head Doppler

3 Consider this sonographic image:

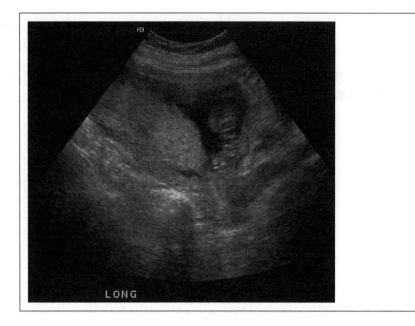

It most likely represents:

A. Low-lying placenta

B. Central placenta previa

C. Focal myometrial contraction

D. Over-distended urinary bladder

4 What would be the most likely clinical presentation for larger, retroplacental abruptions?

A. Painless vaginal bleeding

B. Painful vaginal bleeding

C. Painful vaginal bleeding with severe uterine contractions

D. Painless vaginal bleeding with severe uterine contractions

5 Risk factors for placental abruption include:

A. Maternal hypertension and smoking

B. Trauma and drugs (e.g., cocaine abuse)

C. Maternal vascular disease

D. All of the above

6 Review this image:

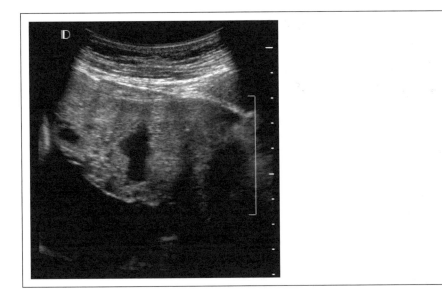

It most likely represents:

A. Placenta accreta

B. Placenta previa and an accreta

C. Placental abruption

D. Over-distended urinary bladder

7 Placental thickness greater than 5–7 cm may be associated with:

A. Rh incompatibility

B. IUGR

C. Pre-eclampsia

D. Pregestational diabetes mellitus

8 Premature calcification in the placenta may be observed in:

A. Gestational diabetes mellitus

B. Rh incompatibility

C. Fetal cardiopulmonary diseases

D. Maternal smoking

9 Consider this sonogram:

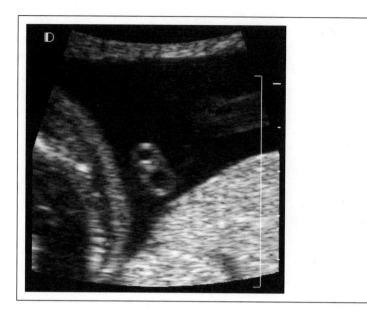

Findings associated with this image include all of the following EXCEPT:

A. Intrauterine growth restriction

B. Gastroschisis

C. Omphalocele

D. VATER or VACTERL

10 In the absence of a heart beat, a failed pregnancy would be considered most likely if:

A. The yolk sac is not visible by the time the gestational sac is 6 mm by endovaginal sonography

B. The yolk sac is not visible by the time the gestational sac is 15 mm by transabdominal sonography

C. The embryo is not visible when the gestational sac is > 16 mm by endovaginal sonography

D. The embryo is not visible when the gestational sac is > 20 mm by transabdominal sonography

11 A heart rate of 75 bpm in a 6-week embryo would indicate:

A. Normal cardiac activity

B. Failed pregnancy

C. Normal bradycardia

D. Impending demise

12 An emergency room patient presents with vaginal bleeding, a positive beta hCG, and a last menstrual period (LMP) 9 weeks ago. Based on this history and the ultrasound findings, the most likely diagnosis would include:

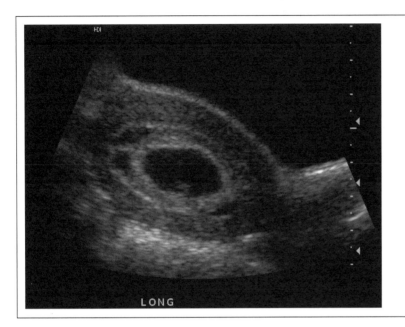

A. Placental abruption

B. Subchorionic hemorrhage

C. Subependymal hemorrhage

D. Placenta previa

13 An echogenic mass in the base of the umbilical cord in a 9-week embryo most likely represents:

A. Normal physiologic gut herniation that should resolve by the 10th menstrual week

B. Normal physiologic gut herniation that should resolve by the 14th menstrual week

C. Gastroschisis

D. Omphalocele

14 Consider the following first trimester ultrasound image:

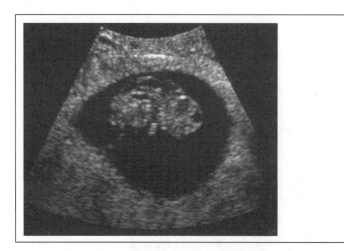

This sonogram:

A. Is considered abnormal if the nuchal sonolucency is > 3 mm

B. Is considered abnormal if the nuchal sonolucency is > 6 mm

C. Is considered to be normal

D. Should resolve by the 25th week of gestation

15 The following sonogram is of a 9-week gestation:

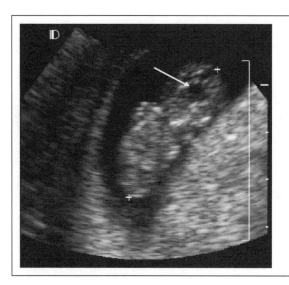

It demonstrates:

A. Hydrocephalus

B. Choroid plexus cyst

C. Rhombencephalon

D. Encephalocele

16 The most common implantation site for an ectopic pregnancy is:

   A. The ampullary portion of the fallopian tube

   B. The interstitial portion of the fallopian tube

   C. The isthmus of the fallopian tube

   D. Intra-abdominal

17 Review the sonogram below:

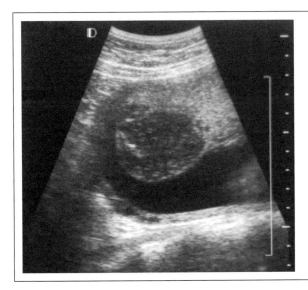

This sonogram most likely represents:

   A. Chorioangioma

   B. Focal myometrial contraction

   C. Placenta accreta

   D. Placenta succenturiate

18 Risk factors for ectopic pregnancy include all of the following EXCEPT:

   A. Prior pelvic inflammatory disease

   B. Prior ectopic pregnancies

   C. Prior D&C

   D. Infertility therapy

19 The classic clinical triad for an ectopic pregnancy is:

   A. Pain, mass, and vaginal bleeding

   B. Pain, cervical motion tenderness, and positive beta hCG

   C. Pain, vaginal bleeding, and elevated AFP

   D. Pain, positive beta hCG, and elevated alpha-fetoprotein

20 Consider this sonogram:

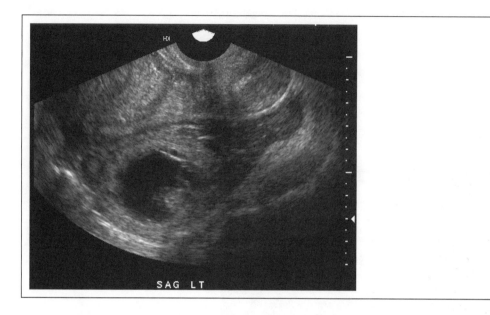

It most likely represents:

A. An ectopic pregnancy

B. A missed abortion

C. A molar pregnancy

D. Chorioangioma

21 Up to 6 weeks' gestation, the hCG level normally:

A. Doubles every 2 days

B. Doubles every 3 days

C. Doubles every day

D. Triples every other day

22 An emergency room physician would like to do an ultrasound on a gravida 4, para 3, ab 0 (G4P3A0), 35-year-old female, whose last menstrual period was 4–5 weeks ago. Ultrasound would most likely visualize a gestational sac by endovaginal sonography when the beta hCG is:

A. 300–400 mIU/ml IRP (International Reference Preparation)

B. 1000–2000 mIU/ml IRP (International Reference Preparation)

C. 1600–1800 mIU/ml IRP (International Reference Preparation)

D. 2000–2500 mIU/ml IRP (International Reference Preparation)

23 In the first trimester the gestational sac grows approximately:

A. 1 cm every day

B. 0.5 cm every day

C. 4 mm every day

D. 0.8 mm every day

24 By transabdominal sonography an intrauterine gestational sac measures 30 mm. The yolk sac and crown-rump length are not seen. This sonographic presentation is most consistent with:

A. A normal early pregnancy

B. A failed pregnancy

C. An ectopic pregnancy

D. A twin pregnancy

25 Placental insufficiency is NOT associated with:

A. Maternal hypertension or pre-eclampsia

B. Trisomy 21

C. Intrauterine infections

D. Twin-twin transfusion

26 Causes for oligohydramnios include all of the following EXCEPT:

A. Renal agenesis

B. Premature rupture of membranes

C. Intrauterine growth restriction

D. Duodenal atresia

27 Oligohydramios could be diagnosed when the amniotic fluid index (AFI) is:

A. <5–7 cm 4 quadrant

B. >9–10 cm 4 quadrant

C. <3 cm single pocket

D. <4 cm single pocket

28 This finding is noted on both sides of the fetal abdomen:

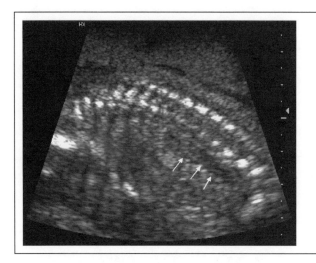

The most likely diagnosis would include:

A. Adrenal masses—neuroblastoma

B. Renal agenesis

C. Normal kidneys

D. Adrenal hyperplasia

29 Review this image:

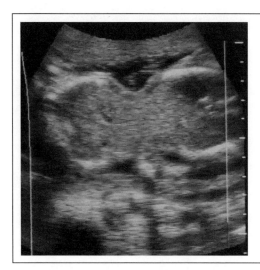

It most likely demonstrates:

A. A normal third trimester abdomen that is squashed

B. An oblique view through the abdomen

C. Omphalopagus conjoined twins

D. Thoracopagus conjoined twins

30 A majority of conjoined twins are attached at:

A. The chest (thoracopagus)

B. The abdomen (omphalopagus)

C. The chest and abdomen (thoraco-omphalopagus)

D. The head (craniopagus)

31 A majority of conjoined twins are:

A. Monochorionic monoamniotic

B. Monochorionic diamniotic

C. Dichorionic diamniotic

D. Males

32 Monochorionic monoamniotic pregnancies have a higher incidence of all of the following EXCEPT:

A. Umbilical cord entanglement

B. Conjoining

C. Nuchal cord and cord prolapse

D. Clubfeet

33 In the case of twin-twin transfusion:

A. The larger twin has oligohydramnios, while the smaller twin has polyhydramnios.

B. The larger twin can be hydropic with polyhydramnios, while the smaller twin can have oligohydramnios.

C. The donor twin is larger, while the recipient is smaller.

D. None of the above

34 Nausea, fainting, and sweating may be experienced by a pregnant patient during an ultrasound procedure. The sonographer should:

A. Allow the symptoms to pass.

B. Call a code.

C. Have the patient hyperventilate to get more oxygen in her system.

D. Roll the patient on her left side and place a cool cloth on her head and neck.

35 Biparietal diameter/head circumference (BPD/HC) should be obtained on an image of the fetal head that contains:

   A. Cerebellum, thalami, and cerebral peduncles

   B. Cavum septi pellucidum, thalami, and third ventricle

   C. Cerebellum, thalami, and cavum septi pellucidum

   D. Cavum septi pellucidum, thalami, and fourth ventricle

36 The most accurate measurement predicting fetal age is:

   A. The third trimester biparietal diameter (BPD)

   B. The first trimester crown-rump length (CRL)

   C. The first trimester femur length (FL)

   D. The third trimester abdominal circumference (AC)

37 To obtain the most accurate mean sac diameter (MSD) measurement, the sonographer should:

   A. Obtain the largest diameter

   B. Add the largest length, width, and A-P dimension

   C. Add the largest length, width, and A-P dimension and divide by 3

   D. Add the largest length, width, and A-P dimension and divide by 2

38 Crown-rump length (CRL) measurement should include the:

   A. Fetal leg buds

   B. Head to rump measurement

   C. Yolk sac

   D. Amnion

39 The embryonic period of development ends after the:

   A. 8th menstrual week

   B. 10th menstrual week

   C. 12th menstrual week

   D. First trimester

40 Organogenesis is complete by:

   A. 8 menstrual weeks

   B. 16 menstrual weeks

   C. 18 menstrual weeks

   D. 20 menstrual weeks

41 The fetal kidneys begin to contribute significantly to the amniotic fluid by:

A. 8 weeks

B. 16 weeks

C. 20 weeks

D. 24 weeks

42 A cephalic index of ~60% would suggest the head shape to be:

A. Dolichocephalic

B. Brachycephalic

C. Normal

D. Kleeblatschadel

43 Consider these sonograms:

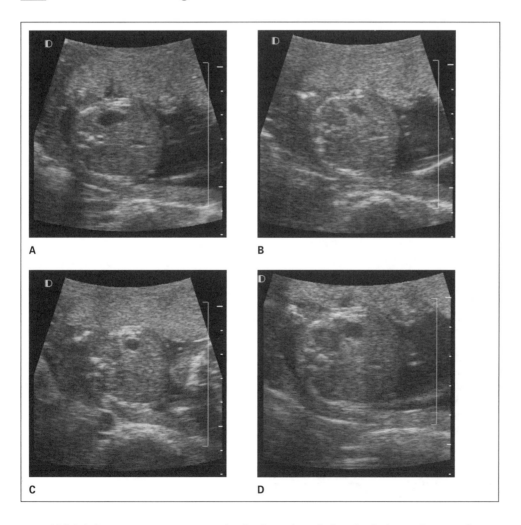

Which image most accurately depicts the abdominal circumference?

A. A B. B

C. C D. D

44 Review this sonogram:

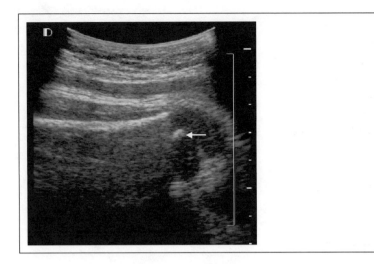

The arrow is pointing to:

A. The proximal tibial epiphysis

B. The proximal femoral epiphysis

C. The distal femoral epiphysis

D. The diaphysis

45 Cystic hygroma is most closely associated with:

A. Meckel's syndrome

B. Chiari malformation

C. Turner's syndrome

D. Trisomy 13

46 You obtain the following sonogram:

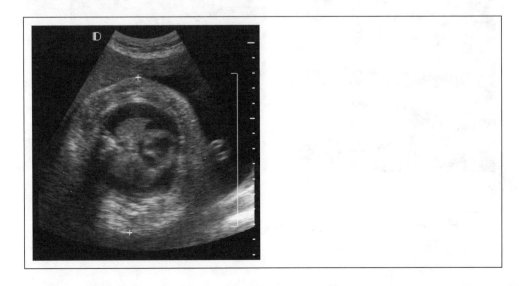

This image could be associated with all the following EXCEPT:

A. Cystic hygroma

B. Rh incompatibility

C. Cardiac anomalies

D. Duodenal atresia

47 You obtain the following image:

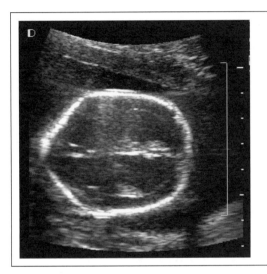

This sonogram most likely represents the:

A. Strawberry sign

B. Banana sign

C. Lemon sign

D. Linguini sign

48 The fetus whose sonogram appears in question 47 also has a spinal abnormality most commonly located:

A. Anywhere along the spine

B. In the C-spine

C. In the T-spine

D. In the L-spine

49 The most common neural tube defect is:

A. Spina bifida

B. Encephalocele

C. Myelomeningocele

D. Anencephaly

50 This abnormal finding on the sonogram may be associated as part of a triad that includes:

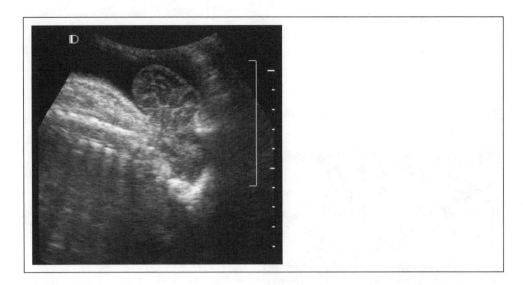

A. Encephalocele, MCDK, polydactyly = Meckel's syndrome

B. Cystic hygroma, streak ovaries, ascites = Turner's syndrome

C. Vertebral, anal atresia, TE fistula = VATER syndrome

D. PCKD, polydactyly, cystic hygroma = Edward's syndrome

51 You obtain the following sonogram:

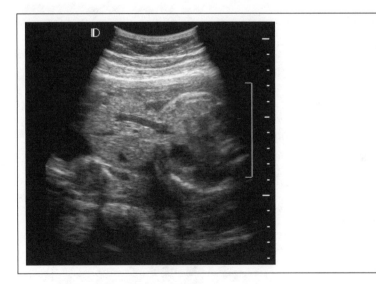

This image demonstrates:

A. Omphalocele

B. Conjoined twins

C. Gastroschisis

D. Chorioangioma

52 Consider this sonogram:

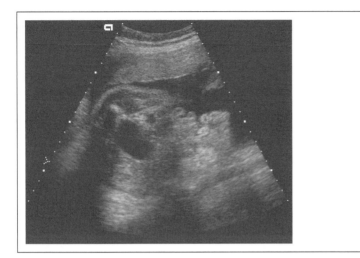

It most likely represents:

A. Gastroschisis

B. Omphalocele

C. Chorioangioma

D. Conjoined twins

53 You obtain the following image:

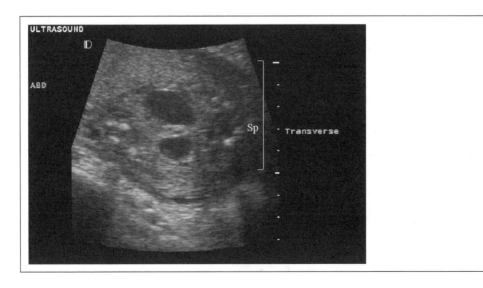

This sonogram most likely demonstrates:

A. A normal stomach variant

B. "Double bubble" sign associated with duodenal atresia

C. Normal stomach with adjacent umbilical vein

D. Normal stomach with adjacent gallbladder

54 Sonographic findings possibly observed in association with the fetus shown in question 53 include:

A. Endocardial cushion defect

B. Short femurs

C. Echogenic intracardiac foci

D. All of the above

55 The fetus whose image appears in question 53 most likely has:

A. Normal chromosomes

B. Trisomy 21

C. Turner's syndrome

D. Meckel's syndrome

56 A molar pregnancy can be associated with all the following EXCEPT:

A. Cystadenomas

B. Increased beta hCG

C. Hyperemesis gravidarum

D. Theca-lutein cysts

57 You obtain this sonogram:

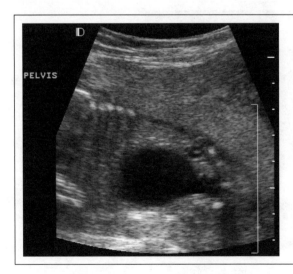

The image most likely demonstrates:

A. Normal urinary bladder

B. Ovarian cyst

C. "Keyhole" sign

D. "Double bubble" sign

58 The fetus whose sonogram appears in question 57 most likely has:

A. Posterior urethral valve obstruction

B. Duodenal atresia

C. Ovarian cyst

D. Meckel's diverticulum

59 Review the following echocardiogram:

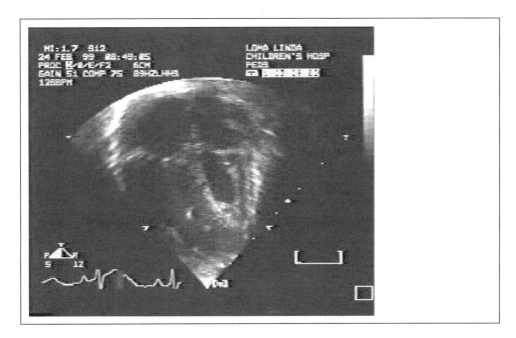

What is the most likely diagnosis?

A. Truncus arteriosus

B. Ventricular septal defect

C. Tetralogy of Fallot

D. Hypoplastic left ventricle

60 You obtain this sonogram of a fetal chest anomaly:

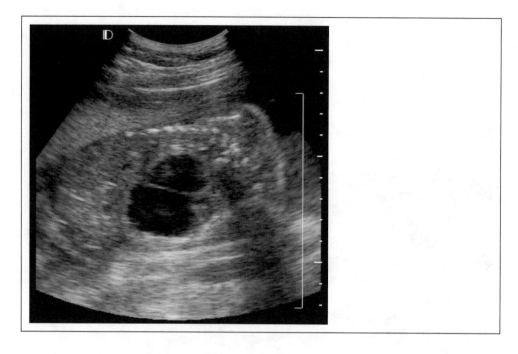

The most likely diagnosis is:

A. Cystic adenomatoid malformation type I-II

B. Cystic adenomatoid malformation type III

C. Pulmonary sequestration

D. Congenital diaphragmatic hernia (CDH)

61 A differential diagnosis for cystic adenomatoid malformation (CAM) type III would include:

A. Cystic adenomatoid malformation type I

B. Pulmonary sequestration

C. Congenital diaphragmatic hernia

D. Branchial cleft cyst

62 The most common location for congenital diaphragmatic hernia (CDH) is through the:

A. Foramen of Morgagni anterior-medially

B. Foramen of Bochdalek posterior-laterally and left

C. Meckel's diverticulum

D. Posterior right foramina

63 These sonograms show a fetus that has:

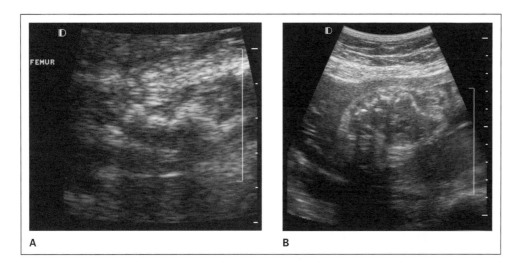

A. Achondrogenesis

B. Thanatophoric dwarfism

C. Osteogenesis imperfecta

D. Hypophosphatasia

64 History and physical findings associated with placenta accreta may include all of the following EXCEPT:

A. Vaginal bleeding

B. History of previous cesarean section

C. Prior history of an IUD

D. Hematuria

65 Biochemical markers associated with a higher incidence of Down syndrome include all of the following EXCEPT:

A. Decreased level of unconjugated estriol

B. Decreased levels of maternal serum alpha-fetoprotein (MS-AFP)

C. Decreased levels of human chorionic gonadotropin (hCG)

D. Elevated levels of human placental lactogen (hPL)

66 Trisomy 13 may be associated with all of the following EXCEPT:

A. Holoprosencephaly

B. Cleft lip and palate

C. Cardiac defects

D. Encephalocele

67 A key feature of trisomy 18 is:

A. Polydactyly

B. Holoprosencephaly

C. "Rocker bottom" feet

D. "Double bubble" associated with duodenal atresia

68 Sonographic findings associated with elevated alpha-fetoprotein include all of the following EXCEPT:

A. Multiple gestations

B. Open neural tube defects

C. Abdominal wall defects

D. Down syndrome

69 Sonographic findings associated with low alpha-fetoprotein include all of the following EXCEPT:

A. Trisomy 18

B. Trisomy 21

C. Miscarriages or failed pregnancies

D. Myelomeningocele

70 Images of this pregnancy demonstrated the following finding on both sides of the placenta:

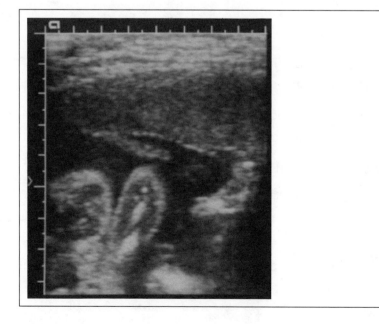

This finding most likely represents:

A. Amniotic bands

B. Circumvallate placenta

C. Synechiae

D. Nonfused amnion

Gynecology

71 The following sonogram is from a 24-year-old patient who has pelvic pain.

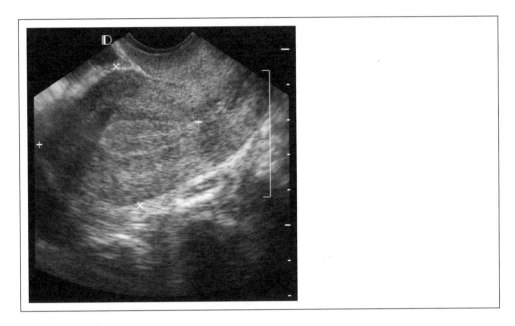

Sonographically, the endometrium appears to be consistent with:

A. Proliferative phase

B. Secretory phase

C. Menstrual phase

D. Endometrial hyperplasia

72 The following pelvic sonogram is from a patient who has a beta hCG of 200,000:

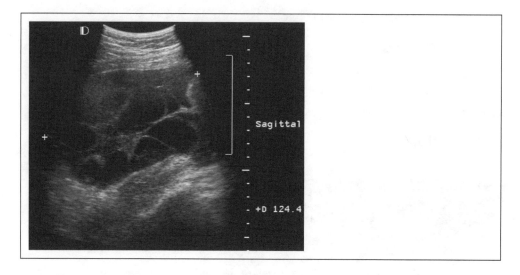

This image most likely represents:

A. Thecoma

B. Cystic teratoma

C. Corpus luteal cyst

D. Theca-lutein cyst

73 The following sonogram is from a 35-year-old patient with abdominal pain and abdominal mass with swelling.

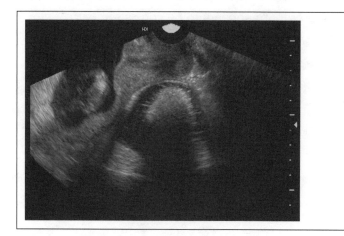

This image most likely represents:

A. Dermoid

B. Cystadenoma

C. Loop of bowel

D. Leiomyoma

74 Leiomyomas present with:

A. Pelvic pain

B. Urinary frequency or urgency

C. Rectal pressure—constipation

D. All of the above

75 Causes of postmenopausal thickening of the endometrium include all of the following EXCEPT:

A. Endometrial carcinoma

B. Endometrial hyperplasia

C. Uterine polyp

D. Uterine adenomyosis

76 Concerning the size of ovarian cysts in menstruating women:

A. Ovarian cysts < 3 cm are most likely to resolve spontaneously.

B. Ovarian cysts 3–5 cm require follow up within approximately 6–8 weeks.

C. Ovarian cysts > 10 cm rarely resolve and have a higher malignancy potential requiring surgical removal.

D. All of the above

77 Corpus luteum cysts usually resolve in a pregnancy by:

A. 12 weeks

B. 16 weeks

C. 20 weeks

D. 24 weeks

78 Theca-lutein cysts regress after molar evacuation:

A. Immediately

B. After 1 month

C. After 2–4 months

D. Rarely and require surgical removal

79 Sonographic findings of hyperstimulated ovaries may include:

A. Enlarged, multiloculated, cystic ovaries bilaterally

B. Ascites

C. Pleural effusions

D. All of the above

80 You obtain this pelvic sonogram from an infertile patient with a history of painful menses:

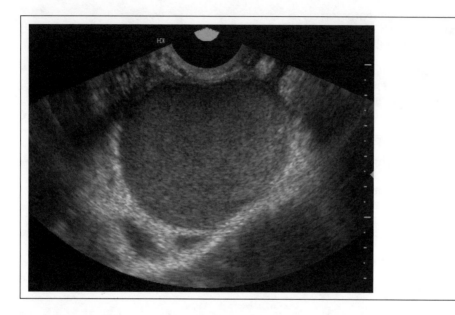

What is the most likely diagnosis?

A. Cystadenoma

B. Endometrioma

C. Dermoid

D. Fibroma

81 The most common germ cell tumor of the ovary in women ages 20–30 is:

A. Cystadenoma

B. Teratoma or dermoid

C. Leiomyoma

D. Androblastoma

82 Meig's syndrome includes all of the following EXCEPT:

A. Pleural effusion

B. Thecoma

C. Fibroma

D. Ascites

83 A 45-year-old female has a history of colon cancer. A solid ovarian mass in this patient would most likely be a:

A. Fibroma

B. Krukenberg tumor

C. Thecoma

D. Cystadenoma

84 All of the following are true regarding endometrial cancer EXCEPT:

A. It is more common than cervical cancer in the USA.

B. It commonly presents with postmenopausal vaginal bleeding.

C. It is associated with tamoxifen and estrogen-replacement therapy.

D. It is more common in African-American women.

85 A postmenopausal patient presents with vaginal bleeding. Endometrial thickness can be considered normal at:

A. 4 mm

B. 6 mm

C. 8 mm

D. 9 mm

86 Endometrial polyps:

A. Can commonly be seen sonographically in the lower uterine segment

B. Can best be evaluated by endovaginal sonography (EVS) alone

C. Appear sonographically as a thickened, echogenic, endometrial stripe

D. Occur commonly in women in their thirties.

87 You obtain the following pelvic ultrasound:

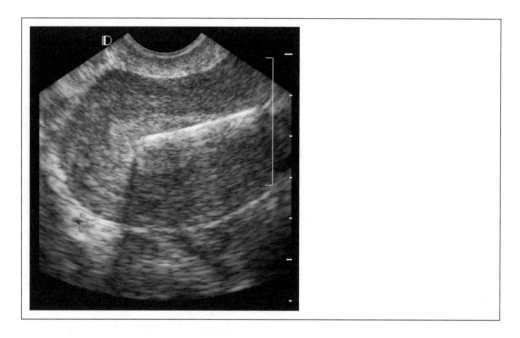

This image most likely demonstrates:

A. Calcified submucosal fibroid

B. Calcified subserosal fibroid

C. Normal calcifications in the endometrium

D. Intrauterine contraceptive device

88 Consider this sonogram:

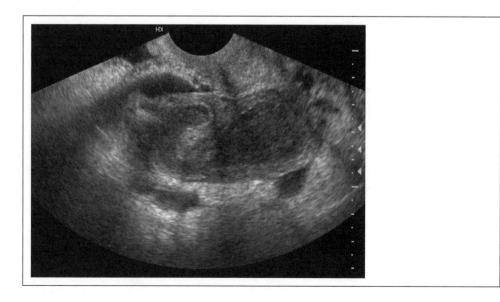

What is the most likely diagnosis?

A. Tubal ovarian abscess

B. Fibroma

C. Subserosal fibroid

D. Theca-lutein cyst

89 Factors decreasing the opportunity for conception include:

A. Sexually transmitted diseases

B. Advanced maternal age

C. Endocrine disorders

D. All of the above

90 The role of ultrasound in the evaluation of infertility patients includes all the following EXCEPT:

A. To evaluate the number of follicles present

B. To follow ovulation induction

C. To follow endometrial changes during therapy

D. To follow hormone levels

91 Which of the following disorders are associated with infertility?

A. Stein-Leventhal syndrome

B. Asherman's syndrome

C. Hypothalamic or pituitary diseases

D. All of the above

92 Normal ovarian diameters in the adult female are approximately:

A. $1 \times 2 \times 3$ cm

B. $3 \times 3 \times 3$ cm

C. $4 \times 4 \times 4$ cm

D. $2 \times 4 \times 3$ cm

93 You obtain the following sonogram:

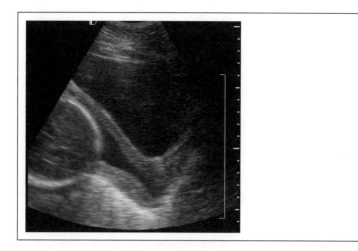

The most likely diagnosis is:

A. Ovarian cyst

B. Incompetent cervix

C. Submucosal fibroid

D. Hydrometrocolpos

94 Leiomyomas most commonly occur in:

A. African-American population

B. Asian population

C. European population

D. Australian population

95 The following sonogram is from a 50-year-old female who presents with "bloating" over the past few months without nausea, vomiting, fever, or pelvic pain:

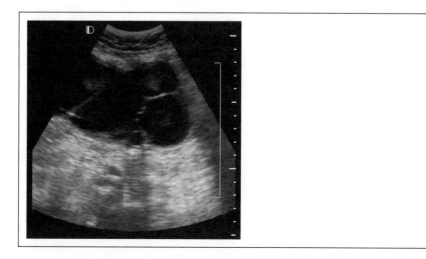

The most likely diagnosis is:

A. Pelvic inflammatory disease (PID)

B. Cystadenoma

C. Loculated ascites

D. Degenerating subserosal fibroid

96 Gestational trophoblastic disease (GTD) occurs most commonly in:

A. African-American population

B. Asian population

C. European population

D. Australian population

97 Possible sonographic findings associated with a patient taking tamoxifen include:

A. Endometrioma

B. Thickened, irregular endometrium

C. Cystadenoma

D. Bilaterally enlarged cystic ovaries

98 You obtain the following sonogram from a postmenopausal patient who has vaginal bleeding:

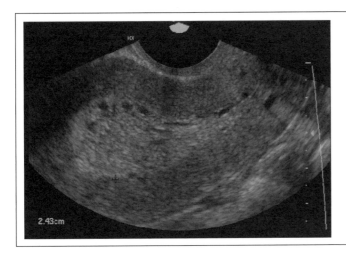

These findings most likely represent:

A. Multiple polyps

B. Adenomyosis

C. Endometrial hyperplasia

D. Subserosal leiomyoma

99 This sonogram is obtained from a patient with imperforate hymen.

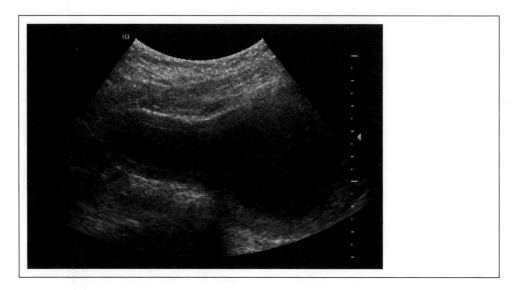

The most likely diagnosis is:

A. Endometritis

B. Hydrometrocolpos

C. Adenomyosis

D. Urethral obstruction

100 If a uterine malformation is detected on sonogram, the sonographer should also scan which organ?

A. Liver

B. Spleen

C. Gallbladder

D. Kidney

Answers

Obstetrics

1 C is correct: *Intrauterine growth restriction (IUGR)*. Answers A, B, and C are most likely associated with placentas > 5 cm in thickness. IUGR is most commonly associated with placental insufficiency. Thin placentas are commonly associated with IUGR, maternal hypertension, toxemia, chromosomal anomalies, severe intrauterine infections, and pregestational diabetes. [Spirt BA, Gordon LP: Sonographic evaluation of the placenta. In Rumack CM, Wilson SR, Charboneau JW (eds): *Diagnostic Ultrasound,* 2nd edition. St. Louis, Mosby-YearBook, 1998, p 1342.]

2 B is correct: *Abnormally high-resistance cord and low-resistance head Doppler.* Under normal circumstances the arterial umbilical cord Doppler is low-resistance, while the middle cerebral artery (MCA) Doppler is high-resistance in character. The two umbilical arteries take blood away from the fetus to the numerous channels within the placenta. This "open pool" provides the low-resistance bed and Doppler signal seen in the cord. With intrauterine growth restriction, the increased flow to the head reflects "brain sparing," with blood being redirected from the vital abdominal organs to the head. In intrauterine growth restriction, MCA Doppler becomes low-resistance, while the cord flow becomes highly resistive. [Tekay A, Campbell S: Doppler ultrasonography in obstetrics. In Callen PW (ed): *Ultrasonography in Obstetrics and Gynecology,* 4th edition. Philadelphia, WB Saunders, 2000, pp 687–691.]

3 A is correct: *Low-lying placenta.* Low-lying placentas are located within 2 cm to the internal cervical os. Surgical intervention, such as c-section, would not be required with ultrasound findings of a low-lying placenta. [Harris RD, Alexander RD: Ultrasound of the placenta and umbilical cord. In Callen PW (ed): *Ultrasonography in Obstetrics and Gynecology,* 4th edition. Philadelphia, WB Saunders, 2000, p 607.]

4 C is correct: *Painful vaginal bleeding with severe uterine contractions.* Pain, vaginal bleeding, and uterine contractions are more severe when the uterine placental separation is greater. Abruption occurs with an incidence of ~0.5–1% with the sensitivity of ultrasound detection of abruption ~50%. Pain experienced by the patient is usually directly related to the placental site. The classic triad, unfortunately, occurs infrequently. [Harris RD, Alexander RD: Ultrasound of the placenta and umbilical cord. In Callen PW (ed): *Ultrasonography in Obstetrics and Gynecology,* 4th edition. Philadelphia, WB Saunders, 2000, p 611.]

5 D is correct: *All of the above.* Pre-eclampsia is also another potential associate of placental abruption. [Harris RD, Alexander RD: Ultrasound of the placenta and umbilical cord. In Callen PW (ed): *Ultrasonography in Obstetrics and Gynecology,* 4th edition. Philadelphia, WB Saunders, 2000, p 612.]

6 A is correct: *Placenta accreta.* Placenta accreta is an abnormal placental attachment in which the chorionic villi are in direct contact with the myometrium. Sonographically, the hypoechoic myometrium will appear thinned or absent with adjacent, irregular sonolucencies in the placenta. Placenta previa commonly occurs with accretas. Further invasion can be categorized according to the level of invasion. Encroachment into the serosa is called *increta*. Penetration through the uterine wall and into the urinary bladder (*percreta*) can cause hematuria and can risk the lives of the mother and fetus. Small areas of placental invasion (<2 cm) may not adhere at delivery. [Harris RD, Alexander RD: Ultrasound of the placenta and umbilical cord. In Callen PW (ed): *Ultrasonography in Obstetrics and Gynecology,* 4th edition. Philadelphia, WB Saunders, 2000, p 613.]

7 A is correct: *Rh incompatibility.* Placental hydrops is due to fluid overload of the fetus, usually from high cardiac output. Blood disorders such as Rh incompatibility, anemia, and infections, as well as such conditions as twin-twin transfusion, placental hemorrhage, and gestational diabetes are often associated with thick placentas. [Harris RD, Alexander RD: Ultrasound of the placenta and umbilical cord. In Callen PW (ed): *Ultrasonography in Obstetrics and Gynecology,* 4th edition. Philadelphia, WB Saunders, 2000, p 599.]

8 D is correct: *Maternal smoking.* The amount of placental calcification is associated with the level of calcium in the maternal bloodstream. Premature development of calcium is most commonly associated with smoking. Other associations of accelerated calcification deposition include maternal hypertension and intrauterine growth restriction, low maternal parity, low maternal age, and late summer–early fall births. Mothers who have thrombotic disorders who were placed on heparin and aspirin prophylactics were also found to have increased calcifications. [Harris RD, Alexander RD: Ultrasound of the placenta and umbilical cord. In Callen PW (ed): *Ultrasonography in Obstetrics and Gynecology,* 4th edition. Philadelphia, WB Saunders, 2000, p 602.]

9 B is correct: *Gastroschisis.* Gastroschisis is not associated with such anomalies as single umbilical artery in the cord. However, single umbilical artery could be associated with intrauterine growth restriction central nervous system, cardiac, or renal anomalies, trisomy 13, 18, vertebral/anal/tracheoesophageal/renal anomalies spinal complex (VATER), and sirenomelia. [Spirt BA, Gordon LP: Sonographic evaluation of the placenta. In Rumack CM, Wilson SR, Charboneau JW: *Diagnostic Ultrasound,* 2nd edition. St. Louis, Mosby-YearBook, 1998, p 1340.]

10 C is correct: *The embryo is not visible when the gestational sac is < 16 mm by endovaginal sonography.* The fetal yolk sac should be seen on endovaginal sonography by the time the mean sac diameter (MSD) is 8 mm (5.5 weeks) and on transabdominal sonography when MSD > 20 mm (7 weeks). By endovaginal sonography the embryo should exhibit heart activity by the time it measures 4–5 mm at 6–6.5 weeks with a MSD of 13–18 mm. Transabdominally, a fetal heartbeat should be seen by the time MSD is 25 mm (8 weeks). [Laing FC, Frates MC: Ultrasound evaluation during the first trimester of pregnancy. In Callen PW (ed): *Ultrasonography in Obstetrics and Gynecology*, 4th edition. Philadelphia, WB Saunders, 2000, p 120.]

11 D is correct: *Impending demise.* Cardiac activity is seen as early as 5–6 weeks.

Doubilet and Benson reported that heart rates < 80 bpm in embryos with crown-rump length (CRL) < 5 mm were universally associated with subsequent demise. [Lyons EA, Levi CS, Dashefsky SM: The first trimester. In Rumack CM, Wilson SR, Charboneau JW: *Diagnostic Ultrasound*, 2nd edition. St. Louis, Mosby-YearBook, 1998, p 994.]

Normal range	100–115 bpm	5–6 weeks
	140 bpm	9 weeks
At-risk range	<100 bpm	<6.2 weeks
	<120 bpm	6.3–7.0 weeks

[Laing FC, Frates MC: Ultrasound evaluation during the first trimester of pregnancy. In Callen PW (ed): *Ultrasonography in Obstetrics and Gynecology*, 4th edition. Philadelphia, WB Saunders, 2000, p 132.]

12 B is correct: *Subchorionic hemorrhage.* Another potential cause for first trimester bleeding is failed pregnancy. Implantation of the gestational sac may also cause normal vaginal spotting. [Laing FC, Frates MC: Ultrasound evaluation during the first trimester of pregnancy. In Callen PW (ed): *Ultrasonography in Obstetrics and Gynecology*, 4th edition. Philadelphia, WB Saunders, 2000, p 126.]

13 B is correct: *Normal physiologic gut herniation that should resolve by the 14th menstrual week.* Normal physiologic gut herniation presents between 8 and 10 weeks. The bowel normally herniates into the umbilical cord at the beginning of 8th week, appearing as a small echogenic mass (6–9 mm) when the crown-rump length (CRL) is approximately 17–20 mm. The midgut rotates 90 degrees counterclockwise and returns into the abdomen by the 12th–14th menstrual week. [Angtuaco TL: Fetal anterior abdominal wall defect. In Callen PW (ed): *Ultrasonography in Obstetrics and Gynecology*, 4th edition. Philadelphia, WB Saunders, 2000, p 492.]

14 A is correct: *Is considered abnormal if the nuchal sonolucency is > 3 mm.* Nuchal sonolucency < 3 mm can normally be observed in the first trimester (10–14 weeks) as part of the normal lymphatic development. Resolution should occur by 18–20 weeks gestation. First trimester nuchal sonolucency is considered abnormal when the fluid persists into the mid-late second trimester or if septations are present. Measurements are made in the sagittal plane from the occipital bone to subcutaneous interface and is abnormal if > 3 mm. Aneuploidies associated with nuchal thickening include trisomy 21, trisomy 18, and Turner's syndrome. [Laing FC, Frates MC: Ultrasound evaluation during the first trimester of pregnancy. In Callen PW (ed): *Ultrasonography in Obstetrics and Gynecology,* 4th edition. Philadelphia, WB Saunders, 2000, p 140.]

15 C is correct: *Rhombencephalon.* The rhombencephalon is a normal cranial cystic space seen until 8–10 weeks. It represents the normal hindbrain that later becomes the fourth ventricular space as the cerebellum develops. It should not be confused with hydrocephalus.

16 A is correct: *The ampullary portion of the fallopian tube.* Between 95% and 97% of ectopic pregnancies occur in the fallopian tubes. The most common sites in descending order include the following:

- Ampullary—most common at 75–80%
- Isthmal—second most common
- Interstitial (cornual)—rare at 2–4%, but most dangerous
- Fimbria—very rare at 5%
- Intra-abdominal—rare
- Ovary—0.5–1.0%
- Cervix—0.1%

[Levine D: Ectopic pregnancy. In Callen PW (ed): *Ultrasonography in Obstetrics and Gynecology,* 4th edition. Philadelphia, WB Saunders, 2000, p 919.]

17 A is correct: *Chorioangioma.* Chorioangioma is the most common benign neoplasm of the placenta, consisting of a vascular mass arising from chorionic tissue. Most chorioangiomas have no clinical significance or sequelae, but those larger than 5 cm have a 30% rate of maternal or fetal complications: polyhydramnios, congestive heart failure/cardiomegaly, fetal death, preterm labor, intrauterine growth restriction, previa

CASE STUDIES FOR SELF-ASSESSMENT 331

and abruption, pre-eclampsia, anemia, and congenital anomalies. Sonographically, chorioangioma appears as a well-circumscribed, rounded, predominantly hypoechoic lesion near the chorionic surface, often near the cord insertion site. There may be hyperechoic foci reflecting prior hemorrhage, infarction, or fibrosis.

18 C is correct: *Prior D&C*. Risk factors also associated with ectopic pregnancies include prior tubal surgery, intrauterine contraceptive device (IUCD), advanced maternal age. [Levine D: Ectopic pregnancy. In Callen PW (ed): *Ultrasonography in Obstetrics and Gynecology,* 4th edition. Philadelphia, WB Saunders, 2000, p 912.] [Lyons EA, Levi CS, Dashefsky SM: The first trimester. In Rumack CM, Wilson SR, Charboneau JW: *Diagnostic Ultrasound,* 2nd edition. St. Louis, Mosby-YearBook, 1998, p 999.]

19 A is correct: *Pain, mass, and vaginal bleeding.* Other signs and symptoms along with the classic clinical triad for an ectopic pregnancy include amenorrhea, adnexal tenderness, cervical excitation pain, and abdominal pain.

20 A is correct: *An ectopic pregnancy.* Long-axis endovaginal view of the normal uterus demonstrates an empty endometrium with a posterior, extrauterine gestational sac containing a fetus.

21 A is correct: *Doubles every 2 days.* The hCG level normally doubles every 2 days and peaks at 6 weeks at 100 IU/ml. By the eighth week after the last menstrual period, hCG levels start to plateau. [Allen T, Cervantes F: Sonographic assessment of ectopic pregnancy. In Berman MC, Cohen HL: *Obstetrics and Gynecology,* 2nd edition. Philadelphia, Lippincott, 1997, p 195, 224.] [Appendix A: Measurements frequently used to estimate gestational age and fetal biometry. In Callen PW (ed): *Ultrasonography in Obstetrics and Gynecology,* 4th edition. Philadelphia, WB Saunders, 2000, Table A-6, p 1023.]

22 B is correct: *1000–2000 mIU/ml IRP (International Reference Preparation) by EVS.* [Laing FC, Frates MC: Ultrasound evaluation during the first trimester of pregnancy. In Callen PW (ed): *Ultrasonography in Obstetrics and Gynecology,* 4th edition. Philadelphia, WB Saunders, 2000, p 137.]

23 D is correct: *0.8 mm every day.* In the first trimester the gestational sac grows approximately 0.8 mm every day.

24 B is correct: *A failed pregnancy.* Crown-rump length should be seen by 25 mm mean sac diameter by transabdominal sonography (TAS) or 18 mm by endovaginal sonography (EVS).

25 D is correct: *Twin-twin transfusion.* Causes for placental insufficiency include the following:

- Maternal hypertension or pre-eclampsia
- Maternal disorders (e.g., collagen vascular disease, chronic renal or heart disease, maternal diabetes mellitus, metabolic disorders, Rh incompatibility)
- Poor maternal nutrition or weight gain (<50 kg)
- Maternal drug or alcohol abuse or teratogenic exposure
- High altitude
- Intrauterine infections

Chromosomal intrauterine growth restriction associations include:

- Trisomy 21—Down syndrome
- <26 Weeks—triploidy
- >26 weeks—trisomy 18

26 D is correct: *Duodenal atresia.* Oligohydramnios (a diminished or absent amount of amniotic fluid) can be caused by the decreased amount of urine output from the fetal genitourinary system. Potential genitourinary etiologies include renal agenesis, infantile polycystic kidney disease, bilateral ureteropelvic junction obstruction, and bilateral multicystic dysplastic kidneys, and outlet obstruction of the urinary bladder with posterior urethral valves. Oligohydramnios may also be caused by maternal events or disorders such as premature rupture of membrane or placental insufficiency causing intrauterine growth restriction and post-term pregnancies. Gastrointestinal anomalies such as duodenal atresia decrease the volume of amniotic fluid that may be ingested by the fetus and are more likely to be associated with polyhydramnios.

27 A is correct: *<5–7 cm 4 quadrant.* By definition the amniotic fluid index (AFI) is obtained by adding 4 A-P quadrant measurements. [Hadlock FP, Vincoff NS: Sonographic evaluation of fetal lung maturity. In Callen PW (ed): *Ultrasonography in Obstetrics and Gynecology,* 4th edition. Philadelphia, WB Saunders, 2000, p 642.]

28 B is correct: *Renal agenesis.* Unfolding of the adrenal glands represents absence of the kidneys within the renal fossa. This elongation is often referred to as the "lying down" or long, flat adrenal sign. Bilateral renal agenesis, oligohydramnios, and the bell-shaped thorax are often associated with Potter's syndrome.

29 C is correct: *Omphalopagus conjoined twins.*

30 C is correct: *The chest and abdomen (thoraco-omphalopagus).*

31 A is correct: *Monochorionic monoamniotic.*

With conjoined twins:

- All are monochorionic monoamniotic.
- Membrane development occurs >8 days after fertilization.
- Incidence is 1 in 50,000–200,000 pregnancies.
- There is 3:1 are female dominance.
- Polyhydramnios occurs in 50–75% of cases.
- 75% will be thoracopagus or omphalopagus.

32 D is correct: *Clubfeet.* They also have a higher incidence of malpresentation.

33 B is correct: *The larger twin can be hydropic with polyhydramnios, while the smaller twin can have oligohydramnios.* The larger twin can be hydropic with polyhydramnios and is usually the recipient twin, while the smaller, donor twin can have oligohydramnios.

34 D is correct: *Roll the patient on her left side and place a cool cloth on her head and neck.* Maternal hypotension occurs as a result of decreased venous return secondary to inferior vena cava compression from the pregnancy. Relief to the patient occurs by turning the patient on her left side until the symptoms subside.

35 B is correct: *Cavum septi pellucidum, thalami, and third ventricle.* Biparietal diameter (BPD) is best measured from "leading edge to leading edge." This requires caliper placement on the highly reflective calvarium, both on the outer surface on the most superficial side toward the transducer and on the inner table on the contralateral side. The grayish scalp region is not to be included in the measurement.

36 B is correct: *The first trimester crown-rump length (CRL).* Multiple studies have demonstrated that the first trimester biparietal diameter (BPD) is an accurate predictor of menstrual age but is not more accurate than the CRL and adds little, if anything, to the age estimate based on the CRL. Studies also demonstrate that the accuracy of the method in predicting menstrual age was 3–5 days. Once the menstrual dates have been established in the first trimester, most recommend not altering them.

37 C is correct: *Add the largest length, width, and A-P dimension and divide by 3.* The most accurate measurement of the mean sac diameter (MSD) is obtained by imaging the largest sac diameter then measuring length, width, and A-P dimension and dividing by 3. If the mean sac diameter is very round, two measurements can be taken and divided by 2. None of the trophoblast is to be included in the measurement.

38 B is correct: *Head to rump measurement.* The most accurate crown-rump length measurement is taken not to include the yolk sac or amnion, but to obtain only a measurement with the crown-rump length as extended as possible. Several measurements should be taken and the average used.

39 B is correct: *10th menstrual week.* The embryonic period ends at the beginning of the 9th week of development or at the end of the 10th menstrual week. At this time it is most appropriately termed the fetus.

40 A is correct: *8 menstrual weeks.* Organogenesis is completed by 8 menstrual weeks, after which point there is less risk of major structural anomalies.

41 B is correct: *16 weeks.* At approximately 16 weeks the kidneys begin to play an important role in contributing to the amniotic fluid. Before then the placenta plays a more dominant role.

42 A is correct: *Dolichocephalic.* A "dolichocephalic" or "scaphocephalic" head is shaped like a football.

43 A is correct: *A.* In order to obtain the most accurate abdominal circumference, the abdomen should be as round as possible, with the spine on the opposite side of the umbilical vein in a "hockey stick" appearance. The stomach will also be visualized many times. The kidneys should not be visualized, because this position is too low, and the umbilical vein should not be short, as this appearance is most likely the result of imaging vein tangentially. B contains kidney, C does not demonstrate the umbilical vein, and D also demonstrates the kidney and a shortened umbilical vein.

44 C is correct: *The distal femoral epiphysis.*

45 C is correct: *Turner's syndrome.* Cystic hygromas are associated with chromosomal abnormalities—most commonly Turner's syndrome—and with the development of hydrothoraces and generalized hydrops as a consequence of a more generalized malformation of the lymphatic system. When diffuse anasarca is associated with cystic hygroma, the condition is referred to as *lymphangiectasis* and is virtually always lethal.

46 D is correct: *Duodenal atresia.* Because of the severity of this disease and its consequences, nonimmune hydrops fetalis (NIHF) is a classic disorder in prenatal medicine. NIHF represents a late stage of redistribution of body fluids among the intravascular and interstitial compartments caused by different pathogenic mechanisms. Fetal regulation of fluid distribution may also be influenced by the placental circulation, which receives approximately 40% of the fetal combined cardiac output.

47 C is correct: *Lemon sign.* The lemon sign represents frontal bossing and is associated with spina bifida.

48 D is correct: *In the L-spine.* The lemon sign is most commonly associated with L-spine spina bifida.

49 D is correct: *Anencephaly.* Anencephaly occurs in about 1 in 1000 births and sonographically should not be diagnosed before 14 menstrual weeks. Classically, sonography demonstrates absence of the cranial vault above the level of the orbits as well as absence of the cerebral hemispheres. An amorphous mass representing cerebral tissue may be seen floating from the vault in the amniotic fluid. Two common abnormalities associated with anencephaly include polyhydramnios and such spinal defects as dysraphism.

50 A is correct: *Encephalocele, MCDK, polydactyly = Meckel's syndrome.* The encephalocele visualized here can be associated with Meckel's syndrome.

51 A is correct: *Omphalocele.* An omphalocele is a defect in the anterior abdominal wall, with extrusion of abdominal contents into the base of the umbilical cord. The herniated mass is covered by a parietal peritoneum and amnion, with Wharton jelly intervening between the two membrane layers. The incidence of associated anomalies in omphaloceles is reported to be as high as 50–88%, with chromosomal anomalies found in 40–60%. To differentiate omphalocele and gastroschisis, it must be established whether or not there is a membrane covering the herniated contents and if it is herniated into the umbilical cord.

52 A is correct: *Gastroschisis.* Gastroschisis commonly occurs on the right side of the abdomen, does not have a membrane covering the defect, and is not associated with nongastrointestinal anomalies.

53 B is correct: *"Double bubble" sign associated with duodenal atresia.* The "double bubble" sign is representative of duodenal atresia and can be associated with Down syndrome.

54 D is correct: *All of the above.* All of the above can be associated with trisomy 21 (Down syndrome), which can be associated with duodenal atresia, as noted above.

55 B is correct: *Trisomy 21.*

56 A is correct: *Cystadenomas.* All except cystadenomas are associated with a molar pregnancy. Higher than normal levels of circulating hCG induce the intense nausea and vomiting associated with hyperemesis gravidarum as well as the growth of the ovarian cysts bilaterally that develop into the theca-lutein cysts.

57 C is correct: *"Keyhole sign."*

58 A is correct: *Posterior urethral valve obstruction.* The "keyhole sign" is associated with posterior urethral valve obstruction, which can result in bilateral hydronephrosis.

59 D is correct: *Hypoplastic left ventricle.*

60 A is correct: *Cystic adenomatoid malformation type I-II.* Cystic adenomatoid malformation (CAM) Stocker type I-II is sonographically recognized by the multiple macroscopic cysts versus the more solid-appearing cystic adenomatoid malformation type III. The cystic appearance of congenital diaphragmatic hernia (CDH) can be differentiated from cystic adenomatoid malformation because of peristalsis of the bowel in the chest along with a small abdominal circumference.

61 B is correct: *Pulmonary sequestration.* Cystic adenomatoid malformation (CAM) type III contains microscopic cysts that sonographically appear solid and echogenic like pulmonary sequestration. The key way to differentiate this solid chest mass from a CAM type III would be to find and demonstrate by color Doppler imaging an anomalous blood supply going into the chest mass.

Pulmonary sequestrations are pathologically divided into intralobar and extralobar forms. Both are separated from the normal tracheobronchial tree. Most investigators believe that an extralobar sequestration results from the growth of an anomalous or supernumerary lung bud that derives its blood supply from the primitive splanchnic vessels surrounding the foregut.

62 B is correct: *Foramen of Bochdalek posterior-laterally and left.*

63 C is correct: *Osteogenesis imperfecta.* Osteogenesis imperfecta typically can present sonographically with multiple fractures and concave ribs, resulting in pulmonary hypoplasia.

64 C is correct: *Prior history of an IUD.* Placenta accreta often occurs with placenta previa and can be associated with vaginal bleeding. Prior cesarean section or other causes of uterine scarring causes partial or complete absence of the decidua basalis into which the placenta can attach and invade. [Harris RD, Alexander RD: Ultrasound of the placenta and umbilical cord. In Callen PW (ed): *Ultrasonography in Obstetrics and Gynecology,* 4th edition. Philadelphia, WB Saunders, 2000, p 613.]

65 C is correct: *Decreased levels of human chorionic gonadotropin (hCG).*

66 D is correct: *Encephalocele.* The incidence of trisomy 13 (Patau's syndrome) is 1 in 5000 births. It is the most severe of the three common autosomal trisomies. There are multiple anomalies of the brain, face, extremities, and heart. In particular, alobar holoprosencephaly is a common finding that is often associated with severe midline facial defects, including hypotelorism, cyclopia, midline clefts, microphthalmia, and absence of the nose.

Other anomalies associated with trisomy 13:

Intracranial

- Microcephaly
- Enlarged posterior fossa
- Agenesis of the corpus callosum
- Ventriculomegaly (9%)

Cardiac

- Echogenic intracardiac foci (30% of fetuses)
- Cardiac defects (i.e., hypoplastic left heart 21% of cases)

Extremities

- Polydactyly
- Radial aplasia

Abdominal

- Omphalocele (one-third of cases)
- Enlarged, echogenic kidneys similar to polycystic kidneys (30%)

67 C is correct: *"Rocker bottom" feet.* Trisomy 18, or *Edward's syndrome,* is associated with multiple, severe structural abnormalities that mostly involve the heart, extremities, face, and brain. Affected fetuses are often miscarried or die in utero.

Sonographic manifestations of trisomy 18:

First trimester:

- Increased incidence of nuchal thickening

Second trimester:

- Onset of IUGR
- Strawberry-shaped skull, single umbilical artery (SUA), and hydronephrosis.

Other structural abnormalities

- Abnormal cisterna magna
- Dandy-Walker malformation
- Meningomyeloceles
- Ventriculomegaly
- Limb abnormalities: preaxial upper limb reduction and clenched hands with overlapping fingers
- GI abnormalities: omphalocele and diaphragmatic hernia
- Facial abnormalities: low-set "pixie" ears, microphthalmos, hypertelorism, micrognathia, and cleft lip and palate

68 D is correct: *Down syndrome.* Alpha-fetoprotein (AFP) is produced by the fetal liver and yolk sac and is a sensitive indicator for structural fetal defects. Increased levels of alpha-fetoprotein are more commonly seen in the amniotic fluid and maternal serum with the following "open defects":

Neural defects:

- Anencephaly
- Spina bifida
- Open encephalocele

Abdominal wall defects:

- Omphalocele
- Gastroschisis

Other multiple causes for elevated alpha-fetoprotein include:

Situations involving hemorrhage:

- Fetal-maternal hemorrhage
- Placental abruption
- Rh sensitization

Renal disorders causing proteinuria:

- Congenital nephrosis
- Infantile polycystic kidney disease (IPKD)
- Bilateral renal agenesis

Maternal masses:

- Hepatic tumors
- Ovarian tumors

Fetal causes:

- Fetal demise
- Multiple gestation
- Triploidy

69 D is correct: *Myelomeningocele.* Trisomy 18, trisomy 21 (Down syndrome), and miscarriages are all associated with decreased alpha-fetoprotein. Myelomeningocele—an "open defect"—is usually associated with spina bifida, causing an increased level of alpha-fetoprotein to "spill" from the fetal system into the amniotic fluid.

70 B is correct: *Circumvallate placenta.* Circumvallate placenta is an abnormality of placental shape in which the chorioamniotic membranes circumferentially roll away from the placental edge toward the center. This thickened ridge of tissue is sometimes accompanied by placental hemorrhage or infarction. The classic ultrasound appearance is an irregular, rolled-up edge of the placenta, which may mimic a placental sheet, band, or shelf.

Gynecology

71 A is correct: *Proliferative phase.* Sonographically, the uterine endometrium progressively changes from a thin stripe in the early proliferative phase to a thicker hypoechoic endometrium later in the proliferative phase (as in this picture). The endometrium is more echogenic in the secretory phase.

72 D is correct: *Theca-lutein cyst.* Theca-lutein cysts increase in size as a result of the elevated levels of circulating hCG in the bloodstream. This systemic circulation causes both of the ovaries to enlarge, forming multiloculated cysts that may hemorrhage, torse, or even rupture. The levels of hCG gradually begin to decrease when the trophoblastic tissue is evacuated from the uterus, and the theca-lutein cysts regress over 2–4 months.

73 A is correct: *Dermoid.* A dermoid cyst is composed of well-differentiated derivatives of three germ layers: ectoderm, mesoderm, and endoderm. (It is frequently partly cystic and consists of a variety of different tissues.) Dermoids are often discovered as an incidental finding. Symptoms when present are usually abdominal pain, abdominal mass or swelling, and abnormal uterine bleeding. The most common complication is torsion. Sonographic appearance varies: calcified structures as well as fluid-fluid levels, "tip of the iceberg," and complex to cystic appearances.

74 D is correct: *All of the above.* Leiomyomas (fibroids) clinically may also be associated with low back or leg discomfort, irregular periods, and spotting. Depending on the size of the leiomyoma pressing on the adjacent structures, the resulting clinical presentation will vary.

75 D is correct: *Uterine adenomyosis.* Endometrial thickening > 8 mm may be associated with endometrial cancer, hyperplasia, or polyp. Endometrial thickening in the postmenopausal patient depends on whether or not the patient is taking hormones. Endometrial thickness is always considered abnormal when the endometrium is > 8 mm. Adenomyosis is a diffuse condition, with thickening of the myometrium, not the endometrium.

76 D is correct: *All of the above*. Follicular cysts normally enlarge and rupture at 18–23 mm. Ruptured follicles become the corpus lutea, which regress into the corpus albicans if pregnancy occurs. As mentioned above, cysts 3–5 cm in diameter should be followed to see if they increase in size or change in internal architecture.

77 B is correct: *16 weeks*. The corpus luteum can increase in size up to 2–3 cm. If pregnancy occurs, the corpus luteal cyst produces progesterone to support the pregnancy and then usually resolves by the 16th week of pregnancy.

78 C is correct: *After 2–4 months*. As previously noted, theca-lutein cysts increase in size according to the level of circulating hCG in the bloodstream. The levels of hCG gradually begin to decrease when the trophoblastic tissue is evacuated from the uterus, with regression of the theca-lutein cysts lasting up to 2–4 months.

79 D is correct: *All of the above*. All of the above may be associated with ovarian hyperstimulation syndrome (OHS) as a result of changes in the blood volume, coagulation, and concentration and the impairment of renal function.

80 B is correct: *Endometrioma*. Endometriosis is the presence of endometrial tissue outside the uterus. At the time of each menstrual cycle the tissue responds to hormones, and bleeding occurs outside the uterus, resulting in endometriomas. Endometriomas are associated with infertility and painful menses. Sonographic findings of these endometriomas, or "chocolate cysts," can range from anechoic cystic masses to cystic masses containing low-level echoes. Cystadenomas and dermoids do not usually contain fine, low-level echoes, and a fibroma would shadow posteriorly.

81 B is correct: *Teratoma or dermoid*. Germ cell tumors are the second most common class of ovarian tumors, and the most common type of germ cell tumor is teratoma or dermoid.

82 B is correct: *Thecoma*. Fibromas are solid ovarian masses that can be associated with pleural effusion and ascites. These are the three components that make up Meig's syndrome. The pleural effusion and ascites regress after removal of the fibroma.

83 B is correct: *Krukenberg tumor.* Krukenberg tumors are metastatic involvement of the ovary, usually from carcinoma of the gastrointestinal tract (gastric, large intestine, appendix) and occasionally as metastasis from the breast. Bilaterally enlarged, solid appearing ovaries should be highly suspicious for Krukenberg's tumor since most primary ovarian cancers are cystic in appearance.

84 D is correct: *It is more common in African-American women.* Endometrial cancer is *not* more common in African-American women. It is more common in Jewish women and is associated with endometrial hyperplasia.

85 A is correct: *4 mm.* Endometrial stripe thickness of 8 mm is considered by many to be the cutoff normal range in a postmenopausal woman. However, if the woman is bleeding, the normal range is usually considered to be < 5 mm, to improve sensitivity for detection for endometrial cancer.

86 C is correct: *Appear sonographically as a thickened, echogenic, endometrial stripe.* Endometrial polyps can further be evaluated by sonohysterography by demonstrating a stalk. Polyps commonly occur in the uterine fundus and present in perimenopausal women between the ages of 40 and 49. Symptoms include menorrhagia or excessive menstrual bleeding.

87 D is correct: *Intrauterine contraceptive device.* Intrauterine contraceptive devices (IUCD or IUD) are echogenic, highly reflective material with posterior shadowing. Their shape reflects their type (i.e., Copper "T," Copper "7," Lippes loop). Normally IUDs should be centrally located within the endometrium.

88 A is correct: *Tubal ovarian abscess.* Salpingitis is a common manifestation of pelvic inflammatory disease (PID). In the early stages the fallopian tube may become scarred and blocked and contain pus (pyosalpinx). In chronic pelvic inflammatory disease, serous fluid replaces the pus (hydrosalpinx). Sonographically, the infected salpinges can have thick internal walls, appear tubular or "football shaped," and may or may not contain internal echoes. Cystic masses found in the pelvis must be distinguished from the ovary.

Pelvic inflammatory disease is a general description of diffuse infection that may individually or globally involve the endometrium (endometritis), uterine muscle (myometritis), and areas surrounding the uterus (parametritis). Most commonly, pelvic inflammatory disease affects the fallopian tubes (salpingitis) and ovaries (oophoritis). Prior pelvic inflammatory disease increases the risk of a subsequent ectopic pregnancy by 6–10 times. Twenty percent of patients who have salpingitis become infertile. [Hall R: Pelvic inflammatory disease and endometriosis. In Berman MC, Cohen HL: *Obstetrics and Gynecology,* 2nd edition. Philadelphia, Lippincott, 1997, p 173.]

89 D is correct: *All of the above.* Infertility affects 1 in 7 American couples, and its prevalence is increasing. Approximately 40% of the time the cause is attributable to the female, 40% to the male, and 20% to combined factors. Traditionally the causes of infertility are divided into cervical, endometrial/uterine, tubal, peritoneal, ovulatory, and male factors.

90 D is correct: *To follow hormone levels.* Ultrasound would also assist in the confirmation of a gestation after the above course of treatment.

91 D is correct: *All of the above.* Stein-Leventhal is associated with polycystic ovary syndrome, which is an endocrine disorder. Asherman's syndrome is intrauterine adhesions in the endometrium that sonographically may appear as calcifications from the synechiae. Hypothalamus or pituitary diseases affect the endocrine system on which ovulatory and endometrial changes depend.

92 A is correct: *1 × 2 × 3 cm.* This is considered the average normal size of the ovary and can vary slightly.

93 B is correct: *Incompetent cervix.* Incompetent cervix affects 1% of pregnant patients. Although it is more commonly listed as a cause of recurrent pregnancy loss, it has become an important contributor to perinatal morbidity and mortality. There is general consensus that if the cervical length is 20 mm or less, it is an indication of cervical incompetence. The presence of funneling, spontaneous or induced, does enhance the diagnosis.

94 A is correct: *African-American population.* Leiomyomas are most common in African-American women.

95 B is correct: *Cystadenoma.* The history indicates that we are dealing with a 50-year-old female with bloating or possible increased girth. She does not have an infectious history to suggest pelvic inflammatory disease, nor does she have pelvic pain to suggest a fibroid. The pelvic sonogram suggests a large cystic, septated mass, which is most indicative of cystadenoma.

96 B is correct: *Asian population.* Fibroids or leiomyomas are most commonly associated with the African-American population. The European and Australian populations do not have a higher predisposition for gestational trophoblastic disease. The Asian population, particularly in the Far East, has been found to have a higher incidence of gestational trophoblastic disease.

97 B is correct: *Thickened irregular endometrium.* Transvaginal sonography (TVS) and endo-vaginal sonography (EVS) show thickened irregular cystic endometrium. Cystic changes in the subendometrial area without epithelial disease have also been documented.

98 C is correct: *Endometrial hyperplasia.* Endometrial hyperplasia is the most common cause of vaginal bleeding in both pre- and postmenopausal women, resulting from unopposed estrogen stimulation. The proliferation manifests as a pronounced endometrial stripe on ultrasound. It may be indistinguishable from an endometrial polyp or carcinoma. The diagnosis is usually confirmed by endometrial biopsy.

99 B is correct: *Hydrometrocolpos.* When imperforate hymen is present in a menstruating female, there is obstruction of flow of menses, which is then present in the vagina and/or uterus.

100 D is correct: *Kidney.* An increased incidence of renal anomalies is associated with uterine malformations.

AIUM Guidelines for Performing Routine Obstetrical Examinations

APPENDIX A

Guidelines for Performance of the Antepartum Obstetric Ultrasound Examination

The following are proposed guidelines for the antepartum obstetrical ultrasound examination. The document consists of three parts:

Part I   Equipment and Documentation Guidelines

Part II Guidelines for First Trimester Sonography

Part III Guidelines for Second and Third Trimester Sonography

These guidelines have been developed for use by practitioners performing obstetric ultrasound studies. They represent minimum guidelines for the performance and documentation of obstetrical sonograms. A limited examination may, however, be performed in clinical emergencies or if used as a follow-up to a complete examination. In certain cases, particularly those in which a purpose of the study is to identify, characterize, or exclude structural congenital anomalies, an additional targeted examination may be necessary. Adherence to the following guidelines will increase the chance of detecting many fetal abnormalities, but even with more detailed examinations, it is not possible to detect all fetal anomalies.

Part I Equipment and Documentation

Equipment

These studies should be conducted with real-time equipment, using an abdominal and/or vaginal approach. A transducer of appropriate frequency should be used. Fetal ultrasound should be performed only when there is a valid medical reason. The lowest possible ultrasonic exposure settings should be used to gain the necessary diagnostic information.

Comment:

(1) Real-time sonography is necessary to confirm the presence of fetal life through observation of cardiac activity and active movement.

(2) The choice of transducer frequency is a balance between beam penetration and resolution. With modern equipment, 3 to 5 MHz abdominal transducers allow sufficient penetration in most patients while providing adequate resolution. A lower-frequency transducer may be needed to provide adequate penetration for abdominal imaging in an obese patient. Vaginal scanning is usually performed at a frequency of 5 to 7.5 MHz.

Documentation

Adequate documentation of the study is essential for quality patient care. This should include a permanent record of the ultrasound images, incorporating whenever possible, the measurement parameters and anatomic findings proposed in the following sections of this document. Images should be appropriately labeled with the examination date, patient identification, and, if appropriate, image orientation. A report of the ultrasound findings should be included in the patient's medical record. Retention of the ultrasound examination should be consistent both with the clinical need and with relevant legal and local health care facility requirements.

Part II Guidelines for First Trimester Sonography

Overall Comment: Scanning in the first trimester may be performed abdominally, vaginally, or by using both methods. If an abdominal examination is performed and fails to provide diagnostic information, a vaginal scan should be done when possible. Similarly, if a vaginal scan is performed and fails to image all areas needed for diagnosis, an abdominal scan should be performed.

1 The uterus and adnexa should be evaluated for the presence of a gestational sac. If a gestational sac is seen, its location should be documented. The presence or absence of an embryo should be noted and the crown rump length recorded.

Comment:

(1) The crown rump length is a more accurate indicator of gestational age than gestational sac diameter. If the embryo is not identified, the gestational sac should be evaluated for the presence of a yolk sac. The estimate of gestational age should then be based on either the mean diameter of the gestational sac or on the morphology and contents of the gestational sac.

(2) Identification of a yolk sac or an embryo is definitive evidence of a gestational sac. Caution should be used in making definitive diagnosis of gestational sac before the development of such structures. Without these findings, an intrauterine fluid collection can sometimes represent a pseudogestational sac associated with ectopic pregnancy.

(3) During the late first trimester, biparietal diameter and other fetal measurements may also be used to establish fetal age.

2 Presence or absence of cardiac activity should be reported.

Comment:

(1) Real-time observation is critical for this diagnosis.

(2) With vaginal scans, cardiac motion should be appreciated by a crown rump length of 5 mm or greater. If an embryo less than 5 mm in length is seen with no cardiac activity, a follow-up scan may be needed to evaluate for fetal life.

3 Fetal number should be documented.

Comment: Multiple pregnancies should be reported only in those instances where multiple embryos are seen. Occasionally, more than one sac-like structure may be seen early in pregnancy and incorrectly thought to represent multiple gestations, owing to incomplete fusion between the amnion and chorion or to elevation of the chorionic membrane by intrauterine hemorrhage.

4 Evaluation of the uterus, adnexal structures, and cul-de-sac should be performed.

Comment:

(1) This will allow recognition of incidental findings or potential clinical significance. The presence, location, and size of myomas and adnexal masses should be recorded. The cul-de-sac should be scanned for presence or absence of fluid. If there is fluid in the cul-de-sac, the flanks and subhepatic space should be scanned for intraabdominal fluid.

(2) Because differentiation of normal pregnancy from abnormal pregnancy and ectopic pregnancy can be difficult, the correlation of serum hormonal levels with ultrasound findings is often helpful.

Part III Guidelines for Second and Third Trimester Sonography

1 Fetal life, number, presentation, and activity should be documented.

Comment:

(1) Abnormal heart rate and/or rhythm should be reported.

(2) Multiple pregnancies require the documentation of additional information: number of gestational sacs, number of placentas, presence or absence of a dividing membrane, fetal genitalia (if visible), comparison of fetal sizes, and comparison of amniotic fluid volume on each side of the membrane.

2 An estimate of amniotic fluid volume (increased, decreased, normal) should be reported.

Comment: Physiologic variation with stage of pregnancy should be considered in assessing the appropriateness of amniotic fluid volume.

3 The placental location, appearance, and its relationship to the internal cervical os should be recorded. The umbilical cord should be imaged.

Comment:

(1) It is recognized that apparent placental position early in pregnancy may not correlate well with its location at the time of delivery.

(2) An overdistended maternal urinary bladder or a lower uterine contraction can give the examiner a false impression of placenta previa.

(3) Abdominal, transperineal, or vaginal views may be helpful in visualizing the internal cervical os and its relationship to the placenta.

4 Assessment of gestational age should be accomplished at the time of the initial scan, using a combination of cranial measurement, such as the biparietal diameter or head circumference, and limb measurement such as the femur length.

Comment:

(1) Third trimester measurements may not accurately reflect gestational age. If one or more previous studies have been performed, the gestational age at the time of the current examination should be based on the earliest examination that permits accurate measurement of crown rump length, biparietal diameter, head circumference, and/or femur length by the equation: current fetal age = estimated age at time of initial study + number of weeks elapsed since first study.

(2) Measurements of structurally abnormal fetal body parts (such as the head in a fetus with hydrocephalus or the limbs in a fetus with a skeletal dysplasia) should not be used in the calculation of estimated gestational age.

4a The standard reference level of measurement of the biparietal diameter is an axial image that includes the thalamus.

Comment: If the fetal head is dolichocephalic or brachycephalic, the biparietal diameter measurement may be misleading. Occasionally, computation of the cephalic index, a ratio of the biparietal diameter to fronto-occipital diameter, will be needed to make this determination. In such situations, other measurements of head size, such as the head circumference, may be necessary.

4b Head circumference is measured at the same level as the biparietal diameter, around the outer perimeter of the calvarium.

4c Femur length should be routinely measured and recorded after the 14th week of gestation.

Comment: As with head measurements, there is considerable biologic variation in normal femur lengths late in pregnancy.

5 Fetal weight should be estimated in the late second and third trimesters and requires the measurement of abdominal diameter or circumference.

5a Abdominal circumference should be determined on a true transverse view, preferably at the level of the junction of the left and right portal veins.

Comment: Abdominal circumference measurement is necessary to estimate fetal weight and may allow detection of growth restriction and macrosomia.

5b If previous fetal biometric studies have been performed, an estimate of the appropriateness of interval growth should be given.

6 Evaluation of the uterus (including the cervix) and adnexal structures should be performed.

Comment: This will allow recognition of incidental findings of potential clinical significance. The presence, location, and size of myomas and adnexal masses should be recorded. It is frequently not possible to image the maternal ovaries during the second and third trimesters. Vaginal or transperineal scanning may be helpful in evaluating the cervix when the fetal head prevents visualization of the cervix by transabdominal scanning.

7 The study should include, but not necessarily be limited to, assessment of the following fetal anatomy: cerebral ventricles, posterior fossa (including cerebellar hemispheres and cisterna magna), four-chamber view of the heart (including its position within the thorax), spine, stomach, kidneys, urinary bladder, fetal umbilical cord insertion site, and intactness of the anterior abdominal wall. Although not considered part of the minimum required examination, when fetal position permits, it is desirable to examine other areas of the anatomy.

Comment:

(1) It is recognized that not all malformation of the preceding organ systems can be detected using ultrasonography.

(2) These recommendations should be considered a minimal guideline for the fetal anatomic survey. Occasionally, some of these structures will not be well visualized, as occurs when fetal position, low amniotic fluid volume, or maternal body habitus limits the sonographic examination. When this occurs, the report of the ultrasound examination should include a notation delineating structures that were not well seen.

(3) Suspected abnormalities may require a targeted evaluation of the area(s) of concern.

AIUM Guidelines for the Gynecological Examination

APPENDIX B

Guidelines for Performance of the Ultrasound Examination of the Female Pelvis

The following are proposed guidelines for ultrasound evaluation of the female pelvis. The document consists of two parts:

Part I   Guidelines for Equipment and Documentation

Part II Guidelines for Performance of the Ultrasound Examination of the Female Pelvis

These guidelines have been developed to provide assistance to practitioners performing ultrasound studies of the female pelvis. In some cases, additional and/or specialized examinations may be necessary. While it is not possible to detect every abnormality, adherence to the following will maximize the probability of detecting most of the abnormalities that occur.

Part I Guidelines for Equipment and Documentation

Equipment

Ultrasound examination of the female pelvis should be conducted with a real-time scanner, preferably using sector or curved linear transducers. The transducer or scanner should be adjusted to operate at the highest clinically appropriate frequency, realizing that there is a trade-off between resolution and beam penetration. With modern equipment, studies performed from the anterior abdominal wall can usually use frequencies of 3.5 MHz or higher, although a lower frequency transducer may occasionally be necessary to provide adequate penetration in an obese patient. Scans performed from the vagina should use frequencies of 5 MHz or higher.

Care of the Equipment

All probes should be cleaned after each patient examination. Vaginal probes should be covered by a protective sheath prior to insertion. Following each examination, the sheath should be disposed and the probe wiped clean and appropriately disinfected. The type of antimicrobial solution and the methodology for disinfection depends on manufacturer and infectious disease recommendations.

Documentation

Adequate documentation is essential for high quality patient care. A permanent record of the ultrasound examination and its interpretation should be kept by the facility performing the study. Images of all appropriate areas, both normal and abnormal, should be recorded. Variations from normal size should be accompanied by measurements. Images are to be appropriately labeled with the examination date, facility name, patient identification, image orientation, and whenever possible, the organ or area imaged. A report of the ultrasound findings should be included in the patient's medical record. Retention of the permanent record of the ultrasound examination should be consistent both with the clinical need and with the relevant legal and local health care facility requirements.

Part II Guidelines for Performance of the Ultrasound Examination of the Female Pelvis

The following guidelines describe the examination to be performed for each organ and anatomic region in the female pelvis. All relevant structures should be identified by the abdominal and/or vaginal approach. If an abdominal examination is performed and fails to provide the necessary diagnostic information, a vaginal scan should be done when possible. Similarly, if a vaginal scan is performed and fails to image all areas needed for diagnosis, an abdominal scan should be performed. In some cases, both an abdominal and a vaginal scan may be needed.

General Pelvic Preparation

For a pelvic sonogram performed from the abdominal wall, the patient's urinary bladder should, in general, be distended adequately to displace small bowel and its contained gas from the field of view. Occasionally, overdistention of the bladder may compromise evaluation. When this occurs, imaging should be repeated after the patient partially empties the bladder.

For a vaginal sonogram, the urinary bladder is preferably empty. The vaginal transducer may be introduced by the patient, the sonographer, or the physician. A female member of the physician's or hospital's staff should be present, when possible, as a chaperone in the examining room during vaginal sonography.

Uterus

The vagina and uterus provide anatomic landmarks that can be used as reference points when evaluating the pelvic structures. In evaluating the uterus, the following should be documented: (a) uterine size, shape, and orientation; (b) the endometrium; (c) the myometrium; and (d) the cervix.

Uterine length is evaluated on a long axis view as the distance from the fundus to the cervix. The depth of the uterus (anteroposterior dimension) is measured on the same long axis view from its anterior to posterior walls, perpendicular to its long axis. The width is measured on the axial or coronal view.

Abnormalities of the uterus should be documented. The endometrium should be analyzed for thickness, focal abnormality, and the presence of fluid or mass in the endometrial cavity. Assessment of the endometrium should allow for normal variations in the appearance of the endometrium expected with phases of the menstrual cycle and with hormonal supplementation. The myometrium and cervix should be evaluated for contour changes, echogenicity, and masses.

The endometrial thickness measurement should include both layers, measured anterior to posterior, in the sagittal plane. Any fluid within the endometrial cavity should be excluded from this measurement.

Adnexa (Ovaries and Fallopian Tubes)

When evaluating the adnexa, an attempt should be made to identify the ovaries first since they can serve as a major point of reference for assessing the presence of adnexal pathology. Although their location is variable, the ovaries are most often situated anterior to the internal iliac (hypogastric) vessels, lateral to the uterus, and superficial to the obturator internus muscle. The ovaries should be measured and ovarian abnormalities should be documented. Ovarian size can be determined by measuring the ovary in three dimensions (width, length, and depth), on views obtained in two orthogonal planes. It is recognized that the ovaries may not be identifiable in some women. This occurs most frequently after menopause or in patients with a large leiomyomatous uterus.

The normal fallopian tubes are not visualized in most patients. The para-adnexal regions should be surveyed for abnormalities, particularly fluid-filled or distended tubular structures that may represent dilated fallopian tubes.

If an adnexal mass is noted, its relationship to the uterus and ipsilateral ovary should be documented. Its size and echopattern (cystic, solid, or mixed; presence of septations) should be determined. Doppler ultrasound may be useful in select cases to identify the vascular nature of pelvic structures.

Cul-De-Sac

The cul-de-sac and bowel posterior to the uterus may not be clearly visualized. This area should be evaluated for the presence of free fluid or mass. When free fluid is detected, its echogenicity should be assessed. If a mass is detected, its size, position, shape, echopattern (cystic, solid, or complex), and its relationship to the ovaries and uterus should be documented. Identification of peristalsis can be helpful in distinguishing a loop of bowel from a pelvic mass. In the absence of peristalsis, differentiation of normal or abnormal loops of bowel from a mass may, at times, be difficult. A transvaginal examination may be helpful in distinguishing a suspected mass from fluid and feces within the normal rectosigmoid. An ultrasound water enema study or a repeat examination after a cleansing enema may also help distinguish a suspected mass from bowel.

Application for CME Credit

APPENDIX C

Objectives of this Activity

How to Obtain CME Credit

Applicant Information

Evaluation—You Grade Us!

CME Quiz

. . . .

Introduction

Ob/Gyn Sonography: An Illustrated Review is a continuing medical educational (CME) activity approved for 12 hours of credit by the Society of Diagnostic Medical Sonography and may be used by more than one person (see *Note* on following page).

This credit may be applied as follows:

1 Sonographers and technologists may apply these hours toward the CME requirements of the ARDMS, ARRT, and/or CCI, as well as to the CME requirements of ICAVL for technologists and sonographers in ICAVL-accredited facilities.

2 Physicians may apply a certain maximum number of SDMS-approved credit hours toward the CME requirements of the ICAVL for accreditation of diagnostic facilities. (Be sure to confirm current requirements with the pertinent organizations.) Physicians who are registered sonographers or technologists may apply all of these hours toward the CME requirements of the ARDMS, ARRT, and/or CCI. SDMS-approved credit is not applicable toward the AMA Physician's Recognition Award.

If you have any questions about CME requirements that affect you, please contact the responsible organization directly for current information. CME requirements can and sometimes do change.

NOTE

The original purchaser of this CME activity is entitled to submit this CME application for an administrative fee of $39.50. Please enclose a check payable to Davies Publishing Inc. with your application or a 16-digit credit card number and expiration date. Others may also submit applications for CME credits by completing the activity as explained above and enclosing an administrative fee of $49.50. The CME administrative fee helps to defray the cost of processing, evaluating, and maintaining a record of your application and the credit you earn. We also directly notify the ARDMS of CME credit you earn from us. Fees may change without notice. For the current fee, call us at 626-792-3046, e-mail us at **cme@DaviesPublishing.com**, or write to us at the address on the next page. We will be happy to help!

Objectives of the Activity

Upon completion of this educational activity, you will be able to:

1. Describe and identify normal and abnormal fetal and female pelvic anatomy and physiology.

2. Describe how, when, and why ultrasonography is applied in the practice of obstetrics and gynecology.

3. Differentiate normal from abnormal obstetrical and gynecologic sonographic findings and explain the correlations between these findings and pertinent laboratory and imaging studies.

4. Describe how, when, and why fetal and gynecological measurements are made.

5. Explain the role of medical genetics in the practice of obstetrics and gynecology.

6. Describe the diseases, disorders, complications, and coexisting disorders of the female reproductive system, pregnancy, and antepartum and postpartum fetus.

7. Explain how to prepare for, perform, and explain the techniques of sonographic examination in the practice of obstetrics and gynecology.

How To Obtain CME Credit

1 To apply for credit, please do all of the following:

2 Read and study the book and complete the interactive exercises it contains.

3 Photocopy and then complete this questionnaire and CME quiz and the evaluation form below.

4 Make copies of the completed forms and quiz for your records and then return the originals (i.e., the photocopied forms with your original writing) to the following address for processing:

Davies Publishing, Inc.
Attn: CME Coordinator
32 South Raymond Avenue, Suite 4
Pasadena, California 91105-1935

or fax to:

1-626-792-5308

Applicant Information

Name

Current credentials + SSN

Home address

City/State/Zip

Telephone/Facsimile   eMail address

ARDMS #   ARRT #   SDMS#

Signature certifying your completion of the activity

Answer Sheet

Circle the correct answer below and return this sheet to Davies Publishing Inc.

1. A B C D	15. A B C D	29. A B C D
2. A B C D	16. A B C D	30. A B C D
3. A B C D	17. A B C D	31. A B C D
4. A B C D	18. A B C D	32. A B C D
5. A B C D	19. A B C D	33. A B C D
6. A B C D	20. A B C D	34. A B C D
7. A B C D	21. A B C D	35. A B C D
8. A B C D	22. A B C D	36. A B C D
9. A B C D	23. A B C D	37. A B C D
10. A B C D	24. A B C D	38. A B C D
11. A B C D	25. A B C D	39. A B C D
12. A B C D	26. A B C D	40. A B C D
13. A B C D	27. A B C D	
14. A B C D	28. A B C D	

Evaluation—You Grade Us!

Please let us know what you think of *Ob/Gyn Sonography: An Illustrated Review*. Participating in this quality survey is a requirement for CME applicants, and it benefits future readers by ensuring that current readers are satisfied and, if not, that their comments and opinions are heard and taken into account. Your opinions count!

1 Why did you purchase *Ob/Gyn Sonography: An Illustrated Review*? (Circle primary reason.)

REGISTRY REVIEW   COURSE TEXT   CLINICAL REFERENCE   CME ACTIVITY

2 Have you used *Ob/Gyn Sonography: An Illustrated Review* for other reasons, too? (Circle all that apply.)

REGISTRY REVIEW   COURSE ACTIVITY   CLINICAL REFERENCE   CME ACTIVITY

3 To what extent did *Ob/Gyn Sonography: An Illustrated Review* meet its stated objectives and your needs? (Circle one.)

GREATLY   MODERATELY   MINIMALLY   INSIGNIFICANTLY

4 The content of *Ob/Gyn Sonography: An Illustrated Review* was (circle one):

JUST RIGHT   TOO BASIC   TOO ADVANCED

5 The quality of the questions and explanations was mainly (circle one):

EXCELLENT   GOOD   FAIR   POOR

6 The manner in which *Ob/Gyn Sonography: An Illustrated Review* presents the material is mainly (circle one):

EXCELLENT   GOOD   FAIR   POOR

7 If you used this book to prepare for the registry exam, did you also use other materials or take any exam-preparation courses?

NO   YES (PLEASE SPECIFY WHAT MATERIALS AND COURSES)

_____

_____

8 If you used this book for a course, please name the course, the instructor's name, the name of the school or program, and any other textbooks you may have used:

COURSE/INSTRUCTOR/SCHOOL OR PROGRAM:

_____

_____

OTHER TEXTBOOKS:

_____

_____

9 What did you like best about *Ob/Gyn Sonography: An Illustrated Review*?

_____

_____

_____

10 What did you like least about *Ob/Gyn Sonography: An Illustrated Review*?

_____

_____

_____

11 If you used *Ob/Gyn Sonography: An Illustrated Review* to prepare for the ARDMS exam in OB/GYN, did you pass?

YES   NO   HAVEN'T YET TAKEN IT

12 May we quote any of your comments in our catalogs or promotional material?

Yes　　No　　Further comment . . .

_____
_____
_____
_____
_____
_____
_____
_____
_____
_____
_____
_____

CME Quiz

Please answer the following questions after you have completed the CME activity. There is one best answer for each question. Circle it on the answer sheet that appears on the previous page.

1 Larger retroplacental abruptions are most likely to present as:

   A. Painless vaginal bleeding with severe uterine contractions

   B. Painful vaginal bleeding

   C. Painful vaginal bleeding with severe uterine contractions

   D. Painless vaginal bleeding

2 When placental thickness exceeds 5 to 7 cm, you suspect:

   A. IUGR

   B. Pregestational diabetes mellitus

   C. Rh incompatibility

   D. Pre-eclampsia

3 You are imaging a 9-week embryo and note an echogenic mass in the base of the umbilical cord. This finding most likely represents:

   A. Omphalocele

   B. Normal physiologic gut herniation that should resolve by the 10th menstrual week

   C. Gastroschisis

   D. Normal physiologic gut herniation that should resolve by the 14th menstrual week

4 In ectopic pregnancy the most common implantation site is:

   A. The isthmus of the fallopian tube

   B. The ampullary portion of the fallopian tube

   C. Intra-abdominal

   D. The interstitial portion of the fallopian tube

5 The heart rate of a 6-week embryo is 75 bpm, indicating:

   A. Impending demise

   B. Normal cardiac activity

   C. Failed pregnancy

   D. Normal bradycardia

6 All of the following are risk factors for ectopic pregnancy EXCEPT:

   A. Prior D&C

   B. Prior ectopic pregnancies

   C. Prior pelvic inflammatory disease

   D. Infertility therapy

7 Approximately how much does the gestational sac grow each day during the first trimester?

   A. 0.5 cm

   B. 0.8 mm

   C. 1 cm

   D. 4 mm

8 Normally, up to 6 weeks' gestation, the level of hCG:

   A. Triples every other day

   B. Doubles every day

   C. Doubles every 2 days

   D. Doubles every 3 days

9 Placental insufficiency is associated with all of the following EXCEPT:

   A. Trisomy 21

   B. Intrauterine infections

   C. Twin-twin transfusion

   D. Maternal hypertension or pre-eclampsia

10 Oligohydramnios may be caused by any of the following EXCEPT:

   A. Duodenal atresia

   B. Intrauterine growth restriction

   C. Premature rupture of membranes

   D. Renal agenesis

11 Most conjoined twins are joined at the:

   A. Abdomen (omphalopagus)

   B. Chest and abdomen (thoraco-omphalopagus)

   C. Head (craniopagus)

   D. Chest (thoracopagus)

12 In monochorionic monoamniotic pregnancies there is a higher incidence of all of the following EXCEPT:

A. Conjoining

B. Umbilical cord entanglement

C. Clubfeet

D. Nuchal cord and cord prolapse

13 The measurement that most accurately predicts fetal age is:

A. The first trimester femur length (FL)

B. The third trimester abdominal circumference (AC)

C. The third trimester biparietal diameter (BPD)

D. The first trimester crown-rump length (CRL)

14 During an ultrasound exam of a pregnant woman she experiences nausea, fainting, and sweating. What should you do?

A. Call a code.

B. Allow the symptoms to pass.

C. Roll the patient onto her left side and place a cool cloth on her head and neck.

D. Have the patient hyperventilate to get more oxygen in her system.

15 In cases of twin-twin transfusion:

A. The donor twin is larger, while the recipient is smaller.

B. The larger twin has oligohydramnios, while the smaller twin has polyhydramnios.

C. The larger twin can be hydropic with polyhydramnios, while the smaller twin can have oligohydramnios.

D. None of the above.

16 Which of the following should be included in the crown-rump length (CRL) measurement?

A. Yolk sac

B. Amnion

C. Fetal leg buds

D. Head to rump measurement

17 When does the embryonic stage of development end?

  A. First trimester

  B. 12th menstrual week

  C. 10th menstrual week

  D. 8th menstrual week

18 When do the fetal kidneys begin to contribute significantly to the amniotic fluid?

  A. 24 weeks

  B. 20 weeks

  C. 16 weeks

  D. 8 weeks

19 With which of the following conditions is cystic hygroma most closely associated?

  A. Turner's syndrome

  B. Meckel's syndrome

  C. Chiari malformation

  D. Trisomy 13

20 A cephalic index of ~60% would suggest the head shape to be:

  A. Brachycephalic

  B. Dolichocephalic

  C. Kleeblatschadel

  D. Normal

21 At what point is organogenesis complete?

  A. 20 menstrual weeks

  B. 18 menstrual weeks

  C. 16 menstrual weeks

  D. 8 menstrual weeks

22 What is the most common neural tube defect?

  A. Spina bifida

  B. Anencephaly

  C. Myelomeningocele

  D. Encephalocele

23 Molar pregnancies can be associated with all of the following EXCEPT:

   A. Theca-lutein cysts

   B. Hyperemesis gravidarum

   C. Increased beta hCG

   D. Cystadenomas

24 Congenital diaphragmatic hernias most commonly are located through the:

   A. Posterior right foramina

   B. Meckel's diverticulum

   C. Foramen of Morgagni anterior-medially

   D. Foramen of Bochdalek posterior-laterally and left

25 Which of the following is NOT associated with placenta accreta?

   A. Hematuria

   B. Vaginal bleeding

   C. Prior history of an IUD

   D. History of previous cesarean section

26 Which one of the following is NOT associated with trisomy 13?

   A. Encephalocele

   B. Cardiac defects

   C. Cleft lip and palate

   D. Holoprosencephaly

27 Low alpha-fetoprotein is associated with all of the following EXCEPT:

   A. Myelomeningocele

   B. Miscarriages or failed pregnancies

   C. Trisomy 18

   D. Trisomy 21

28 What is a key feature of trisomy 18?

   A. Holoprosencephaly

   B. "Double bubble" associated with duodenal atresia

   C. Polydactyly

   D. "Rocker bottom" feet

29 Which of the following biochemical markers is NOT associated with a higher incidence of Down syndrome?

   A. Decreased levels of human chorionic gonadotropin (hCG)

   B. Elevated levels of human placental lactogen (hPL)

   C. Decreased level of unconjugated estriol ($\mu E3$)

   D. Decreased levels of maternal serum alpha-fetoprotein (MS-AFP)

30 A solid ovarian mass in a 45-year-old female with a history of colon cancer most likely is a:

   A. Krukenberg tumor

   B. Cystadenoma

   C. Thecoma

   D. Fibroma

31 What is the most common germ cell tumor of the ovary in women ages 20–30?

   A. Leiomyoma

   B. Cystadenoma

   C. Androblastoma

   D. Teratoma or dermoid

32 Corpus luteum cysts usually resolve in a pregnancy by:

   A. 24 weeks

   B. 20 weeks

   C. 16 weeks

   D. 12 weeks

33 Postmenopausal thickening of the endometrium is caused by all of the following EXCEPT:

   A. Uterine polyp

   B. Endometrial hyperplasia

   C. Uterine adenomyosis

   D. Endometrial carcinoma

34 The presenting symptom(s) of leiomyomas is (are):

   A. Urinary frequency or urgency

   B. Pelvic pain

   C. Rectal pressure—constipation

   D. All of the above

35 The normal endometrial thickness of a postmenopausal patient who presents with vaginal bleeding is:

   A. 9 mm

   B. 8 mm

   C. 6 mm

   D. 4 mm

36 Which of the following statements about endometrial polyps is TRUE?

   A. Sonographically they appear as a thickened, echogenic, endometrial stripe.

   B. They occur commonly in women in their thirties.

   C. They are commonly seen sonographically in the lower uterine segment.

   D. They are best evaluated by endovaginal sonography (EVS) alone.

37 Which of the following factors diminish the odds for conception?

   A. Endocrine disorders

   B. Sexually transmitted diseases

   C. Advanced maternal age

   D. All of the above

38 Disorders associated with infertility include:

   A. Asherman's syndrome

   B. Hypothalamic or pituitary diseases

   C. Stein-Leventhal syndrome

   D. All of the above

39 Which statement about endometrial cancer is NOT true?

    A. It commonly presents with postmenopausal vaginal bleeding.

    B. It is more common in African-American women.

    C. It is more common than cervical cancer.

    D. It is associated with tamoxifen and estrogen-replacement therapy.

40 The normal dimensions of the ovary in an adult female are:

    A. 2 × 4 × 3 cm

    B. 4 × 4 × 4 cm

    C. 3 × 3 × 3 cm

    D. 1 × 2 × 3 cm

Bibliography

Suggested Reading

Berman MC, Cohen HL: *Diagnostic Medical Sonography: A Guide to Clinical Practice Obstetrics and Gynecology,* 2nd Edition. Philadelphia, Lippincott, 1997.

Callen P: *Ultrasonography in Obstetrics and Gynecology,* 4th Edition. St. Louis, Saunders, 2000.

Fleisher AC, Manning FA, Jeanty P, Romero R: *Sonography in Obstetrics and Gynecology: Principles and Practice,* 5th Edition. New York, McGraw Hill Professional, 1996.

McGahan JP, Goldberg BB: *Diagnostic Ultrasound: A Logical Approach.* Philadelphia, Lippincott Williams & Wilkins, 1998.

Moore KL, Persaud TVN: *The Developing Human: Clinically Oriented Embryology,* 7th Edition. Philadelphia, Saunders, 2003.

Nyberg DA, McGahan JP, Pretorius DH, et al: *Diagnostic Imaging of Fetal Anomalies.* Philadelphia, Lippincott Williams Wilkins, 2003.

Rumack CM, Wilson SR, Charboneau W: *Diagnostic Ultrasound,* 2nd Edition, Volume 2. St. Louis, Mosby, 1998.

References

1. Nicolaides K, Campbell S: Diagnosis of fetal abnormalities by ultrasound. In Milunsky A (ed): *Genetic Disorders and the Fetus: Diagnosis, Prevention and Treatment,* 2nd edition. New York, Plenum Press, 1986, pp 521–570.
2. Guidelines for Performance of the Antepartum Obstetric Examination. JUM 15:185, 1996.
3. Yeh H-C, Goodman JD, Carr L, et al: Intradecidual sign: An ultrasound criterion of early intrauterine pregnancy. *Radiology* 161:463–467, 1986.
4. Doubilet PM, Benson CB: Embryonic heart rate in the early first trimester: What rate is normal? *J Ultrasound Med* 14:431–434, 1995.
5. Wilcox AJ, Weinberg CR, O'Connor JF, et al: Incidence of early loss of pregnancy. *N Engl J Med* 319:189–194, 1988.
6. Bateman BG, Felder R, Kolp LA, et al: Subclinical pregnancy loss in clomiphene citrate treated women. *Fertil Steril* 57:25–27, 1992.
7. Snijders RJM, Noble P, Sebire N, et al: UK multicentre project on assessment of risk of trisomy 21 by maternal age and fetal nuchal-translucency thickness at 10–14 weeks gestation. *The Lancet* 352:343–346, 1998.
8. van Vugt JMG, van Zalen-Sprock RM, Kostense PJ: First-trimester nuchal translucency: A risk analysis on fetal chromosome abnormality. *Radiology* 200:537–540, 1996.
9. Hidalgo H, Bowie J, Rosenberg ER, et al: In utero sonographic diagnosis of fetal cerebral anomalies. *AJR* 139:143–148, 1982.
10. Fiske CE, Filly RA: Ultrasound evaluation of the normal and abnormal fetal neural axis. *Radiol Clin North Am* 20:285–296, 1982.
11. Pasto ME, Kurtz AB: The prenatal examination of the fetal cranium, spine, and central nervous system. *Semin Ultrasound CT MR* 5:170, 1984.
12. Filly RA: Ultrasonography. In Harrison MR, Golbus MS, Filly RA (eds): *The Unborn Patient: Prenatal Diagnosis and Treatment.* Orlando, Florida: Grune & Stratton, 1984, pp 33–123.
13. Carrasco CR, Stierman ED, Harnsberger HR, et al: An algorithm for prenatal ultrasound diagnosis of congenital CNS abnormalities. *J Ultrasound Med* 4:163–168, 1985.
14. Edwards MSD, Filly RA: Diagnosis and management of fetal disorders of the central nervous system. In Hoffman HJ, Epstein F (eds): *Disorders of the Developing Nervous System; Diagnosis and Treatment.* Boston, Blackwell Scientific Publications, 1986, pp 55–73.
15. Parulekar SG: Sonography of normal fetal bowel. *J Ultrasound Med* 10:211–220, 1991.
16. Harris RD, Alexander, RB: Ultrasound of the placenta and umbilical cord. In Callen P (ed). *Ultrasonography in Obstetrics and Gynecology,* 4th edition. Philadelphia, Saunders, 2000, pp 597–626.
17. Tindall VR, Scott JS: Placental calcification: A study of 3,025 singleton and multiple pregnancies. *J Obstet Gynecol Br Commonw* 72:356–373, 1965.
18. Spirt BA, Cohen WN, Weinstein HM: The incidence of placental calcification in normal pregnancies. *Radiology* 142:707–711, 1982.
19. Benirsche K, Kaufman P: *Pathology of the Human Placenta,* 2nd edition. New York, Springer-Verlag, 1990.
20. Jassani MN, Brennan JN, Merkatz IR: Prenatal diagnosis of single umbilical artery by ultrasound. *J Clin Ultrasound* 8:447–448, 1980.
21. Persutte WH, Hobbins J: Single umbilical artery: A clinical enigma in modern prenatal diagnosis. *Ultrasound Obstet Gynecol* 6:216–222, 1995.
22. Cohen HL, Shapiro ML, Haller JO, et al: The multivessel umbilical cord: An antenatal indicator of possible conjoined twinning. *J Clin Ultrasound* 20:278–282, 1992.
23. Miser WF: Outcome of infants born with nuchal cords. *J Fam Pract* 34:441–445, 1992.
24. Larson JD, Rayburn WF, Crosby S, et al: Multiple nuchal cord entanglements and intrapartum complications. *Am J Obstet Gynecol* 173:1228–1231, 1995.
25. Fink IJ, Filly RA: Omphalocele associated with umbilical cord allantoic cyst: Sonographic evaluation in utero. *Radiology* 149:473–476, 1983.
26. Frazier HA, Guerrieri JP, Thomas RL, et al: The detection of a patent urachus and allantoic cyst of the umbilical cord on prenatal ultrasonography. *J Ultrasound Med* 11:117–120, 1992.
27. Weissman A, Jakobi P, Bronshtein M, et al: Sonographic measurements of the umbilical cord and vessels during normal pregnancies. *J Ultrasound Med* 13:11–14, 1994.
28. Skibo LK, Lyons EA, Levi CS: First-trimester umbilical cord cysts. *Radiology* 182:719–722, 1992.
29. Jauniaux E, Donner C, Thomas C, et al: Umbilical cord pseudocyst in trisomy 18 [see comments]. *Prenat Diagn* 8:557–563, 1988.
30. Ballas S, Gitstein S, Kharasch J: Fetal heart rate variation with umbilical hematoma. *Postgrad Med J* 61:753, 1985.
31. de Crespigny LC, Cooper D, McKenna M: Early detection of intrauterine pregnancy with ultrasound. *J Ultrasound Med* 7:7–10, 1988.
32. Benson CB, Doubilet PM: Fetal measurements: Normal and abnormal fetal growth. In Rumack CM, Wilson SR, Charboneau JW (eds): *Diagnostic Ultrasound,* 2nd edition. St. Louis, Mosby-Year Book, 1998, p 1014.
33. Gray DL, Songster GS, Parvin CA, et al: Cephalic index: A gestational age-dependent biometric parameter. *Obstet Gynecol* 74:600–603, 1989.

34. Doubilet PM, Greenes RA: Improved prediction of gestational age from fetal head measurements. *AJR* 142:797–800, 1984.
35. Benson CB, Doubilet PM: Sonographic prediction of gestational age: Accuracy of second- and third-trimester fetal measurements. *AJR* 157:1275–1277, 1991.
36. Lubchenco LO, Hansman C, Boyd E, et al: Intra-uterine growth as estimated from liveborn birth-weight data at 24 to 42 weeks of gestation. *Pediatrics* 37:403–408, 1966.
37. Scott KE, Usher R: Fetal malnutrition: Its incidence, causes, and effects. *Am J Obstet Gynecol* 94:951–963, 1966.
38. Williams RL, Creasy RK, Cunningham GC, et al: Fetal growth and perinatal viability in California. *Obstet Gynecol* 59:624–632, 1982.
39. Hadlock FP, Harrist RB: In utero analysis of fetal growth: A sonographic weight standard. *Radiology* 181:129–133, 1991.
40. Hadlock FP, Harrist RB, Carpenter RJ, et al: Sonographic estimation of fetal weight. The value of femur length in addition to head and abdomen measurements. *Radiology* 150:535–540, 1984.
41. Benson CB, Boswell SB, Brown DL, et al: Improved prediction of intrauterine growth retardation with use of multiple parameters. *Radiology* 168:7–12, 1988.
42. Benirschke K, Kim CK: Multiple pregnancy. Part 1. *N Engl J Med* 288:1276–1284, 1973.
43. Hrubec Z, Robinette CD: The study of human twins in medical research. *N Engl J Med* 310:435–441, 1984.
44. Luke B: The changing pattern of multiple births in the United States: Maternal and infant characteristics, 1973 and 1990. *Obstet Gynecol* 84:101–106, 1994.
45. Ghai V, Vidyasagar D: Morbidity and mortality factors in twins. An epidemiologic approach. *Clin Perinatol* 15:123–140, 1988.
46. Crane JP: Sonographic evaluation of multiple pregnancy. *Semin Ultrasound CT MR* 5:144–156, 1984.
47. Naeye RL, Tafari N, Judge D, et al: Twins: Causes of perinatal death in twelve United States cities and one African city. *Am J Obstet Gynecol* 131:267–272, 1978.
48. Benirschke K, Kim CK: Multiple pregnancy. Part 1. *N Engl J Med* 288:1276–1284, 1973.
49. Milham Jr S: Pituitary gonadotrophin and dizygotic twinning. *Lancet* 2(7359):566, 1964.
50. White C, Wyshak G: Inheritance in human dizygotic twinning. *N Engl J Med* 271:1003–1005, 1964.
51. Moore KL: The placenta and fetal membranes. In Moore KL, Persaud TVN, Schmitt W (eds): *The Developing Human: Clinically Oriented Embryology,* 6th edition. Philadelphia, Saunders, 1998, pp 104–130.
52. Hertzberg BS, Kurtz AB, Choi HY, et al: Significance of membrane thickness in the sonographic evaluation of twin gestations. *AJR* 148:151–153, 1987.
53. Townsend RR, Simpson GF, Filly RA: Membrane thickness in ultrasound prediction of chorionicity of twin gestations. *J Ultrasound Med* 7:327–332, 1988.
54. Winn HN, Gabrielli S, Reece EA, et al: Ultrasonographic criteria for the prenatal diagnosis of placental chorionicity in twin gestations. *Am J Obstet Gynecol* 161(part 1):1540–1542, 1989.
55. Finberg HJ: The "twin peak" sign: Reliable evidence of dichorionic twinning. *J Ultrasound Med* 11:571–577, 1992.
56. Weissman A, Achiron R, Lipitz S, et al: The first-trimester growth-discordant twin: An ominous prenatal finding. *Obstet Gynecol* 84:110–114, 1994.
57. Vintzileos AM, Rodis JF: Growth discordance in twins. In Divon MY (ed): *Abnormal Fetal Growth*. New York, Elsevier, 1991, pp 289.
58. Benson CB, Doubilet PM: Ultrasound of multiple gestations. *Semin Roentgenol* 26:50–62, 1991.
59. Storlazzi E, Vintzileos AM, Campbell WA, et al: Ultrasonic diagnosis of discordant fetal growth in twin gestations. *Obstet Gynecol* 69:363–367, 1987.
60. Divon MY, Girz BA, Sklar A, et al: Discordant twins: A prospective study of the diagnostic value of real-time ultrasonography combined with umbilical artery velocimetry. *Am J Obstet Gynecol* 161:757–760, 1989.
61. Spellacy WN: Multiple pregnancies. In Scott JR, DiSaia PJ, Hammond CB, et al (eds): *Danforth's Obstetrics and Gynecology,* 7th edition. Philadelphia, Lippincott, 1994, pp 333–341.
62. Hagay ZJ, Mazor M, Leiberman JR, et al: Management and outcome of multiple pregnancies complicated by the antenatal death of one fetus. *J Reprod Med* 31:717–720, 1986.
63. Levi CS, Lyons EA, Lindsay DJ, et al: The sonographic evaluation of multiple gestation pregnancy. In Fleischer AC, Romero R, Manning FA, et al (eds): *The Principles and Practice of Ultrasonography in Obstetrics and Gynecology,* 4th edition. East Norwalk, CT, Appleton & Lange, 1991, pp 359–380.
64. Patten RM, Mack LA, Nyberg DA, et al: Twin embolization syndrome: Prenatal sonographic detection and significance. *Radiology* 173:685–689, 1989.
65. Benirschke K: The contribution of placental anastomoses to prenatal twin damage. *Hum Pathol* 23:1319–1320, 1992.
66. Pretorius DH, Mahony BS: Twin gestations. In Nyberg DA, Mahony BS, Pretorius DH (eds): *Diagnostic Ultrasound of Fetal Anomalies: Text and Atlas*. Chicago, Year Book Medical Publishers, 1990, pp 592–622.
67. Filly RA, Goldstein RB, Callen PW: Monochorionic twinning: Sonographic assessment. *AJR* 154:459–469, 1990.
68. Finberg HJ: Ultrasound evaluation in multiple gestation. In Callen PW (ed): *Ultrasonography in Obstetrics and Gynecology,* 3rd edition. Philadelphia, Saunders, 1994, pp 102–128.
69. Benson CB, Bieber FR, Genest DR, et al: Doppler demonstration of reversed umbilical blood flow in an acardiac twin. *J Clin Ultrasound* 17:291–295, 1989.
70. Benirschke K, des Roches Harper V: The acardiac anomaly. *Teratology* 15:311–316, 1977.

71. Pretorius DH, Leopold GR, Moore TR, et al: Acardiac twin report of Doppler sonography. *J Ultrasound Med* 7:413–416, 1988.
72. Benirschke K, Kim CK: Multiple pregnancy. Part 1. *N Engl J Med* 288:1276–1284, 1973.
73. Ferris TF: Toxemia and hypertension. In Burrow GM, Ferris TF (eds.): *Medical Complications during Pregnancy*, 3rd edition. Philadelphia, Saunders, 1988.
74. Mari G, Adrignolo A, Abuhamad AZ, et al: Diagnosis of fetal anemia with Doppler ultrasound in the pregnancy complicated by maternal blood group immunization. *Ultrasound Obstet Gynecol* 5:400–405, 1995.
75. Albanese CT, Jennings RW, Filly RA, et al: Endoscopic fetal tracheal occlusion: Evolution of techniques. *Pediatr Endosurg Innov Tech* 2:47, 1998.
76. Harrison MR, Mychaliska GB, Albanese CT, et al: Correction of congenital diaphragmatic hernia in utero. IX. Fetuses with poor prognosis (liver herniation and low lung-to-head ratio) can be saved by fetoscopic temporary tracheal occlusion. *J Pediatr Surg* 33:1017–1022, 1998; discussion, p 1022.
77. Okitsu O, Mimura T, Nakayama T, et al: Early prediction of preterm delivery by transvaginal ultrasonography. *Ultrasound Obstet Gynecol* 2:402–409, 1992.
78. Cousins L: Cervical incompetence: A time for reappraisal. *Clin Obstet Gynecol* 23:467–479, 1980.
79. Stromme WB, Haywa EW: Intrauterine fetal death in the second trimester. *Am J Obstet Gynecol* 85:223, 1963.
80. Singer MS, Hockman M: Incompetent cervix in a hormone-exposed offspring. *Obstet Gynecol* 51:625–626, 1978.
81. Hertzberg B, Bowie J: Ultrasound of postpartum uterus, prediction of retained placental tissue. *J Ultrasound Med* 10:451–456, 1991.
82. Gibbs RS, Rodgers PJ, Castaneda YS, et al: Endometritis following vaginal delivery. *Obstet Gynecol* 56:555–558, 1980.
83. Willson JR: The conquest of cesarean section related infections: A progress report. *Obstet Gynecol* 72[II]:519–532 Review, 1988.
84. Hanemann N, Mohr J: Antenatal fetal diagnosis in the embryo by means of biopsy with extra embryonic membranes. *Bull Eur Soc Hum Genet* 2:23, 1968.
85. Kullander S, Sandahl V: Fetal chromosome analysis after transcervical placental biopsy during early pregnancy. *Acta Obstet Gynecol Scand* 52:355–359, 1973.
86. Tiatung Hospital of Anshan Steel Works Department of Obstetrics and Gynaecology: Fetal sex prediction by sex chromatin of chorionic villi cells during early pregnancy. *Chin Med J* 1:117–126, 1975.
87. Kazy Z, Rozovsky IS, Bakharev VA: Chorion biopsy in early pregnancy: A method of early prenatal diagnosis for inherited disorders. *Prenat Diagn* 2:39, 1982.
88. Canadian Collaborative CVS-Amniocentesis Clinical Trial Group: Multicentered randomized clinical trial of chorionic villus sampling and amniocentesis. First Report. *Lancet* i:2–6, 1989.
89. National Institute of Child Health and Human Development: The safety and efficacy of chorionic villus sampling for early prenatal diagnosis of cytogenetic abnormalities. *N Engl J Med* 320:609–617, 1989.
90. Jeanty P, Dramaix-Wilmet MS, Van Gansbeke D, et al: Fetal ocular biometry by ultasound. *Radiology* 143:513–516, 1982.
91. Myrianthopoulos N: Epidemiology of central nervous system malformations. In Vinken PJ, Bruyn GW (eds): *Handbook of Clinical Neurology*. Amsterdam, Elsevier, 1977, p 139.
92. Mahony BS, Nyberg DA, Hirsch JH, et al: Mild idiopathic lateral ventricular dilatation in utero: Sonographic evaluation. *Radiology* 169:715–721, 1988.
93. Hertzberg BS, Lile R, Foosaner DE, et al: Choroid plexus-ventricular wall separation in fetuses with normal-sized cerebral ventricles at sonography: Postnatal outcome. *AJR* 163:405–410, 1994.
94. Green JJ, Hobbins JC: Abdominal ultrasound examination of the first trimester fetus. *Am J Obstet Gynecol* 159:165–175, 1988.
95. Devries PA: The pathogenesis of gastroschisis and omphalocele. *J Pediatr Surg* 15:245–251, 1980.
96. Hoyme HE, Higginbottom MC, Jones KL: The vascular pathogenesis of gastroschisis: Intrauterine interruption of the omphalomesenteric artery. *J Pediatr* 98:662–663, 1981.
97. Timor-Tritsch IE, Warem WP, Peisner DB, et al: First-trimester midgut herniation: A high frequency transvaginal sonographic study. *Am J Obstet Gynecol* 161:831–833, 1989.
98. Shah HR, Patwa PC, Pandya JB, et al: Case report: Antenatal ultrasound diagnosis of a case of "pentalogy of Cantrell" with common cardiac chambers. *Ind J Radiol Imag* 10:2:99–101, 2000.
99. Herva R, Karinen-Jaaskelainen M: Amniotic adhesion malformation syndrome: Fetal and placental pathology. *Teratology* 19:11, 1984.
100. Kino Y: Clinical and experimental studies of the congenital constriction band syndrome, with an emphasis on its etiology. *J Bone Joint Surg Am* 57:636–643, 1987.
101. Teresita TL: Fetal anterior abdominal wall defect. In Callen PW (ed): *Ultrasonography in Obstetrics and Gynecology*, 4th edition. Philadelphia, Saunders, 2000, p 506.
102. Levi A, Findler M, Dolfin T, et al: Intrapericardial extralobar pulmonary sequestration in a neonate. *Chest* 98:1014–1015, 1990.
103. Granum P, Bracken M, Silverman R, et al: Assessment of kidney size in normal gestation by comparison of kidney circumference to abdominal circumference. *Am J Obstet Gynecol* 136:249–254, 1980.
104. Potter EL: Bilateral absence of ureters and kidneys. A report of 50 cases. *Obstet Gynecol* 25:3–12, 1965.
105. Dunnick NR, McCallum RW, Sandler CM: Congenital anomalies. In *Textbook of Uroradiology*. Baltimore, Williams and Wilkins, 1991, pp 15–18.

106. Hill LM: Ultrasound of fetal gastrointestinal tract. In Callen PW (ed): *Ultrasonography in Obstetrics and Gynecology*, 4th edition. Philadelphia, Saunders, 2000, p 458.
107. Hill LM: Ultrasound of fetal gastrointestinal tract. In Callen PW (ed): *Ultrasonography in Obstetrics and Gynecology*, 4th edition. Philadelphia, Saunders, 2000, p 460.
108. Fonkalsrud EW, de Lorimier AA, Hays MD: Congenital atresia and stenosis of the duodenum. A review compiled from the members of the surgical section of the American Academy of Pediatrics. *Pediatrics* 43:79–83, 1969.
109. Hancock BJ, Wiseman NE: Congenital duodenal obstruction: The impact of an antenatal diagnosis. *J Pediatr Surg* 24:1027–1031, 1989.
110. Boute A, Muller F, Nezelof C, et al: Prenatal diagnosis in 200 pregnancies with a 1-in-4 risk of cystic fibrosis. *Hum Genet* 74:288–297, 1986.
111. Szeifert GT, Szabo M, Papp Z: Morphology of cystic fibrosis at 17 weeks of gestation (letter to the editor). *Clin Genet* 28:561–565, 1985.
112. Hill LM: Ultrasound of fetal gastrointestinal tract. In Callen PW (ed): *Ultrasonography in Obstetrics and Gynecology*, 4th edition. Philadelphia, Saunders, 2000, p 465.
113. Orioli I, Castilla EE, Barbosa-Neto JG, et al: The birth prevalence rates for the skeletal dysplasias. *J Med Genet* 23:328–332, 1986.
114. Camera G, Mastroiacovo P: Birth prevalence of skeletal dysplasias in the Italian multicentric monitoring system for birth defects. In Bartsocas CS, Papadatos CJ (eds): *Skeletal Dysplasias*. New York, Alan R. Liss, 1982, pp 442–449.
115. Weldner BM, Persson PH, Aivarsson S: Prenatal diagnosis of dwarfism by ultrasound screening. *Arch Dis Child* 60:1070–1072, 1985.
116. Connor JM, Connor RA, Sweet EM, et al: Lethal neonatal chondrodysplasias in the west of Scotland 1970–1983 with a description of a thanato-phoric, dysplasialike, autosomal recessive disorder, Glasgow variant. *Am J Med Genet* 22:243–253, 1985.
117. Houston CS, Optiz JM, Spranger J, et al: The camptomelic syndrome: Review, report of 17 cases, and follow-up on the currently 17 year old boy first reported by Maroteauz et al in 1971. *Am J Med Genet* 15:3–28, 1983.
118. Jones KL: *Smith's Recognizable Patterns of Human Malformation*. Philadephia, Saunders, 1997, pp 324, 325.
119. Chung CS, Nemechek RW, Larsen IJ, et al: Genetic and epidemiological studies of clubfoot in Hawaii: General and medical considerations. *Human Hered* 19:321–342, 1969.
120. Ianniruberto A: Management of fetal cardiac structural abnormalities. *Fetal Ther* 1:89–91, 1986.
121. Hoffman JIE: Incidence of congenital heart disease. II. Prenatal incidence. *Pediatr Cardiol* 16:155–165, 1995.
122. Hoffman JIE, Christianson R: Congenital heart disease in a cohort of 19,502 births with long-term follow-up. *Am J Cardiol* 42:640–647, 1978.
123. Hoffman JIE: Incidence of congenital heart disease. I. Postnatal incidence. *Pediatr Cardiol* 16:103–113, 1995.
124. Brown DL, Emerson DS, Cartier MS, et al: Congenital cardiac anomalies: Prenatal sonographic diagnosis. *AJR* 153:109–114, 1989.
125. Moss AJ, Adams FH, Emmanouilides GC: *Moss and Adams Heart Disease in Infants, Children, and Adolescents: Including the Fetus and Young Adult*, 5th edition. Lippincott, Williams and Wilkins, 1995, p 555.
126. Benecerraf BR, Barss VA, Laboda LA: A sonographic sign for the detection in the second trimester of the fetus with Down's syndrome. *Am J Obstet Gynecol* 153:49, 1985.
127. American Institute in Medicine (AIUM) Technical Bulletin, Ultrasound Med 17:601–607, 1998.
128. Oberhoffer R, Cook C, Lang D, et al: Correlation between echocardiographic and morphological investigations of lesions of the tricuspid valve diagnosed during fetal life. *Br Heart J* 68:580–585, 1992.
129. Hornberger LK, Sahn DJ, Kleinman CS, et al: Tricuspid valve disease with significant tricuspid insufficiency in the fetus: Diagnosis and outcome. *J Am Coll Cardiol* 17:167–173, 1991.
130. Oberhoffer R, Cook AC, Lang D, et al: Correlation between echocardiographic and morphological investigations of lesions of the tricuspid valve diagnosed during fetal life. *Br Heart J* 68:580–585, 1992.
131. Robertson DA, Silverman NH: Ebstein's anomaly: Echocardiographic and clinical features in the fetus and neonate. *J Am Coll Cardiol* 14:1300–1307, 1989.
132. Sharland GK, Chita SK, Allan LD: Tricuspid valve dysplasia or displacement in intra-uterine life. *J Am Coll Cardiol* 17:944–949, 1991.
133. Freedom RM, Dische MR, Rowe RD: The tricuspid valve in pulmonary atresia and intact ventricular septum. *Arch Pathol Lab Med* 102:28–31, 1978.
134. Zuberbuhler JP, Anderson RH: Morphological variations in pulmonary atresia with intact ventricular septum. *Br Heart J* 41:281–288, 1979.
135. Roberson HA, Silverman NH, Zuberbuhler JR: Congenitally enlarged tricuspid orifice: Its differentiation from Ebstein's malformation in association with pulmonary atresia with an intact ventricular septum. *Pediatr Cardiol* 11:86–90, 1990.
136. Watson H: Natural history of Ebstein's anomaly of tricuspid valve in childhood and adolescence. An international cooperative study of 505 cases. *Br Heart J* 36:417–427, 1974.
137. Keith JD: Congenital mitral atresia. In Keith JD, Rowe RD, Vlad P (eds): *Heart Disease in Infancy and Childhood*, 3rd edition. New York, Macmillan, 1978, pp 549–553.
138. Friedman S, Murphy L, Ash R: Congenital mitral atresia with hypoplastic non-functioning left heart. *Am J Dis Child* 90:176–188, 1955.
139. Lev M, Arcilla R, Rimolde HJA, et al: Premature narrowing or closure of the foramen ovale. *Am Heart J* 65:638–647, 1963.
140. Bankl H: Particular malformations: Congenital malformations of the heart and great vessels. In *Synopsis of Pathology, Embryology and Natural History*. Baltimore, Urban and Schwarzenberg, 1977, pp 155–159.

141. Benacerraf BR, Saltzman DH, Sanders SP: Sonographic signs suggesting the prenatal diagnosis of coarctation of the aorta. *J Ultrasound Med* 8:65–69, 1989.
142. Benacerraf BR, Pober BR, Sanders SP: Accuracy of fetal echocardiography. *Radiology* 165:847–849, 1987.
143. Collett RW, Edwards JE: Persistent truncus arteriosus: A classification according to anatomic types. *Surg Clin North Am* 29:1245–1270, 1947.
144. Van Praagh R, Van Praagh S: The anatomy of common aorticopulmonary trunk (truncus arteriosus communis) and its embryologic implications: A study of 57 necropsy cases. *Am J Cardiol* 16:406–423, 1965.
145. Allan LD, Crawford DC, Anderson RH: Spectrum of congenital heart disease detected echocardiographically in prenatal life. *Br Heart J* 54:523–526, 1984.
146. Sadler TW: Cardiovascular system. In Sadler TW (ed): *Langman's Medical Embryology*, 6th edition. Baltimore, Williams & Wilkins, 1990, pp 179–227.
147. Webb GD, McLaughlin PR, Gow RM, et al: Transposition complexes. *Cardiol Clin* 11:651–664, 1993.
148. Thompson WE, Nichols DG, Ungerleider RM: Double-outlet right ventricle and double-outlet left ventricle. In Nichols DG, Cameron DE, Greeley WJ, et al (eds): *Critical Heart Disease in Infants and Children*. St Louis, Mosby-Year Book, 1995, pp 623–646.
149. Sanders SP, Bierman FZ, Williams RG: Conotruncal malformations: Diagnosis in infancy using subxiphoid 2-dimensional echocardiography. *Am J Cardiol* 50:1361–1367, 1982.
150. Snider AR, Serwer GA: Abnormalities of ventriculoarterial connection. In Snider AR, Serwer GA (eds): *Echocardiography in Pediatric Heart Disease*. St. Louis, Mosby-Year Book, 1990, pp 190–194.
151. Higgins CB, Silverman NH, Kersting-Sommerhoff B, et al: Atrioventricular septal (canal) defects. In Higgins CB, Silverman NH, Kersting-Sommerhoff B, et al (eds): *Congenital Heart Disease: Echocardiography and Magnetic Resonance Imaging*. New York, Raven Press, 1990, pp 135–150.
152. Dennis MA, Appareti K, Manco-Johnson ML: The echocardiographic diagnosis of multiple fetal cardiac tumors. *J Ultrasound Med* 4:327–329, 1985.
153. Corno A, de Simone G, Catena G, et al: Cardiac rhabdomyoma: Surgical treatment in the neonate. *J Thorac Cardiovasc Surg* 87:725–731, 1984.
154. Moss AJ, Adams FH, Emmanouilides GC: *Moss and Adams Heart Disease in Infants, Children, and Adolescents: Including the Fetus and Young Adult*, 5th edition. Lippincott, Williams and Wilkins, 1995, p 528.
155. Glanc P, Chitayat D, Azouz EM: The fetal musculoskeletal system. In Rumack CM (ed): *Diagnostic Ultrasound*, 2nd edition. St. Louis, Mosby, 1998, p 1228.
156. Benacerraf BR: Ultrasound evaluation of chromosomal abnormalities. In Callen PW (ed): *Ultrasonography in Obstetrics and Gynecology*, 4th edition. Philadelphia, Saunders, 2000, p 52, Table 3-3.
157. Benacerraf BR: Ultrasound evaluation of chromosomal abnormalities. In Callen PW (ed): *Ultrasonography in Obstetrics and Gynecology*, 4th edition. Philadelphia, Saunders, 2000, p 52.
158. Adapted from Bromley B, Lieberman E, Bernaceraf BR: The detection of Down syndrome using a scoring index of sonographic markers and maternal age. *Ultrasound Obstet Gynecol* 10:321–324, 1997.
159. Bernaceraf BR, Harlow B, Frigoletto FD Jr: Hypoplasia of the middle phalanx of the fifth digit: A feature of the second trimester fetus with Down syndrome. *J Ultrasound Med* 9:389–394, 1990.
160. Benaceraf BR: Ultrasound evaluation of chromosomal abnormalities. In Callen PW (ed): *Ultrasonography in Obstetrics and Gynecology*, 4th edition. Philadelphia, Saunders, 2000, p 47.
161. Vintzileos A, Walters C, Yeo L: Absent nasal bone in the prenatal detection of fetuses with trisomy 21 in high-risk population. *Obstet Gynecol* 101:905–908, 2003.
162. Cicero S, Bindra R, Rembouskos G, et al: Integrated ultrasound and biochemical screening for trisomy 21 using fetal nuchal translucency, absent fetal nasal bone, free beta-hCG and PAPP-A at 11 to 14 weeks. *Prenatal Diagn* 23:306–310, 2003.
163. Bunduki V, Ruano R, Miguelez J, et al: Fetal nasal bone length: Reference range and clinical application in ultrasound screening for trisomy 21. *Ultrasound Obstet Gynecol* 21:156–160, 2003.
164. Cicero S, Sonek JD, McKenna DS, et al: Nasal bone hypoplasia in trisomy 21 at 15–22 weeks gestation. *Ultrasound Obstet Gynecol* 21:15–18, 2003.
165. Lee W, DeVore GR, Comstock CH, et al: Nasal bone evaluation in fetuses with Down syndrome during the second and third trimesters of pregnancy. *J Ultrasound Med* 22:55–60, 2002.
166. Bromley B, Lieberman E, Shipp TD, et al: Fetal nose bone length: A marker for Down syndrome in the second trimester. *J Ultrasound Med* 21:1387–1394, 2002.
167. Cicero S, Bindra R, Rembouskos G, et al: Fetal nasal bone length in chromosomally normal and abnormal fetuses at 11–14 weeks of gestation. *J Matern Fetal Neonatal Med* 11:400–402, 2002.
168. Bernaceraf BR, Neuberg D, Bromley B, et al: Sonographic scoring index for prenatal detection of chromosomal abnormalities. *J Ultrasound Med* 11:449–458, 1992.
169. Jones KL: *Smith's Recognizable Patterns of Human Malformations*. Philadelphia, Saunders, 1997, p 30.
170. Benaceraf BR: Ultrasound evaluation of chromosomal abnormalities. In Callen PW (ed): *Ultrasonography in Obstetrics and Gynecology*, 4th edition. Philadelphia, Saunders, 2000, p 57.
171. Davee MA, Weaver DD: Turner syndrome. In Buyse ML (ed): *Birth Defects Encyclopedia*. Cambridge, MA, Blackwell Scientific Publications, 1990, pp 1717–1719.

172. Shehard J, Bean C, Bove B, et al: Long-term survival in a 69XXY triploid male. *Am J Med Genet* 25: 307–312, 1986.
173. Sperling MA: Steroid 21-hydroxylase deficiency. In Buyse ML (ed): *Birth Defects Encyclopedia*. Cambridge, MA, Blackwell Scientific Publications, 1990, pp 1602–1604.
174. Moore KC, Persaud TVN: *The Developing Human: Clinically Oriented Embryology*. Philadelphia, Saunders, 1999, p 336.
175. Pinsky L: Androgen insensitivity, complete. In Buyse ML (ed): *Birth Defects Encyclopedia*. Cambridge, MA, Blackwell Scientific Publications, 1990, pp 117–119.
176. Guellaen G, Casanova M, Bishop C, et al: Human XX males with Y single-copy DNA fragments. *Nature* 307:172–173, 1984.
177. Stephen EH, Chandra A: Updated projections of infertility in the United States: 1995–2025. *Fertil Steril* 70:30–34, 1998.
178. Wiseman DA, Greene CA, Pierson RA: Infertility. In Rumack CM (ed): *Diagnostic Ultrasound,* 2nd edition. St. Louis, Mosby, 1998, p 1413.
179. Society for Assisted Reproductive Technology and The American Society for Reproductive Medicine: Assisted reproductive technology in the United States and Canada: 1994 results generated from the American Society for Reproductive Medicine/Society for Assisted Reproductive Technology Registry. *Fertil Steril* 66:697–705, 1996.
180. Lobo RA: Estrogen replacement: the evolving role of alternative delivery systems. Introduction. *Am J Obstet Gynecol* 173:981, 1995.
181. Lazebnik N, Hill LM, Robinson TM: Transvaginal sonography in a woman treated with megestrol acetate for breast cancer. *J Ultrasound Med* 13:652, 1994.
182. Salem S: The uterus and adnexa. In Rumack CM (ed): *Diagnostic Ultrasound,* 2nd edition. St. Louis, Mosby, 1998, p 529.
183. Richenber J, Cooperberg P: Ultrasound of the uterus. In Callen PW (ed): *Ultrasonography in Obstetrics and Gynecology,* 4th edition. Philadelphia, Saunders, 2000, p 832.
184. Salem S: The uterus and adnexa. In Rumack CM (ed): *Diagnostic Ultrasound,* 2nd edition. St. Louis, Mosby, 1998, p 531.
185. Townsend DE, Fields G, McClausland A, et al: Diagnostic and operative hysteroscopy in the management of persistent post-menopausal bleeding. *Obstet Gynecol* 82:419–421, 1993.
186. Silverberg E, Boring CC, Squres TS: Cancer statistics. *CA Cancer J Clin* 40:9,1990.
187. Salem S: The uterus and adnexa. In Rumack CM (ed): *Diagnostic Ultrasound,* 2nd edition. St. Louis, Mosby, 1998, p 548.
188. Hibbard LT: Adnexal torsion. *Am J Obstet Gynecol* 152:456, 1985.
189. Dill-Macky MJ, Atri M: Ovarian sonography. In Callen PW (ed): *Ultrasonography in Obstetrics and Gynecology,* 4th edition. Philadelphia, Saunders, 2000, p 874.
190. Kurman RJ: *Blaustein's Pathology of the Female Genital Tract,* 4th edition. New York, Springer-Verlag, 1994.
191. Dill-Macky MJ, Atri M: Ovarian sonography. In Callen PW (ed): *Ultrasonography in Obstetrics and Gynecology,* 4th edition. Philadelphia, Saunders, 2000, p 875.
192. Dill-Macky MJ, Atri M: Ovarian sonography. In Callen PW (ed): *Ultrasonography in Obstetrics and Gynecology,* 4th edition. Philadelphia, Saunders, 2000, p 876.
193. Salem S: The uterus and adnexa. In Rumack CM (ed): *Diagnostic Ultrasound,* 2nd edition. St. Louis, Mosby, 1998, p 556.
194. Dill-Macky MJ, Atri M: Ovarian sonography. In Callen PW (ed): *Ultrasonography in Obstetrics and Gynecology,* 4th edition. Philadelphia, Saunders, 2000, p 877.
195. Salem S: The uterus and adnexa. In Rumack CM (ed): *Diagnostic Ultrasound,* 2nd edition. St. Louis, Mosby, 1998, p 556.
196. Salem S: The uterus and adnexa. In Rumack CM (ed): *Diagnostic Ultrasound,* 2nd edition. St. Louis, Mosby, 1998, p 557.
197. Dill-Macky MJ, Atri M: Ovarian sonography. In Callen PW (ed): *Ultrasonography in Obstetrics and Gynecology,* 4th edition. Philadelphia, Saunders, 2000, p 878.
198. Salem S: The uterus and adnexa. In Rumack CM (ed): *Diagnostic Ultrasound,* 2nd edition. St. Louis, Mosby, 1998, p 558.
199. Kurman RJ: *Blaustein's Pathology of the Female Genital Tract,* 4th edition. New York, Springer-Verlag, 1994.
200. Dill-Macky NJ, Atri M: Ovarian sonography. In Callen PW (ed): *Ultrasonography in Obstetrics and Gynecology,* 4th edition. Philadelphia, Saunders, 2000, p 881.
201. Salem S: The uterus and adnexa. In Rumack CM (ed): *Diagnostic Ultrasound,* 2nd edition. St. Louis, Mosby, 1998, p 551.
202. Carlson KJ, Skates SJ, Singer DE: Screening for ovarian cancer. *Ann Intern Med* 121:124, 1994.
203. Jacobs I, Davies AP, Bridges J, et al: Prevalence screening for ovarian cancer in postmenopausal women by CA 125 measurement and ultrasonography. *BMJ* 306:1030, 1993.

Index

Abdominal circumference (AC), 39, 67–70
Abdominal wall abnormalities, 144–152
    amniotic band syndrome, 150–151
    Beckwith-Wiedemann syndrome, 148
    cloacal exstrophy, 151–152
    embryology of the abdominal wall, 144–145
    gastroschisis, 145–146
    limb-body wall complex, 148–150
    omphalocele, 146–147
    pentalogy of Cantrell, 147–148
    potential pitfalls possibly leading to incorrect diagnosis, 152
    sonographic approach to evaluating, 152
Abnormal first trimester (failed pregnancy), 15–16
    complete abortion, 15–16
    threatened abortion, 15
Abnormalities
    of cord formation, 54
    of the fetal head and face, 123–124
    of fetal heart rate and rhythm, 201
    of the fetal neck, 139
    of the fetal skeleton, 177
    of the gestational sac, 16
    of placental shape, 43–45
Abnormalities of genitalia, 169–170
    cryptorchidism, 170
    hydrocele, 169
    hydrometrocolpos, 170
    ovarian cyst, 170
Abnormalities of the uterus, 249
    endometrial evaluation and infertility, 249
    leiomyomas, 249
AC. *See* Abdominal circumference
Acardiac parabiotic twin syndrome, 82
Acardiac twin (TRAP sequence), 88–90
Acetylcholinesterase (ACHE), 118
Achondrogenesis, 184
Achondroplasia, 177
Acoustic cavitation, 290–291
Adenomyosis, 262
Adnexa, 353–354

ADPKD. *See* Autosomal dominant polycystic kidney disease
AF-AFP. *See* Amniotic fluid alpha-fetoprotein
AFI. *See* Amniotic fluid index
AFP. *See* Alpha-fetoprotein
Agenesis corpus callosum, 133
AIUM. *See* American Institute of Ultrasound in Medicine guidelines
Allantois, cord cysts from, 56–57
Alloimmunization, 95–96
Alobar holoprosencephaly, 134
Alpha-fetoprotein (AFP), 116–118, 339
American Institute of Ultrasound in Medicine (AIUM) guidelines, 2, 123, 144, 227
    for gynecological examination, 351–354
    for routine obstetrical examinations, 345–350
Amniocentesis, 2
Amnion, 5, 14, 240
Amnionicity, of twin pregnancy, 81
Amniotic band syndrome, 150–151
Amniotic fluid, 111–113
    fetal pulmonic maturity studies, 113
Amniotic fluid alpha-fetoprotein (AF-AFP), 117
Amniotic fluid index (AFI), 112
Amniotic fluid volume, 111–113
    estimation, 112
    oligohydramnios, 112
    polyhydramnios, 112–113
Amniotic sac, 5
Amniotic sheet, 150–151
Androblastomas, 277
Androgen insensitivity syndrome, 243
Anembryonic pregnancy, 16
Anemic fetus, management of, 97
Anencephaly, 18, 139–140, 335
Angiogenesis, 7
Anovulation, 247
    hypothalamic causes, 247
    pituitary causes, 247
Antepartum/postpartum considerations, 102–109
    cesarean section, 108–109
    postpartum bleeding, 107–108
    postpartum infection, 108
    preterm delivery, 102–103
    ultrasound determination of risk for preterm delivery, 103–107
Anterior arcuate artery, 231

Appendicitis, 218
ARPKD. *See* Autosomal recessive polycystic kidney disease
Arrhenoblastomas, 277
ART. *See* Assisted reproductive technology
Artifacts, 289–290
    refraction, 289–290
    reverberation, 289
Asphyxiating thoracic dystrophy (Jeune syndrome), 187
Assessment of gestational age, 59–71
    first trimester, 60–64
    second and third trimester, 64–71
Assisted reproductive technology (ART), 250–252
    gamete intrafallopian transfer, 252
    in vitro fertilization, 251–252
    zygote intrafallopian transfer, 252
Atrial ventricular septal defects, 193
Atrioventricular canal (AVC), 199–200
Autosomal dominant conditions, 115–116
Autosomal dominant polycystic kidney disease (ADPKD), 166
Autosomal recessive disorders, 115
Autosomal recessive polycystic kidney disease (ARPKD), 162–165
AVC. *See* Atrioventricular canal

Battledore placenta, 56
Beckwith-Wiedemann syndrome, 130, 148, 224
Benign cystic mesothelioma, 269
Beta-human chorionic gonadotropin and sonographic findings, 15
Bilaminar embryonic disc, 5
Bilateral renal agenesis, 167–168
Binocular measurement, 71
Bioeffects, 290–291
    cavitation, 290–291
    thermal heating, 290
Biparietal diameter (BPD), 29, 64–66, 74, 124, 333
Blastocyst, implantation of, 5
Blastocyst cavity, 239
Blighted ovum, 16
Body stalk anomaly, 149

Bowel duplication, 176
BPD. *See* Biparietal diameter
Brachycephaly, 204
Brenner tumors, 273
Broad ligament, 229–230
Bronchogenic cysts, 156–157

CAM. *See* Cystic adenomatoid malformation
Camptomelic dysplasia, 185–186
Cardiac abnormalities, 92, 189–201
    abnormalities of fetal heart rate and rhythm, 201
    atrial ventricular septal defects, 193
    atrioventricular canal, 199–200
    cardiac tumors, 201
    coarctation, 195–196
    double-outlet right ventricle, 199
    Ebstein's anomaly, 193
    hypoplastic left heart syndrome, 194–195
    indications, 189–190
    persistent truncus arteriosus, 197
    single ventricle, 196
    situs abnormalities, 200
    sonographic findings, 190–200
    tetralogy of Fallot, 198–199
    transposition of the great arteries, 197–198
Cardiac activity, in the embryo, 13
Cardiomyopathy (CMP), 199–200
Cardiovascular system, in the embryonic period, 8
Case studies for self-assessment, 293–344
    in gynecology, 317–326, 340–344
    in obstetrics, 295–317, 326–340
Cavitation, 290–291
CDH. *See* Congenital diaphragmatic hernia
Cebocephaly, 126
Cephalic index, 67–68
Cephaloceles, 140–141
Cerebral ventriculomegaly, mild lateral, 131
Cervical cerclage, 107
Cervix, 249, 265–266
Cesarean section, 108–109
Chest masses, 154–155
Cholecystitis, 218
Choledochal cysts, 176

Chondroectodermal dysplasia (Ellis-Van Creveld syndrome), 187
Chorioadenoma destruens, 224
Chorioangioma, 52–53, 330
Choriocarcinoma, 224
Chorion, 5, 240
Chorion frondosum, 17, 81
Chorionic cavity, 5
Chorionic sac, 60
Chorionic villus sampling (CVS), 2, 119–121
   concept/indications, 119
   history, 119
   transabdominal approach, 120–121
   transcervical approach, 119–120
Chorionicity, of twin pregnancy, 81
Choroid plexus cysts, 142–143
Chromosomal abnormality, 118
Circummarginate placenta, 43–44
Circumvallate placenta, 43–44, 340
Classic hydatidiform mole (CHM), 219–221
   with normal twin, 222–223
Clear cell tumors, 273
Clinical aspects of cervical incompetence, 106–107
Cloacal exstrophy, 151–152
Clubfoot deformity, 188
CME. See Continuing medical education
CMN. See Congenital mesoblastic nephroma
CMP. See Cardiomyopathy
CMV. See Cytomegalovirus
CNS malformations, 92
Coarctation, 195–196
Coexisting disorders, 213–224
   complex masses, 216
   cystic masses, 214–216
   maternal disorders presenting primarily with pain and swelling, 218–219
   pelvic masses, 213
   solid masses, 216–217
   trophoblastic disease, 219–224
Colon atresia, 174
Color Doppler, 39, 42, 51, 167, 200
Complete abortion, 15–16
Complete placenta previa, 47
Complex masses, 216
   dermoid cyst, 216
   pelvic kidney, 216
Complications, 73–109
   antepartum/postpartum considerations, 102–109
   fetal therapy, 98–102
   intrauterine growth restriction, 73–80, 146, 203
   maternal illness, 91–98
   multiple gestations, 80–91
Complications of twin pregnancy, 85–91
   acardiac twin (TRAP sequence), 88–90
   conjoined twins, 90–91
   cord entanglement, 90
   twin embolization syndrome, 87–88
   twin-twin transfusion syndrome, 86
Computerized tomography (CT), 289
Conceptus period, 4
Congenital adrenal hyperplasia, 241
Congenital diaphragmatic hernia (CDH), 156–159
Congenital mesoblastic nephroma (CMN), 169
Congenitally corrected transposition, 197–198
Conjoined twins, 90–91
Continuing medical education (CME) application for credit, 355–368
   applicant information, 357
   CME quiz, 361–368
   evaluation of text, 358–360
   objectives, 356
   steps in obtaining, 357
Contraindications, to endovaginal sonography, 236
Conus medullaris, 34
Cord abnormalities, 54–58
   abnormal twists, 55–56
   cord cysts, 56–58
   cord insertion, 56
   cord masses, 58
   structural abnormalities, 54–55
   vascular abnormalities, 54
Cord anatomy, 53–54
Cord cysts, 56–58
   from the allantois, 56–57
   from the omphalomesenteric duct, 56–57
Cord entanglement, 90
Cord insertion, 56
   battledore placenta, 56
   vasa previa, 56
   velamentous insertion, 56
Cord masses, 58
   diffuse abnormalities, 58
   hemangioma, 58
   hematoma, 58
   teratoma, 58
   varix/aneurysm, 58
Cordocentesis, 98–99
Corpus luteum cyst, 214, 267
Cranium, 29–32
CRL. See Crown-rump length
Crown-rump length (CRL), 11, 53, 62–64, 85, 334
Cryptorchidism, 170
CT. See Computerized tomography
Cul de sac, 23, 354
   fluid, 232–233
CVS. See Chorionic villus sampling
Cystadenofibroma, 271
Cystadenoma, 215, 336, 343
Cystic adenomatoid malformation (CAM), 154, 336
Cystic masses, 214–216
   corpus luteum cyst, 214
   hydrosalpinx, 214
   paraovarian cyst, 214–215
   torsion, 215
Cystic teratoma (dermoid cyst), 273–274
Cytomegalovirus (CMV), 138

D-transposition of the great arteries, 197
Dandy-Walker malformation (DWM), 132–133
DC/DA. See Dichorionic diamniotic twins
Decidua basalis, 9, 17, 81
Decidual thickening, 8
Dermoid cyst, 216, 273–274, 340
DES. See Diethylstilbestrol exposure
Diabetes mellitus, 92–94
   cardiac anomalies, 92
   CNS malformations, 92
   gastrointestinal anomalies, 93
   renal and urologic anomalies, 92
Diaphragmatic hernia repair, 100–101
Dichorionic diamniotic (DC/DA) twins, 81
Diethylstilbestrol (DES) exposure, 107, 258
Diffuse abnormalities, 58
Diseases arising from a single gene, 115–116
   autosomal dominant conditions, 115–116
   autosomal recessive disorders, 115
   X-linked diseases, 116
Disorders of ovulation, 246–247, 247
   anovulation, 247
   dysfunctional dominant follicle, 247
   failure of ovulation, 247
Dizygotic twinning (DZ), 81
Double bleb sign, 12
Double decidual sign, 9
Double-outlet right ventricle, 199
Down syndrome, 118, 172, 201–206, 339
   brachycephaly, 204
   duodenal atresia, 205
   echogenic bowel, 203
   echogenic intracardiac focus, 204
   heart defects, 205
   hypoplasia of the middle phalanx of the 5th digit, 204
   iliac angle, 206
   prognosis, 206
   renal pyelectasis, 203
   short femur and/or humerus, 203
   sonographic scoring system for fetal anomalies associated with chromosomal abnormality, 206
   thickened nuchal fold, 202
   underossified nasal bones, 205
DUB. See Dysfunctional uterine bleeding
Duodenal atresia, 172, 205, 332, 335–336
DWM. See Dandy-Walker malformation
Dysfunctional dominant follicle, 247
Dysfunctional uterine bleeding (DUB), 20
Dysgerminoma, 275
DZ. See Dizygotic twinning

Early intrauterine pregnancy, vs. ectopic pregnancy, 21–22
Ebstein's anomaly, 193
Echogenic bowel, 203
   small, 174–176
Echogenic intracardiac focus, 204
Eclampsia, 94
Ectopic pregnancy, 20–23, 331
   early intrauterine pregnancy vs., 21–22
   incidence, 21
   serum beta-human chorionic gonadotropin, 21
   sites of, 22–23
   treatment, 21
Edward's syndrome, 19, 206–207, 338
Ellis-Van Creveld syndrome, 187
Embryo, 13, 63
   cardiac activity, 13
   endovaginal sonography, 13, 17
Embryology, 139, 227–228
   of the abdominal wall, 144–145
Embryology of the fetal face, 124–130
   hypertelorism, 127
   hypotelorism, 124–126
   lips and mouth, 127–129
   macroglossia, 129–130
   micrognathia, 129
   microphthalmia, 127
Embryology of the placenta, 81–82
   dichorionic diamniotic twins, 81
   monochorionic diamniotic twins, 81
   monochorionic monoamniotic twins, 82

Embryonic demise, 16
Embryonic period, 8
Encephalocele, 140–141, 335, 337
Endometrial evaluation, and infertility, 249
Endometrial pathology, 262–265
 endometrial adhesions, 265
 endometrial carcinoma, 264–265
 endometrial hyperplasia, 262–264, 344
 endometritis, 264
Endometriosis, 279, 341
Endometritis, 264
Endometrium, 23, 231–232
Endometroid tumors, 272–273
Endovaginal sonography (EVS), 13, 17, 234
 of the embryo, 13, 17
Equipment and documentation guidelines, for routine obstetrical examinations, 346
Esophageal atresia, 171–172
Ethmocephaly, 126
EVS. See Endovaginal sonography
Examination, performing, 288
Exencephaly/acrania, 139
Extralobar sequestration (ELS), 156
Extrauterine adnexal ring, 23
Extremities, 36–38

Face, 27–29
 anomalies of, 136
Failed pregnancy, 15–16, 332
Failure of ovulation, 247
Fallopian tubes, 231, 248–249, 330, 353–354
Female pelvic organs, development during childhood, 228–229
Female pelvis, gynecological examination guidelines for performance of the ultrasound examination of, 352–354
Female pseudohermaphroditism, 241
Femur length (FL), 67, 70–71
Fertilization, 4–8, 239–240
 cardiovascular system, 8
 gastrointestinal system, 8
 musculoskeletal system, 8
 urogenital system, 8
Fetal abdomen and pelvis, 38–40
 gastrointestinal, 40
 genitourinary, 40
Fetal abnormalities, 17–20, 123–211
 abnormalities of the abdominal wall, 144–152
 abnormalities of the fetal head and face, 123–124
 abnormalities of the fetal neck, 139
 anencephaly, 18

 cardiac abnormalities, 189–201
 embryology of the fetal face, 124–130
 gastrointestinal abnormalities, 170–176
 genitourinary abnormalities, 159–170
 neural tube defects, 139–144
 nuchal translucency, 18–20
 rhombencephalon, 17
 skeletal abnormalities, 177–189
 syndromes, 201–211
 thoracic abnormalities, 152–159
Fetal ascites, 176
Fetal bladder decompression, 101–102
Fetal blood sampling/transfusion, 98–100
 cordocentesis, 98–99
 intraperitoneal fetal transfusion, 100
 intravascular fetal transfusion, 99
Fetal brain and cranium, 130–139
 agenesis corpus callosum, 133
 Dandy-Walker malformation, 132–133
 embryology of, 130
 holoprosencephaly, 133–137
 hydrocephaly, 130–131
 mild lateral cerebral ventriculomegaly, 131
 neural proliferation differentiation, 137–139
 ventriculomegaly, 130–131
Fetal demise, 121, 223, 329
Fetal gallbladder, 176
Fetal intracranial tumors, 143–144
Fetal liver, 176
Fetal pulmonic maturity studies, 113
 lecithin/sphingomyelin ratio, 113
 phosphatidylglycerol, 113
Fetal sex determination, 84
Fetal spleen, 176
Fetal therapy, 98–102
 diaphragmatic hernia repair, 100–101
 fetal bladder decompression, 101–102
 fetal blood sampling/transfusion, 98–100
 selective reduction of multifetal pregnancy, 102
Fetal weight
 estimation of, 74–75
 tables, 74
Fetus, 63
 management of the anemic, 97
Fetus papyraceus, 87
Fibroids, 259–261

Fibroma tumors, 276–277
First trimester assessment of gestational age, 60–64
 crown-rump length, 62–64
 gestational sac, 60–61
 yolk sac, 61–62
First trimester obstetrics, 3–24
 abnormal first trimester (failed pregnancy), 15–16
 ectopic pregnancy, 20–23
 fertilization/embryology, 4–8
 gestational age, 3
 sonographic findings in early intrauterine pregnancy, 8–15
 sonographic findings related to ectopic pregnancy, 23–24
 sonographic signs of abnormal early pregnancy, 16–20
First trimester sonographic determination of chorionicity and amnionicity, 83
First trimester sonography, guidelines for routine obstetrical examinations, 346–347
FL. See Femur length
Fluid, 23
FMC. See Focal myometrial contraction
Focal femoral hypoplasia, 188
Focal limb anomalies, 187–189
 clubfoot deformity, 188
 focal femoral hypoplasia, 188
 radial ray abnormalities, 188
Focal myometrial contraction (FMC), 10, 217
FOD. See Fronto-occipital diameter
Follicle-stimulating hormone (FSH), 237
Follicular cysts, 267
Follicular phase, of menstrual cycle, 237–238
Fronto-occipital diameter (FOD), 68
FSH. See Follicle-stimulating hormone
Functional cysts, 267–270
 corpus luteum cysts, 267
 follicular cysts, 267
 hemorrhagic cysts, 267–268
 theca-lutein cysts, 268–269
Funneling, 106

Gamete intrafallopian transfer (GIFT), 252
Gartner's duct cyst, 266
Gastrointestinal (GI) abnormalities, 40, 93, 170–176
 bowel duplication, 176
 colon atresia, 174
 duodenal atresia, 172
 echogenic small bowel, 174–176
 embryology of, 170–171
 esophageal atresia, 171–172
 fetal ascites, 176

 fetal gallbladder, 176
 fetal liver, 176
 fetal spleen, 176
 meconium ileus, 174
 meconium peritonitis, 174
 nonvisualization of the stomach, 172
 position of the stomach, 171
 small bowel obstruction, 172–174
Gastrointestinal system, in the embryonic period, 8
Gastroschisis, 145–146, 328, 336
Gastrulation, 6
Genetic studies, 115–121
 chorionic villus sampling, 2, 119–121
 diseases arising from a single gene, 115–116
 fetal demise, 121
 maternal serum testing, 116–118
Genitourinary abnormalities, 40, 159–170
 abnormalities of genitalia, 169–170
 associated with in utero exposure to diethylstilbesterol, 107, 258
 bilateral renal agenesis, 167–168
 embryology of, 159
 hydronephrosis, 159–160
 Meckel-Gruber syndrome, 166–167
 neoplasms, 169
 prune belly syndrome, 162
 pyelectasis and aneuploidy, 161
 reflux and ureterovesical junction obstruction, 161
 renal cystic disease, 162–166
 renal duplication, 162
 renal ectopia, 169
 unilateral renal agenesis, 168–169
 ureteropelvic junction obstruction, 160
 urethral obstruction, 161
Germ cell tumors, 273–276
 cystic teratoma (dermoid cyst), 273–274
 dysgerminoma, 275
 immature teratomas, 275
 mature solid teratomas, 275
 struma ovarii, 274
 yolk sac tumor, 275–276
Gestational dating, 3, 64
Gestational diabetes mellitus, 92
Gestational sac, 8–9, 60–61, 328
 decidua basalis, 9, 17, 81
 double decidual sign, 9
 intradecidual sign, 9
Gestational trophoblastic disorder (GTD), 219

GIFT. *See* Gamete intrafallopian transfer
Gonadotropin-releasing hormone agonists (GnRHa), 250
Granulosa cell tumor, 276
Growth and development (embryology), 42
Growth in twin gestations, 85
GTD. *See* Gestational trophoblastic disorder
Gynecological examination guidelines, 351–354
 for equipment and documentation, 351–352
 for performance of the ultrasound examination of the female pelvis, 352–354
Gynecology, 225–283
 case studies for self-assessment, 317–326, 340–344
 infertility, 245–252
 pediatric abnormalities, 241–243
 pelvic anatomy, 227–236
 pelvic pathology, 257–283
 physiology, 237–240
 postmenopausal pelvis, 253–255

HC. *See* Head circumference
hCG. *See* Human chorionic gonadotropin hormone level; Serum beta-human chorionic gonadotropin hormone level
Head circumference (HC), 66–67, 124
Heart, 33–34
 defects of, 205
Hemangioma, 58
Hematocolpos, 243
Hematogenesis, 7
Hematoma, 58
Hematometra, 242
Hemorrhagic cysts, 267–268
Heredity, 81
Heterotaxia, 200
Heterozygous achondroplasia, 185
HLHS. *See* Hypoplastic left heart syndrome
hMG. *See* Human menopausal gonadotropin level
Holoprosencephaly, 124, 126, 133–137
 alobar, 134
 differential diagnoses, 136
 with dorsal cyst, 136
 facial anomalies, 136
 lobar, 134–135
 semilobar, 134
Hormonal replacement, 255
Human chorionic gonadotropin hormone (hCG) level, 61, 118, 239, 337

Human menopausal gonadotropin (hMG) level, 250
Hydranencephaly, 137
Hydrocele, 169
Hydrocephaly, 130–131
Hydrometrocolpos, 170, 344
Hydronephrosis, 159–160, 161
Hydrops, 95, 155–156
Hydrosalpinx, 214
Hypertelorism, 127
Hypoechoic/cystic lesions, 45–46
 in the mid-placental regions, 46
 at the placental myometrial interface, 46
Hypoplasia of the middle phalanx of the 5th digit, 204
Hypoplastic left heart syndrome (HLHS), 194–195, 336
Hypotelorism, 124–126
Hypothalamic causes, of anovulation, 247

Iliac angle, 206
ILS. *See* Intralobar sequestration
Immature teratomas, 275
Imperforate hymen, 266
Implantation of blastocyst, 5
In vitro fertilization, 251–252
Incorrect diagnosis, potential pitfalls possibly leading to, 152
Indications
 for pelvic sonography, 236
 for sonography in infertility, 246
Infantile polycystic kidney disease, 162
Infectious disease control, 288–289
Infertility, 245–252, 343
 assisted reproductive technology, 250–252
 causes of, 246–250
 indications for sonography in, 246
 medications and treatment, 250–251
 work-up, 246
Inflammatory conditions, 280–281
 pelvic inflammatory disease, 280–281
 tubal-ovarian abscess, 280–281
International Reference Preparation (IRP), 15, 331
Intracranial calcifications, 138–139, 144
Intracranial hemorrhage in utero, 144
Intradecidual sign, 9
Intralobar sequestration (ILS), 156
Intraperitoneal fetal transfusion, 100

Intraplacental lesions, 45–46
 hypoechoic/cystic lesions, 45–46
 placental calcifications, 45
Intrathoracic masses, 159
Intrauterine blood, 17
Intrauterine device (IUD), 20, 248, 282, 337, 342
Intrauterine growth restriction (IUGR), 46, 73–80, 146, 203, 326
 conditions associated with, 75, 77
 defined, 73
 fetal weight estimation, 74–75
 fetal weight tables, 74
 percentile values for fetal abdominal circumference, 76
 role of maternal nutrition, 77–79
 scan techniques to evaluate, 75
Intravascular fetal transfusion, 99
Invasive hydatidiform mole (chorioadenoma destruens), 224
IRP. *See* International Reference Preparation
Isoimmunization, 95
Isthmus, 231
IUD. *See* Intrauterine device
IUGR. *See* Intrauterine growth restriction

Jeune syndrome, 187

Karyotyping, 20, 58, 127
Klinfelter syndrome, 243
Krukenberg tumors, 277, 342

L/S. *See* Lecithin/sphingomyelin ratio
L-transposition of the great arteries, 197–198
"Lambda" sign, 84–85
Last menstrual period (LMP), 3
Lateral cerebral ventriculomegaly, mild, 131
LBWC. *See* Limb-body wall complex
Lecithin/sphingomyelin (L/S) ratio, 113
Leiomyomas, 216–217, 249, 259–261, 340
Leiomyosarcomas, 262
Lethal hypophosphatasia, 185
Lethal skeletal dysplasias, 179–185
 achondrogenesis, 184
 lethal hypophosphatasia, 185
 osteogenesis imperfecta type II, 181–184

short-rib polydactyly syndrome, 184–185
 thanatophoric dwarfism, 179–181
LH. *See* Lutenizing hormone
LHR. *See* Lung-head ratio
Limb-body wall complex (LBWC), 148–150
Lips and mouth, 127–129
Lissencephaly, 131
LMP. *See* Last menstrual period
Lobar holoprosencephaly, 134–135
Long cord, 55
Low-lying placenta, 48, 327
Lower extremity deep venous thrombosis, 218
LUF. *See* Luteinized unruptured follicle syndrome
Lung-head ratio (LHR), 101
Luteal phase, of menstrual cycle, 238
Luteinized unruptured follicle syndrome (LUF), 247
Lutenizing hormone (LH), 238

Macroglossia, 129–130
Macrosomia, 93
Magnetic resonance imaging (MRI), 50, 289
Male pseudohermaphroditism, 241
Marginal hemorrhage, 49
Marginal placenta previa, 47
Maternal age and parity, 80
Maternal basal plate infarction, 46
Maternal disorders presenting primarily with pain and swelling, 218–219
 appendicitis, 218
 cholecystitis, 218
 lower extremity deep venous thrombosis, 218
 pyelonephritis, 218
 ureteral calculus, 218–219
Maternal illness, 91–98
 diabetes mellitus, 92–94
 management of the anemic fetus, 97
 maternal hypertension, 94, 328
 maternal isoimmunization (Rh incompatibility), 94–97
Maternal serum alpha-fetoprotein (MS-AFP), elevated, 50, 117, 147
Maternal serum testing, 116–118
 acetylcholinesterase, 118
 alpha-fetoprotein, 116–118
 chromosomal abnormality, 118
 human chorionic gonadotropin, 118
 triple screen, 118
 unconjugated estriol, 118
Mature solid teratomas, 275

MC/DA. *See* Monochorionic diamniotic twins
MC/MA. *See* Monochorionic monoamniotic twins
MCDK. *See* Multicystic dysplastic kidney
Mean sac diameter (MSD), 8, 61, 334
Meckel-Gruber syndrome, 140, 164, 166–167, 210
Meconium ileus, 174
Meconium peritonitis, 174
Medications for infertility, 250–251
  gonadotropin-releasing hormone agonists, 250
  human menopausal gonadotropin, 250
  ovarian hyperstimulation syndrome, 250–251
  sonographic follicular monitoring, 250–251
  ultrasound use in infertility procedures, 250
Megaureter, primary, 161
Megestrol acetate, 255
Membrane presence, 83–84
Menstrual age, 59
Menstrual cycle, 237–238
  follicular phase, 237–238
  luteal phase, 238
  secretory phase, 238
Menstrual weeks, 3, 334
Mesenchyme, 6
Mesosalpinx, 231
Metastatic tumors, 277–278
Metatropic dysplasia, 187
Microcephaly, 138
Micrognathia, 129
Microphthalmia, 127
Mild lateral cerebral ventriculomegaly, 131
Mild osteogenesis imperfecta, 186
Monochorionic diamniotic (MC/DA) twins, 81
Monochorionic monoamniotic (MC/MA) twins, 82, 333
Monozygotic twinning (MZ), 81
Morula stage, 4, 239
MRI. *See* Magnetic resonance imaging
MS-AFP. *See* Maternal serum alpha-fetoprotein
MSD. *See* Mean sac diameter
Mucinous cystadenocarcinoma, 271–272
Mucinous cystadenoma, 271
Mucinous degeneration of the umbilical cord, 57
Multicystic dysplastic kidney (MCDK), 165–166, 335
Multiple gestations, 80–91
  complications of twin pregnancy, 85–91
  embryology/placenta, 81–82

growth in twin gestations, 85
sonographic determination of chorionicity and amnionicity, 82–85
twin pregnancy, 80–81
Musculoskeletal system, in the embryonic period, 8
Myelomeningocele, 141, 339
MZ. *See* Monozygotic twinning

Neoplasms, 169
  congenital mesoblastic nephroma, 169
  neuroblastomas, 169
Neoplastic ovarian masses, 270–277
  germ cell tumors, 273–276
  sex-cord stromal tumors, 276–277
  surface epithelial-stromal tumors, 270–273
Neural proliferation differentiation, 137–139
  hydranencephaly, 137
  intracranial calcifications, 138–139
  microcephaly, 138
  porencephaly, 138
  schizencephaly, 138
Neural tube defects, 139–144
  anencephaly, 139–140
  cephaloceles/encephalocele, 140–141
  choroid plexus cysts, 142–143
  embryology, 139
  exencephaly/acrania, 139
  fetal intracranial tumors, 143–144
  intracranial calcifications, 144
  intracranial hemorrhage in utero, 144
  spinal bifida, 141–142
  vein of Galen aneurysm, 143
Neuroblastomas, 169
Neurulation, 7
Nonneoplastic lesions, 267–270
  functional cysts, 267–270
  ovarian torsion, 269
  paraovarian cysts, 269
  peritoneal inclusion cysts, 269
Nonvisualization of the stomach, 172
Noonan syndrome, 209
Normal adult pelvic anatomy, 229–233
  cul de sac fluid, 232–233
  the uterus, 229–233
Normal cervix, 105–106
Normal sonographic anatomy, 266–267
Notocord, 6
Nuchal translucency, 18–20, 330

Obstetrical examinations, 345–350
  equipment and documentation guidelines, 346
  guidelines for first trimester sonography, 346–347
  guidelines for second and third trimester sonography, 346–347
Obstetrics, 1–224
  American Institute of Ultrasound in Medicine guidelines, 2
  amniotic fluid, 111–113
  assessment of gestational age, 59–71
  case studies for self-assessment, 295–317, 326–340
  coexisting disorders, 213–224
  complications, 73–109
  fetal abnormalities, 123–211
  first trimester, 3–24
  genetic studies, 115–121
  placenta, 41–58
  second/third trimester (normal anatomy), 25–40
Obstructive renal dysplasia, 166
OHS. *See* Ovarian hyperstimulation syndrome
Oligohydramnios, 112, 333
Omphalocele, 146–147, 336
Omphalomesenteric duct, cord cysts from, 56–57
Open spinal bifida, 141
Osteogenesis imperfecta, mild, 186, 337
Osteogenesis imperfecta type II, 181–184
Ovarian artery, 231
Ovarian cancer, 254
Ovarian carcinoma screening, 278
Ovarian cyst, 170
Ovarian hyperstimulation syndrome (OHS), 250–251
Ovarian torsion, 269
Ovaries, 254, 266–278, 353–354
  metastatic tumors, 277–278
  neoplastic ovarian masses, 270–277
  nonneoplastic lesions, 267–270
  normal sonographic anatomy, 266–267
  ovarian carcinoma screening, 278
Ovulation-induction agents, 81

Paraovarian cyst, 214–215, 269
Partial hydatidiform mole (PHM), 209, 221–222
Partial placenta previa, 47
Patient care, preparation and techniques, 285–291
  artifacts, 289–290
  bioeffects, 290–291

infectious disease control, 288–289
  performing the examination, 288
  physical principles, 289
  sonographer's interaction with the patient, 287
  supine hypotension, 288
PCOS. *See* Polycystic ovary syndrome
Pediatric abnormalities, 241–243
  hematocolpos, 243
  hematometra, 242
  precocious puberty, 242
  sexual ambiguity, 241–242
  testicular feminization syndrome, 243
  "wrong gender," 243
  XX male, 243
Pelvic anatomy, 227–236
  contraindications to endovaginal sonography, 236
  development of female pelvic organs during childhood, 228–229
  embryology, 227–228
  indications for pelvic sonography, 236
  normal adult pelvic anatomy, 229–233
  sonographic appearance of normal pelvic organs, 235
  sonographic technique, 234–235
Pelvic inflammatory disease (PID), 20, 280–281
Pelvic kidney, 216
Pelvic pathology, 257–283
  endometriosis, 279
  inflammatory conditions, 280–281
  the ovary, 266–278
  pelvic masses, 213, 281
  polycystic ovary disease, 279–280
  sonographic imaging of contraceptive devices, 282
  upper abdominal findings associated with pelvic disease, 283
  urinary masses, 281
  uterine pathology, 257–266
  vaginal pathology, 266
Pentalogy of Cantrell, 147–148
Percentile values for fetal abdominal circumference, 76
Percutaneous umbilical blood sampling (PUBS), 2
Peritoneal inclusion cysts, 269
Persistent truncus arteriosus, 197
PG. *See* Phosphatidylglycerol
PHM. *See* Partial hydatidiform mole; Pseudo partial hydatidiform mole

Phosphatidylglycerol (PG), 113
Physiology, 237–240, 253–254
    of fertilization, 239–240
        human chorionic gonadotropin, 239
    of the menstrual cycle, 237–238
    of the ovaries, 254
    of pregnancy tests, 239
    of the uterus, 253
PID. See Pelvic inflammatory disease
Pituitary causes, of anovulation, 247
Placenta, 41–58
    abnormalities of placental shape, 43–45
    chorioangioma, 52–53
    growth and development (embryology), 42
    intraplacental lesions, 45–46
    marginal hemorrhage, 49
    placental abruption, 48–49
    placental calcifications, 45
    placental Doppler, 52
    placental grading, 46–47
    placental size and shape, 43
    subchorionic hemorrhage, 49
    umbilical cord, 53–58
Placenta accreta, 49–52, 109, 327
    placenta accreta vera, 50
    placenta increta, 50
    placenta percreta, 50
Placenta membranacea, 44
Placenta previa, 47–48
    complete, 47
    low-lying placenta, 48
    marginal/partial, 47
Placental size and shape, 43
    thick placenta, 43
    thin placenta, 43
Pleural effusion, 154
Polycystic ovary disease, 279–280
Polycystic ovary syndrome (PCOS), 247–248
Polyhydramnios, 112–113, 333
Porencephaly, 138
Posterior arcuate artery, 231
Postmenopausal pelvis, 253–255
    anatomy and physiology, 253–254
    indications for sonography, 254
    pathology, 254–255
    therapy, 255
Postpartum bleeding, 107–108
    primary postpartum hemorrhage, 107–108
    secondary postpartum hemorrhage, 108
Postpartum infection, 108
Potter's syndromes, 163
Pouch of Douglas, 229
Power Doppler, 42
Pre-eclampsia, 94, 327

Pre-existing diabetes mellitus, 92
Precocious puberty, 242
    pseudo, 242
    true, 242
Pregnancy tests, 239
Preterm delivery, 102–103
Primary postpartum hemorrhage, 107–108
Prognosis, 206
Prune belly syndrome, 162
Pseudo partial hydatidiform mole (PHM), 223–224
    Beckwith-Wiedemann syndrome, 224
    fetal demise, 223
Pseudo precocious puberty, 242
Pseudoascites, 176
Pseudomyxoma peritonei, 272
PUBS. See Percutaneous umbilical blood sampling
Pulmonary hypoplasia, 153
Pulmonary sequestration, 156, 337
PW Doppler analysis, 199
Pyelectasis and aneuploidy, 161
Pyelonephritis, 218

Quiz, 361–368

Race factor, 80, 342–344
Rachischisis, 142
Radial ray abnormalities, 188
Radiography, 289
Real-time imaging, 26
Reduction of multifetal pregnancy, selective, 102
Reflux and ureterovesical junction (UVJ) obstruction, 161
Refraction artifact, 289–290
Renal and urologic anomalies, 92
Renal cystic disease, 162–166
    autosomal dominant polycystic kidney disease, 166
    autosomal recessive polycystic kidney disease, 162–165
    multicystic dysplastic kidney, 165–166
    obstructive renal dysplasia, 166
    Potter's syndromes, 163
Renal duplication, 162
Renal ectopia, 169
Renal pyelectasis, 203
Reverberation artifact, 289
Rh incompatibility, 94–97, 328
Rhogam, 95
Rhombencephalon, 17, 330
Rocker-bottom foot, 188, 338
Rostral end of neural tube, 7
Round ligament, 230
Routine obstetrical examinations, 345–350
    equipment and documentation guidelines, 346

    guidelines for first trimester sonography, 346–347
    guidelines for second and third trimester sonography, 346–347

Sacro-uterine ligaments, 230
Schizencephaly, 138
Second and third trimester assessment of gestational age, 64–71
    abdominal circumference, 68–70
    binocular measurement, 71
    biparietal diameter, 64–66
    cephalic index, 67–68
    femur length, 70–71
    gestational dating, 64
    head circumference, 66–67
    pitfalls, 66
    transcerebellar measurement, 71
Second and third trimester complications, 83–85
    fetal sex determination, 84
    membrane presence, 83–84
    "twin peak" or "lambda" sign, 84–85
Second and third trimester obstetrics (normal anatomy), 25–40
    cranium, 29–32
    extremities, 36–38
    face, 27–29
    fetal abdomen and pelvis, 38–40
    heart, 33–34
    spine, 34–36
    thorax, 32–33
Second and third trimester sonographic determination of chorionicity and amnionicity, 83–85
Second and third trimester sonography, guidelines for routine obstetrical examinations, 346–347
Second International Standard (SIS), 15
Secondary postpartum hemorrhage, 108
Secretory phase, of menstrual cycle, 238
Self-assessment, case studies for, 293–344
Semilobar holoprosencephaly, 134
Septal cyst, 46
Septo-optic dysplasia, 135
Serous cystadenocarcinoma, 271
Serous cystadenoma, 270
Sertoli-Leydig tumors, 277
Serum beta-human chorionic gonadotropin hormone (serum hCG) level, 15, 20–21

Sex-cord stromal tumors, 276–277
    fibroma tumors, 276–277
    granulosa cell tumor, 276
    Sertoli-Leydig tumors, 277
    thecoma tumors, 276–277
Sexual ambiguity, 241–242
    congenital adrenal hyperplasia, 241
    female pseudohermaphroditism, 241
    male pseudohermaphroditism, 241
    true hermaphroditism, 242
Short cord, 55
Short femur and/or humerus, 203
Short-limb skeletal dysplasias, 177–179
    fetal examination for, 178–179
    with milder limb shortening, 185
Short-rib polydactyly syndrome, 184–185
Single ventricle, 196
Sirenomelia, 168
SIS. See Second International Standard
Situs abnormalities, 200
Situs inversus, 200
Skeletal abnormalities, 177–189
    abnormal fetal skeleton, 177
    asphyxiating thoracic dystrophy (Jeune syndrome), 187
    camptomelic dysplasia, 185–186
    chondroectodermal dysplasia (Ellis-Van Creveld syndrome), 187
    focal limb anomalies, 187–189
    lethal skeletal dysplasias, 179–185
    metatropic dysplasia, 187
    mild osteogenesis imperfecta, 186
    short-limb skeletal dysplasias, 177–179
Small bowel obstruction, 172–174
Society of Diagnostic Medical Sonography, 355
Solid masses, 216–217
    leiomyomas, 216–217
    ovarian, 217
Sonographer, interaction with the patient, 287
Sonographic appearance of normal pelvic organs, 235
Sonographic determination of chorionicity and amnionicity, 82–85
    first trimester, 83
    second and third trimester, 83–85
Sonographic determination of risk for preterm delivery, 103–107

cervical cerclage, 107
clinical aspects of cervical incompetence, 106–107
normal cervix, 105–106
transabdominal approach, 103–104
transperineal (translabial) approach, 104–105
transvaginal approach, 105
Sonographic findings, 8–15, 190–200
  amnion, 14
  beta-human chorionic gonadotropin and sonographic findings, 15
  decidual thickening, 8
  double bleb sign, 12
  embryo, 13
  endometrium, 23
  extrauterine adnexal ring, 23
  fluid, 23
  gestational sac, 8–9
  related to ectopic pregnancy, 23–24
  yolk sac, 11
Sonographic follicular monitoring, 250–251
Sonographic imaging of contraceptive devices, 282
Sonographic scoring system for fetal anomalies associated with chromosomal abnormality, 206
Sonographic signs of abnormal early pregnancy, 16–20
  abnormal gestational sac, 16
  fetal anomalies, 17–20
  intrauterine blood, 17
Sonography, 152, 234–235, 254–255
  endovaginal, 234
  of the normal lung, 153
  sonohysterography, 235
  transabdominal, 234
  use in infertility procedures, 250
Spinal bifida, 141–142, 335
Spinal bifida occulta, 142
Spinal bifida operta, 141
Spine, 34–36
Stein Leventhal syndrome, 247–248, 343
Stomach
  nonvisualization of, 172
  position of, 171
Structural abnormalities, 54–55
Structural cord abnormalities, 54–55
  abnormal cord formation, 54
  long cord, 55
  short cord, 55
Struma ovarii, 274
Subchorionic hemorrhage, 49, 329
Succenturiate lobe, 45

Supine hypotension, 288
Surface epithelial-stromal tumors, 270–273
  clear cell tumors, 273
  cystadenofibroma, 271
  endometroid tumors, 272–273
  mucinous cystadenocarcinoma, 271–272
  mucinous cystadenoma, 271
  pseudomyxoma peritonei, 272
  serous cystadenocarcinoma, 271
  serous cystadenoma, 270
  transitional cell tumor, 273
Syncytiotrophoblast, formation of, 5, 42, 239–240
Syndromes, 201–211
  Meckel-Gruber syndrome, 210
  triploidy, 209–210
  trisomy 13, 208
  trisomy 18 (Edward's syndrome), 206–207
  trisomy 21 (Down syndrome), 201–206
  Turner syndrome, 208–209

Tamoxifen, 255
TD. See Thanatophoric dwarfism
TDF. See Testes-determining factor
Teratoma, 58, 341
TES. See Twin embolization syndrome
Testes-determining factor (TDF), 243
Testicular feminization syndrome, 243
Tetralogy of Fallot, 198–199
Thanatophoric dwarfism (TD), 177, 179–181
Theca-lutein cysts, 268–269, 340–341
Thecoma tumors, 276–277, 341
Therapy, 255
  hormonal replacement, 255
  megestrol acetate, 255
  tamoxifen, 255
Thermal heating, 290
Thick placenta, 43
Thickened nuchal fold, 202
Thin placenta, 43
Third IRP (3IS), 15
Thoracic abnormalities, 152–159
  bronchogenic cysts, 156–157
  chest masses, 154–155
  congenital diaphragmatic hernia, 156–159
  embryology of, 152–153
  intrathoracic masses, 159
  pleural effusion, 154
  pulmonary hypoplasia, 153
  pulmonary sequestration, 156
  sonography of the normal lung, 153
  tracheal atresia, 156

Thorax, 32–33
Threatened abortion, 15
TOA. See Tubal-ovarian abscess
Torsion, 215
Tracheal atresia, 156
Transabdominal approach, 103–104, 234
  to chorionic villus sampling, 120–121
Transcerebellar measurement, 71
Transcervical approach, to chorionic villus sampling, 119–120
Transitional cell tumor, 273
Transperineal (translabial) approach, 104–105
Transposition of the great arteries, 197–198
  D-transposition, 197
  L-transposition, 197–198
Transvaginal approach, 105
TRAP. See Twin reversed arterial perfusion sequence
Treatment, of ectopic pregnancy, 21
Treatment for infertility, 250–251
  gonadotropin-releasing hormone agonists, 250
  human menopausal gonadotropin, 250
  ovarian hyperstimulation syndrome, 250–251
  sonographic follicular monitoring, 250–251
  ultrasound use in infertility procedures, 250
Triple screen, 118
Triploidy, 209–210
Trisomy 13, 208
Trisomy 18 (Edward's syndrome), 19, 206–207
Trisomy 21 (Down syndrome), 19, 201–206, 336
  brachycephaly, 204
  duodenal atresia, 205
  echogenic bowel, 203
  echogenic intracardiac focus, 204
  heart defects, 205
  hypoplasia of the middle phalanx of the 5th digit, 204
  iliac angle, 206
  prognosis, 206
  renal pyelectasis, 203
  short femur and/or humerus, 203
  sonographic scoring system for fetal anomalies associated with chromosomal abnormality, 206
  thickened nuchal fold, 202
  underossified nasal bones, 205
Trophoblastic disease, 219–224
  choriocarcinoma, 224

  classic hydatidiform mole, 219–223
  invasive hydatidiform mole (chorioadenoma destruens), 224
  partial hydatidiform mole, 221–222
  pseudo partial hydatidiform mole, 223–224
Trophotropism, 56
True hermaphroditism, 242
True precocious puberty, 242
Tubal-ovarian abscess (TOA), 280–281, 342
Turner's syndrome, 19, 208–209, 335
Twin embolization syndrome (TES), 82, 87–88
"Twin peak" sign, 84–85
Twin pregnancy, 80–81
  heredity, 81
  maternal age and parity, 80
  race factors, 80
  use of ovulation-induction agents, 81
Twin reversed arterial perfusion (TRAP) sequence, 88–90
Twin transfusion syndrome, 82
Twin-twin transfusion syndrome, 86, 332

UE3. See Unconjugated estriol
Umbilical cord, 53–58
  cord abnormalities, 54–58
  cord anatomy, 53–54
Umbilical vein, 39
Unconjugated estriol (UE3), 118
Underossified nasal bones, 205
Unilateral renal agenesis, 168–169
UPJ. See Ureteropelvic junction obstruction
Upper abdominal findings associated with pelvic disease, 283
Ureteral calculus, 218–219
Ureteropelvic junction (UPJ) obstruction, 160
Ureterovesical junction (UVJ) obstruction, reflux and, 161
Urethral obstruction, 161, 336
Urinary masses, 281
Urogenital system, in the embryonic period, 8
Uterine artery, 231
Uterine masses, 259–262
  adenomyosis, 262, 340
  leiomyomas, 259–261
  leiomyosarcomas, 262
Uterine pathology, 257–266
  the cervix, 265–266
  congenital malformations, 257–258
  endometrial pathology, 262–265

genital anomalies associated with in utero exposure to diethylstilbesterol, 107, 258
uterine masses, 259–262
Uterus, 229–233, 253, 353
Uterus bicornis bicollis, 257
Uterus bicornis unicollis, 257
Uterus didelphys, 257
Uterus septus, 258
Uterus subseptus, 258
Uterus unicornis unicollis, 258
UVJ. *See* Ureterovesical junction obstruction

Vagina, 231
Vaginal pathology, 266
    Gartner's duct cyst, 266
    imperforate hymen, 266
Varix/aneurysm, 58
Vasa previa, 56
Vascular abnormalities, 54
Vein of Galen aneurysm, 143
Velamentous insertion, 56
Ventriculomegaly, 130–131, 141

"Wrong gender," 243
    androgen insensitivity syndrome, 243
    testicular feminization, 243

X-linked diseases, 116
XX male, 243

Yolk sac, 11, 61–62
    tumor, 275–276

Zygote intrafallopian transfer (ZIFT), 252